Case Studies in Dermatology

Case Studies in Dermatology

Editor: Alina Foster

AMERICAN
MEDICAL PUBLISHERS
www.americanmedicalpublishers.com

AMERICAN
MEDICAL PUBLISHERS
www.americanmedicalpublishers.com

Cataloging-in-Publication Data

Case studies in dermatology / edited by Alina Foster
p. cm.
Includes bibliographical references and index.
ISBN 979-8-88740-620-6
1. Dermatology. 2. Dermatology--Research. 3. Skin--Diseases. 4. Skin--Diseases--Diagnosis.
5. Skin--Diseases--Treatment. I. Foster, Alina.
RL72 .C87 2023
616.5--dc23

American Medical Publishers,
41 Flatbush Avenue,
1st Floor, New York,
NY 11217, USA

ISBN 979-8-88740-620-6 (Hardback)

Contents

Preface

It is often said that books are a boon to mankind. They document every progress and pass on the knowledge from one generation to the other. They play a crucial role in our lives. Thus I was both excited and nervous while editing this book. I was pleased by the thought of being able to make a mark but I was also nervous to do it right because the future of students depends upon it. Hence, I took a few months to research further into the discipline, revise my knowledge and also explore some more aspects. Post this process, I begun with the editing of this book.

Dermatology is a medical specialty which focuses on the skin, hair, nails, and mucous membranes as well as the diagnosis, treatment, and prevention of conditions which affect them. Some of the various skin conditions which are diagnosed and managed within this field are skin infections, eczema, acne, psoriasis, dermatitis, skin cancer and allergic reactions. Skin infections can be classified into bacterial, viral, parasitic or fungal infections. They are generally treated using antibiotics or antifungal medications, to help clear the infection and prevent complications. This area of medicine also deals with cosmetic concerns and performs various procedures, such as chemical peels, laser treatments, injectable fillers, and botox injections, to enhance the appearance of the skin and treat the signs of aging. This book unravels the recent studies in the field of dermatology. It is appropriate for students seeking detailed information in this area of medicine as well as for experts.

I thank my publisher with all my heart for considering me worthy of this unparalleled opportunity and for showing unwavering faith in my skills. I would also like to thank the editorial team who worked closely with me at every step and contributed immensely towards the successful completion of this book. Last but not the least, I wish to thank my friends and colleagues for their support.

Editor

1

Use of Cryopreserved Human Umbilical Cord for Wound Healing of the Nose after Mohs Micrographic Surgery

Kathleen Herne[1] and Robert K. Fabric[2]

[1]Integrated Dermatology of West Palm Beach, West Palm Beach, FL, USA
[2]Department of Surgery in the Division of Plastic Surgery at the Leonard M. Miller School of Medicine, Miami, FL, USA

Correspondence should be addressed to Robert K. Fabric; docfab2000@aol.com

Academic Editor: Tak-Wah Wong

Mohs micrographic surgery (MMS) is microscopically controlled surgery used to treat common skin cancers including primary and recurrent basal cell carcinoma (BCC). Unfortunately, postexcisional MMS wounds, particularly down to periosteum or perichondrium, are susceptible to potentially poor cosmetic outcomes, including wound contracture, hypopigmentation and hyperpigmentation, and contour mismatch. Herein, we report a case to show how adjunctive application of human cryopreserved umbilical cord tissue (UC) may expedite wound healing with improved aesthetic outcome. A 53-year-old Caucasian female with a slight natural lifelong depression between her lower nasal tip alar cartilages suffered from a recurrent BCC mostly of the right nasal tip. After MMS down to the perichondrium, UC was immediately applied to the surgical wound. Prolific granulation developed at one week followed by rapid reepithelialization at two weeks. This resulted in complete closure at four weeks and a pleasing aesthetic nasal tip at 6 weeks. At one year and 5 months after MMS, there continued to be excellent aesthetic outcome as evaluated by surrounding skin color, contour, and texture with a minimal residual scar. In this case, the adjunctive use of cryopreserved human UC accelerated the postsurgical MMS wound healing in the nasal tip particularly in patients with significant comorbidities or are unwilling to undergo a formal surgical reconstruction. This encouraging finding warrants further controlled studies in the future.

1. Introduction

Basal cell carcinoma (BCC) is the most common skin malignancy with an increasing incidence worldwide [1]. The disease primarily affects older Caucasian populations and often appears on the face. Treatment options include topical therapies (fluorouracil and imiquimod), photodynamic therapy, laser treatment, radiation, and surgery [1]. Mohs micrographic surgery (MMS) offers high cure rates with maximal normal tissue preservation in sites at risk for high rates of recurrence. Post-MMS wounds can be managed by primary closure if the wound is small, but if the wound is more extensive, it may require reconstructive surgery with flaps (local or distant) or skin grafts (split or full thickness). Nonetheless, wound healing can be complicated by contracture (including a trapdoor deformity), hypopigmentation, hyperpigmentation, contour mismatch to the surrounding skin, and unsightly scarring of both the surgical and donor sites. The umbilical cord (UC) contains the same histological features as amniotic membrane except that the avascular stroma contains more hyaluronic acid and was selected as an adjunctive therapy for this patient because it had been demonstrated in various types of wounds [2, 3] to elicit anti-inflammatory, antiscarring, and regenerative healing properties.

2. Case Presentation

Three years prior, a 53-year-old Caucasian female presented with a nonhealing lesion on her nose of several months' duration (Figure 1(a)). A shave biopsy revealed BCC, and the site healed within one month (Figure 1(b)). At that time, due to the patient's use of blood thinners for pulmonary emboli,

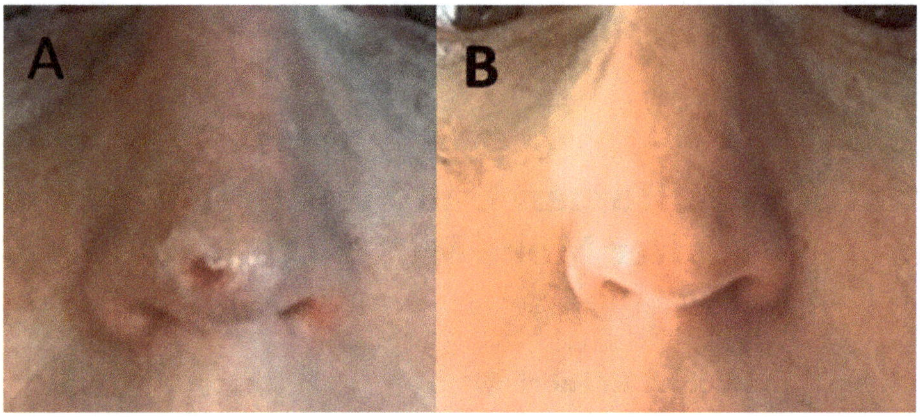

FIGURE 1: Three years prior to the present illness, the primary lesion of the right nasal tip was confirmed as BCC (a) through a shave biopsy on 1/24/2017. Approximately a month later in February (b), the wound was healed, and the patient was started on a full course of imiquimod.

extensive surgical intervention was not indicated; therefore, the patient was placed on a full course of topical imiquimod (Aldara®; Bausch Health, Bridgewater Township, NJ). During this three-year interim, the patient was doing well until a recent slowly enlarging papule appeared at the same site (Figure 2(a)). The patient underwent a shave biopsy (Figures 2(b) and 2(c)) that confirmed the lesion as a recurrent BCC of the nodular infiltrative type.

The patient was advised to undergo MMS. Preoperatively, she consulted with a different plastic surgeon regarding her surgical repair, and his surgical plan depending upon the margins was to use either a skin graft or flap to reconstruct her nasal tip. Rather, based on the reported anti-inflammatory, antiscarring, and regenerative healing properties of UC, the patient was advised and consented with a plan that included MMS followed by the adjunctive use of UC. On the date of the Mohs surgery (Figure 3(a)), two stages were required to obtain tumor-free margins with the resultant wound size of 1.0×1.1 cm which crossed the midline of the nasal tip exposing the perichondrium of the nasal alar cartilage (Figure 3(b)). Immediately after MMS (Figure 3(c)), a UC allograft (NEOX CORD® 1K; Amniox Medical, Miami, FL) was cut to wound size and applied to the wound under a nonadherent moist dressing (Xeroform®; Covidien, Dublin, Ireland), cotton bolster, and adhesive tape (Omnifix, Hartmann USA, Rock Hill). The patient was instructed to leave the dressing in place until each follow-up office visit. By one-week after MMS, the wound displayed prolific high-quality granulation tissue with minimal inflammatory response (Figure 3(d)) without any evidence of infection. Rapid reepithelialization was evident at two weeks (Figure 4(a)), resulting in complete closure at four weeks (Figure 4(b)) and a pleasing aesthetic result in the nasal tip at 6 weeks. It should be noted in the literature that others have left the UC allograft in place for up to 3 weeks. However, in this case, the graft was reapplied with a new UC (NEOX CORD® 1K) allograft during weekly dressing changes of the 4 weeks of wound healing. At one year and 5 months after MMS, there was excellent aesthetic outcome as evaluated by surrounding skin color, contour, and texture with a minimal residual scar (Figures 4(c) and 4(d)).

3. Discussion

This case report highlights a successful aesthetic outcome using cryopreserved UC to accelerate post-MMS wound healing after a sizeable excision down to the perichondrium for a recurrent BCC of the nasal tip. The wound was fully closed within 4 weeks after MMS without any additional surgical intervention. Comparatively, typical healing times for secondary intention of similar wounds could range from 2 to 3 times as long, dependent upon the wound depth, size, and metabolic health of the patient [4]. This adjunctive weekly application of UC negated additional reconstruction, which carries an inherent risk of scarring including a trapdoor deformity, pigment irregularities, telangiectasias, texture and contour mismatch, and scarring associated with donor tissue for flaps or grafts. Similarly, the convexity of the distal third of the nose makes it a less-than-ideal area for quality healing by secondary intention. These wound problems are particularly undesirable on the face especially involving the nose which may generate future aesthetic concerns with its associated emotional overlay.

The UC used herein is a cryopreserved product that preserves hyaluronic acid (HA)-rich extracellular matrix and growth factors/cytokines therein but devitalizes all living cells [2, 5]. It is stored at 4°C to −80°C ready for immediate usage without rehydration. This UC allograft was used in preference of any other type of natal membranes because it is about ten times thicker and contains higher concentrations of biological components than pure amniotic tissue. Furthermore, such UC tissue has successfully been used to heal complex diabetic foot ulcers with evidence of exposed bone, tendon, muscle and/or joint capsule, orthopedic joint problems, spina bifida, radiation-induced wounds, and ischemic wounds [6–11]. The biological effects of UC have been attributed to a unique extracellular matrix component known as Heavy Chain Hyaluronic Acid/Pentraxin-3 complex (HC-HA/PTX3), which modulates the local inflammatory environment by inducing apoptosis of activated inflammatory cells and promotes an antiscarring effect by downregulating transforming growth factor (TGF)-β,

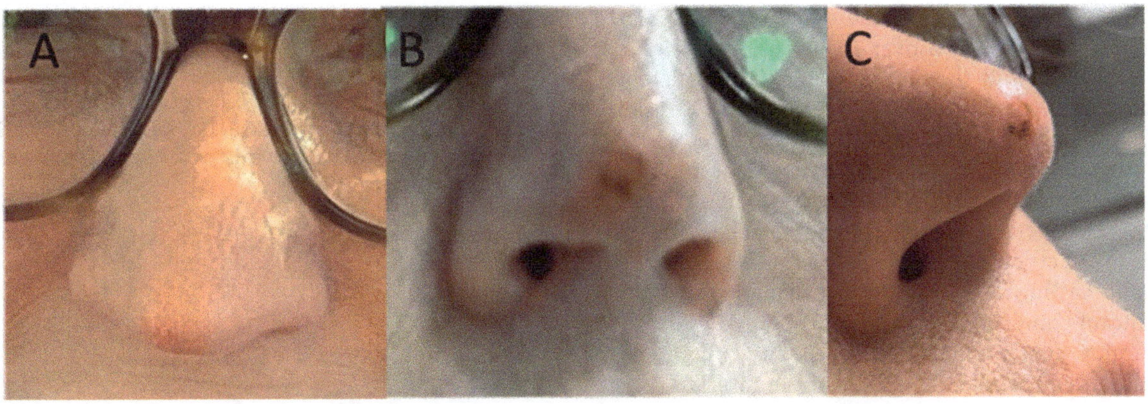

Figure 2: Three years later, the patient presented with a recurrent lesion on the nasal tip on 12/3/2019 (a) confirmed as recurrent BCC following a shave biopsy (b and c).

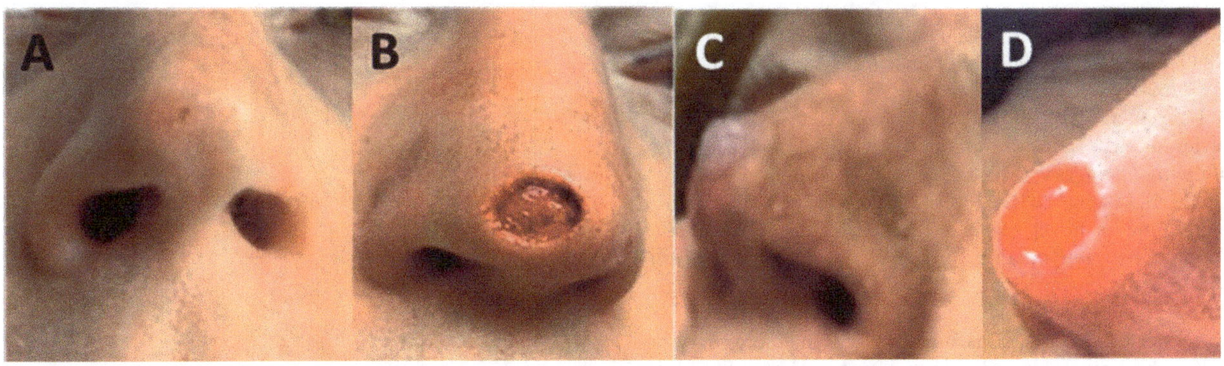

Figure 3: The patient underwent MMS down to the perichondrium on 2/27/2020 ((a) before and (b) immediately after MMS). UC was immediately applied (c), and then, a new piece of UC allograft with nonadherent dressing was applied weekly for the following three weeks with minimal debridement. Prolific granulation tissue was formed by one week, on 3/5/2020 (d).

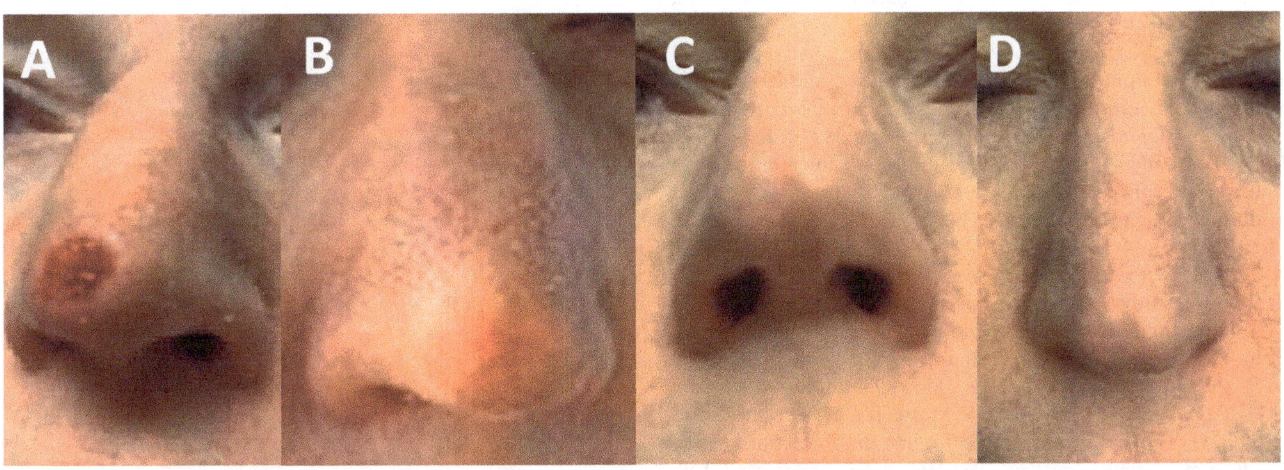

Figure 4: Evident peripheral epithelization from around the edge by two weeks (a); after a final UC graft was applied, the wound was fully reepithelialized and closed at four weeks (b). At one year and 5 months after MMS with UC (c, d) the wound is fully matured revealing a soft nasal tip with matched contour, color, and texture to the surrounding area and maintained the normal nasal tip light reflex.

preventing myofibroblast formation [3]. These regenerative biological actions are in contrast to properties of other available xenografts such as acellular dermis which is primarily used as a mechanical scaffolding that provides a structure for host cell migration and proliferation. This was verified in a head-to-head study, wherein UC was demonstrated to significantly reduce inflammation, reduce cell death, and promote superior cellular organization compared to acellular dermal matrix [12]. The safety of UC has also been demonstrated based on over 65,000 units distributed (per manufacturer) and shown not to increase recurrence after ocular, oral, dermal, and prostate tumor excision. Hence, UC was chosen to use in this case and reduce the known potential risks of conventional treatment including contracture, altered pigmentation, and contour mismatch. Overall, these properties collectively might explain why the adjunctive use of cryopreserved human UC accelerates post-MMS wound healing in the nasal tip particularly in patients with significant comorbidities or are unwilling to undergo a formal surgical reconstruction. This encouraging finding warrants further controlled studies in the future.

References

[1] A. I. Rubin, E. H. Chen, and D. Ratner, "Basal-cell carcinoma," *New England Journal of Medicine*, vol. 353, no. 21, pp. 2262–2269, 2005.

[2] S. Tighe, O. G. Mead, A. Lee, and S. C. G. Tseng, "Basic science review of birth tissue uses in ophthalmology," *Taiwan journal of ophthalmology*, vol. 10, no. 1, pp. 3–12, 2020.

[3] S. C. G. Tseng, "HC-HA/PTX3 purified from amniotic membrane as novel regenerative matrix: insight into relationship between inflammation and regeneration," *Investigative Opthalmology & Visual Science*, vol. 57, no. 5, 8 pages, 2016.

[4] G. D. Becker, L. A. Adams, and B. C. Levin, "Secondary intention healing of exposed scalp and forehead bone after Mohs surgery," *Otolaryngology-Head and Neck Surgery*, vol. 121, no. 6, pp. 751–754, 1999.

[5] M. Cooke, E. K. Tan, C. Mandrycky, H. He, J. O'Connell, and S. C. G. Tseng, "Comparison of cryopreserved amniotic membrane and umbilical cord tissue with dehydrated amniotic membrane/chorion tissue," *Journal of Wound Care*, vol. 23, no. 10, pp. 465–476, 2014.

[6] L. S. M. Chua, J. O'Connell, and S. Kang, "An open label prospective pilot study to evaluate the efficacy of cryopreserved amniotic tissue grafts for chronic non-healing ulcers," *Wounds*, vol. 26, no. 5, pp. E30–E38, 2014.

[7] D. Fernandez, "Cryopreserved amniotic membrane and umbilical cord for a radiation-induced wound with exposed dura: a case report," *Journal of Wound Care*, vol. 28, pp. S4–s8, 2019.

[8] W. J. Caputo, C. Vaquero, A. Monterosa et al., "A retrospective study of cryopreserved umbilical cord as an adjunctive therapy to promote the healing of chronic, complex foot ulcers with underlying osteomyelitis," *Wound Repair and Regeneration*, vol. 24, no. 5, pp. 885–893, 2016.

[9] R. Papanna, S. Fletcher, K. J. Moise Jr., L. K. Mann, and S. C. G. Tseng, "Cryopreserved human umbilical cord for in utero myeloschisis repair," *Obstetrics & Gynecology*, vol. 128, no. 2, pp. 325–330, 2016.

[10] A. Raphael and J. Gonzales, "Use of cryopreserved umbilical cord with negative pressure wound therapy for complex diabetic ulcers with osteomyelitis," *Journal of Wound Care*, vol. 26, pp. S38–S44, 2017.

[11] T. B. Bemenderfer, R. B. Anderson, S. M. Odum, and W. H. Davis, "Effects of cryopreserved amniotic membrane-umbilical cord allograft on total ankle arthroplasty wound healing," *Journal of Foot and Ankle Surgery*, vol. 58, no. 1, pp. 97–102, 2019.

[12] L. K. Mann, J. H. Won, N. J. Trenton et al., "Cryopreserved human umbilical cord versus acellular dermal matrix patches for in utero fetal spina bifida repair in a pregnant rat model," *Journal of Neurosurgery*, vol. 32, no. 2, pp. 321–331, 2019.

Pulse Dye Laser Therapy Successful for Elastosis Perforans Serpiginosa

Giulia Rinaldi,[1] **Alisha Chacko,**[2] **and Samira Batul Syed**[2]

[1]*Guys and St. Thomas' Hospital, NHS Foundation Trust, London, UK*
[2] *Great Ormond Street Hospital, NHS Foundation Trust, London, UK*

Correspondence should be addressed to Giulia Rinaldi; giulia.rinaldi@nhs.net

Academic Editor: Michela Curzio

Background. We describe a case of elastosis perforans serpiginosa and its successful management with PDL laser. *Case Presentation.* A 15-year-old male presented with a history of itchy, raised, red and unsightly lesions on the back of his neck. He was diagnosed with Elastosis Perforans Serpiginosa on tissue biopsy and underwent pulse dye laser therapy over four years with excellent results. *Conclusions.* Our results show that pulse dye laser therapy is a safe and effective treatment for elastosis perforans serpiginosa.

1. Background

Elastosis perforans serpingosa (EPS) is one of four classic perforating disorders including Kyrle's disease, reactive perforating collagenosis and perforating folliculitis [1]. Histological evaluation allows perforating disorders to be classified according to which skin material appears to be eliminated. In EPS, this involves trans epithelial elimination which is characterised by abnormal dermal elastic, other connective tissue, and cellular elements being extruded from the papillary dermis through the epidermis [2]. The pathogenesis of EPS is divided into three subtypes; idiopathic (where no cause can be identified), reactive (associated with connective tissue disorders such as Marfan's, Ehler Danlos, Down's syndrome or osteogenesis imperfecta) and drug-induced (penicillamine being the commonest drug reported) [3, 4]. EPS usually presents as small umbilicated or keratotic erythematous papules which cluster together in a serpiginous pattern around the neck, face or arms. The appearance of EPS is commonest in males under the age of 30.

2. Case Presentation

We present a 15 year old male who was referred with idiopathic EPS presenting as extensive umbilicated papules on his posterior neck present for over 2 years. The patient's main concern was their appearance causing him embarrassment at school.

On examination, he had two localized areas of erythematous umbilicated papules arranged in a serpiginous pattern on both the left and right side of his posterior neck (Figure 1). A biopsy had been performed at his previous centre of care and a diagnosis of EPS was confirmed. An EPS biopsy, as shown on DermNet.nz, shows keratotic debris columns perforating through a hyperplastic epidermis. This can be accentuated using an Elastic-Van Gieson stain that highlights elastic fibres in black (Figure 2) [5].

The patient's main concerns were extreme itch and the unsightly appearance of the lesions. At the time of referral, he had already failed treatment with cryotherapy, topical retinoids and 10% urea cream. The decision was made to treat with pulse dye laser (PDL) therapy.

He received eight treatment sessions over a four year period using pulse dye laser of 585 nm wavelength, the parameters of which are shown in Table 1. He achieved positive results with over 75% clearance of the lesions, a significant reduction in itch and colour and flattening of most of the remaining lesions (Figure 3). No side effects were noted by the patient, parents or laser team. Fifteen years after being discharged the patient has received no further treatments for this condition and he has remained free of new lesions.

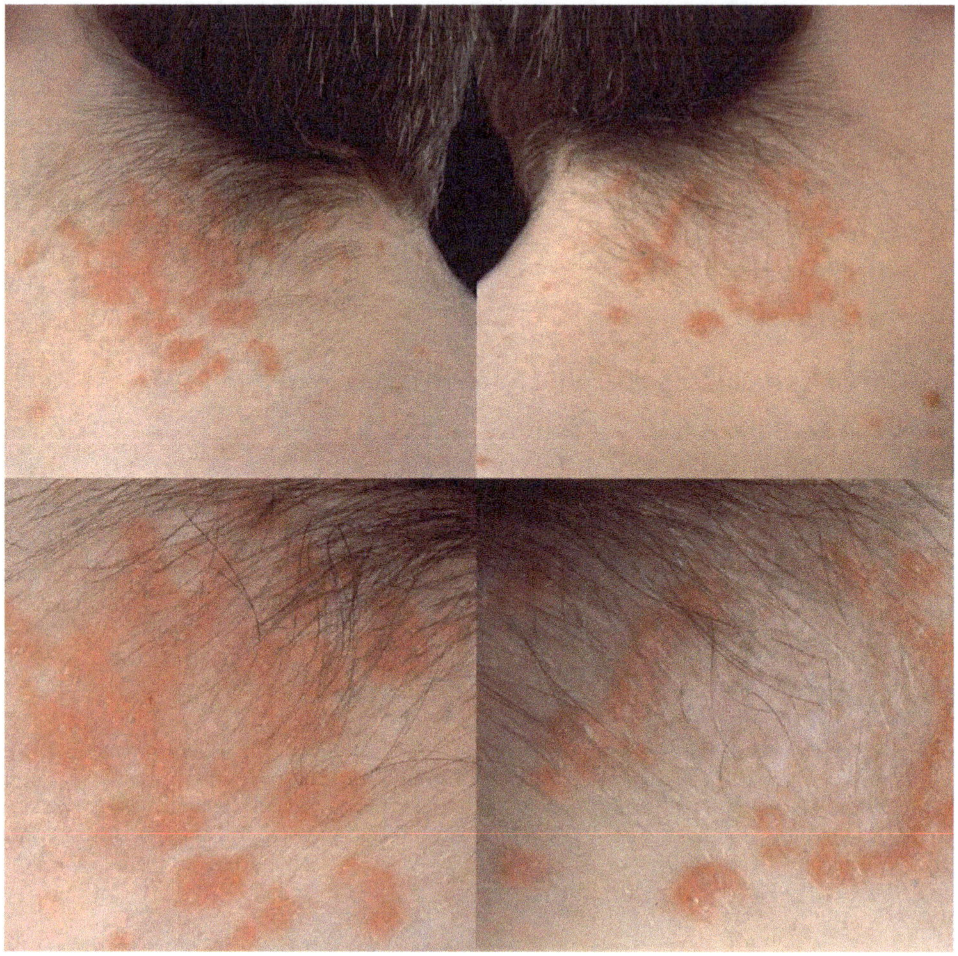

FIGURE 1: Lesions on left & right neck before treatment.

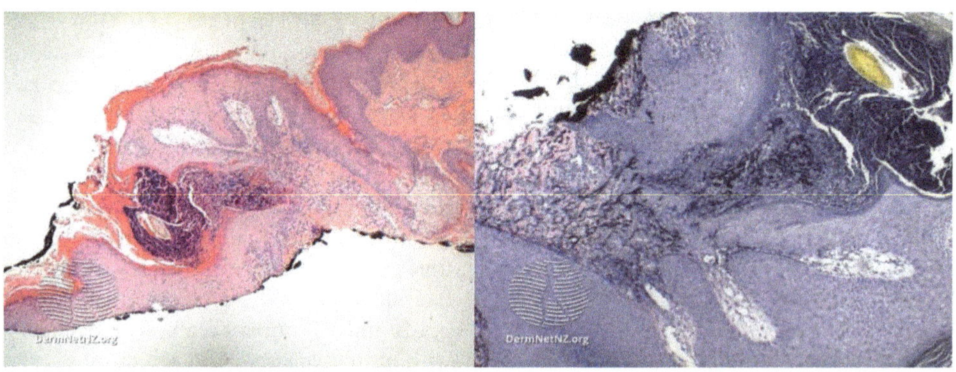

FIGURE 2: EPS biopsy—https://creativecommons.org/licenses/by-nc-nd/3.0/nz/legalcode.

TABLE 1: Laser parameters used to treat our patient.

Probe	7 mm
Laser fluence	8–15 J/cm^2
Pulse duration	0.45–1.5 ms
Maximum pulses	46
Cooling method	Cryogen spray

3. Discussion

EPS remains one of the rarer dermatological perforating disorders for which the exact prevalence remains unestablished. Published cases of EPS mainly focus on the association with possible triggers, for example, Down's syndrome, penicillamine, scabies, osteogenesis imperfecta, and systemic sclerosis [3, 4, 6–8]. For less experienced clinicians it can create a

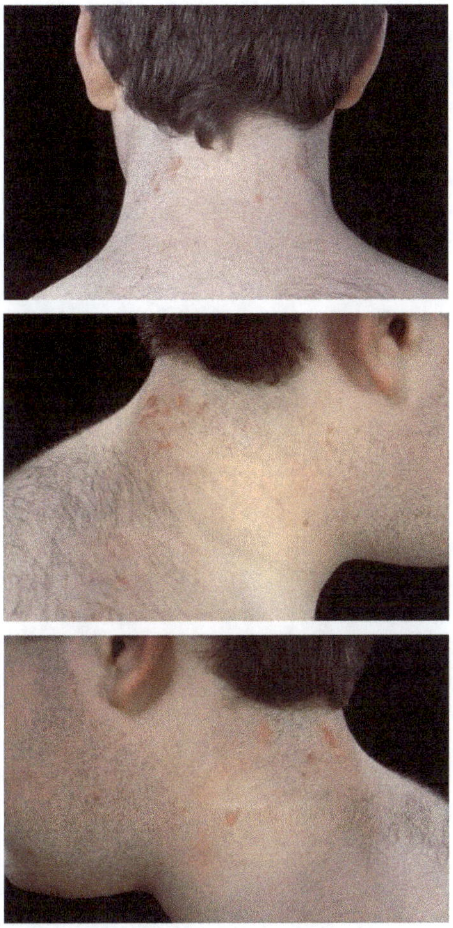

FIGURE 3: Lesions on left and right neck after 7 laser sessions.

diagnostic conundrum and therefore remains best diagnosed via a biopsy and histological examination.

Importantly, EPS remains difficult to treat with minimal published evidence and no consensus on successful treatment methods. Various attempted treatment methods have been reported with many clinicians initially trialling topical steroids and topical retinoids. However these treatments have not shown to be successful [7]. Other treatment options include oral isotretinoin, intralesional steroids, curettage & cautery, and cryotherapy. Similarly these interventions have not been shown to be successful [2, 3, 7, 9]. Experimental treatments such as narrow band UVB, topical imiquimod and tazarotene have shown contradictory results with temporary improvement in certain patients [2, 10]. However in other patients either no improvement was reported or there was rebound flaring upon discontinuation [11, 12].

Over the last three decades laser therapy has emerged as a possible treatment option. One case, reported by Kaufman in the year 2000, demonstrated marked improvement of EPS after PDL therapy (585 nm and fluencies of 6.0–7.0 J/cm^2) [13]. However, we are not aware of any further cases reported. More recently, the use of CO_2 laser has had contradictory results with one case reporting it as successful [11] and two other cases reporting clinically insignificant results and even scarring in one patient [12, 14].

As far as we are aware only one other case, almost 20 years ago, has been reported to use PDL laser therapy for EPS treatment. Our experience confirms Kaufman's initial success with PDL laser for treatment of EPS and encourages other practitioners who encounter EPS to consider this treatment method. Furthermore, we encourage fellow laser practitioners to report their experiences in treating this condition. This would produce a larger evidence base and facilitate the creation of a consensus for the successful treatment of this recalcitrant skin condition.

4. Conclusions

In conclusion, we report a case of idiopathic EPS that was successfully managed with PDL therapy. This is important as it reconfirms that PDL therapy is a safe and effective treatment for EPS.

Consent

Consent was taken from the patient and he was offered to view the final manuscript. This was formally documented in the patient notes.

Authors' Contributions

Samira Batul Syed was involved with the care of the patient. Giulia Rinaldi was involved in the writing of the manuscript. Both Samira Batul Syed and Alisha Chacko reviewed the manuscript. All three authors read and approved the final manuscript version that was submitted.

Acknowledgments

We would like to thank our patient, his family, and our laser team.

References

[1] K. Arora, K. A. Hajirnis, S. Sawant, V. Sabnis, and N. Gaikward, "Perforating disorders of the skin," *Indian Journal of Pathology and Microbiology*, vol. 56, no. 4, pp. 355–358, 2013.

[2] S.-H. Lee, Y. Choi, and S.-C. Kim, "Elastosis perforans serpiginosa," *Annals of Dermatology*, vol. 26, no. 1, pp. 103–106, 2014.

[3] S. Menzies and B. Kirby, "Drug-induced elastosis perforans serpiginosa," *BMJ Case Reports*, 2015.

[4] X.-Y. Yao, G.-D. Wen, C. Zhou et al., "D-penicillamine-induced elastosis perforans serpiginosa," *Chinese Medical Journal*, vol. 130, no. 16, pp. 2013–2014, 2017.

[5] B. Tallon, "Elastosis perforans serpiginosa pathology," 2010, https://dermnetnz.org/topics/elastosis-perforans-serpiginosa-pathology/.

[6] M. Kassardjian, J. Frederickson, J. Griffith, P. Shitabata, and D. Horowitz, "Elastosis perforans serpiginosa in association with scabies mite," *The Journal of Clinical and Aesthetic Dermatology*, vol. 6, no. 10, pp. 36–40, 2013.

[7] R. K. Mehta, N. P. Burrows, C. M. Payne, S. S. Mendelsohn, F. M. Pope, and E. Rytina, "Elastosis perforans serpiginosa and associated disorders," *Clinical and Experimental Dermatology*, vol. 26, no. 6, pp. 521–524, 2001.

[8] N. C. May and R. S. Lester, "Elastosis perforans serpiginosa associated with systemic sclerosis," *Journal of the American Academy of Dermatology*, vol. 6, no. 5, p. 945, 1982.

[9] A. Polańska, M. Bowszyc-Dmochowska, R. W. Żaba, Z. Adamski, A. Reich, and A. Dańczak-Pazdrowska, "Elastosis perforans serpiginosa: a review of the literature and our own experience," *Advances in Dermatology and Allergology*, vol. 33, no. 5, pp. 392–395, 2016.

[10] S. C. Kelly and S. M. Purcell, "Imiquimod therapy for elastosis perforans serpiginosa," *JAMA Dermatology*, vol. 142, no. 7, pp. 829–830, 2006.

[11] A. Kelati, S. Lagrange, F. Le Duff, J.-P. Lacour, and T. Passeron, "Treatment of elastosis perforans serpiginosa using a fractional carbon dioxide laser fractional CO_2 laser treatment of elastosis perforans serpiginosa letters," *JAMA Dermatology*, vol. 153, no. 10, pp. 1063–1064, 2017.

[12] J. D. Outland, T. S. Brown, and J. P. Callen, "Tazarotene is an effective therapy for elastosis perforans serpiginosa," *Archives of Dermatology*, vol. 138, no. 2, pp. 169–171, 2002.

[13] A. J. Kaufman, "Treatment of elastosis perforans serpiginosa with the flashlamp pulsed dye laser," *Dermatologic Surgery*, vol. 26, no. 11, pp. 1060–1062, 2000.

[14] M. Saxena and W. D. Tope, "Response of elastosis perforans serpiginosa to pulsed CO_2, Er:YAG, and dye lasers," *Dermatologic Surgery*, vol. 29, no. 6, pp. 677–678, 2003.

3

Atypical Mycobacterial Infection Arising Amid Corticosteroid Therapy for Livedoid Vasculopathy

John R. Edminister [1], Nicole Dominiak [2], and Lorie D. Gottwald [3]

[1]*University of Toledo College of Medicine and Life Sciences, 3000 Arlington Avenue, Toledo, OH 43614, USA*
[2]*Department of Pathology, University of Toledo Medical Center, 3000 Arlington Avenue, Toledo, OH 43614, USA*
[3]*Department of Dermatology, University of Toledo Medical Center, 3000 Arlington Avenue, Toledo, OH 43614, USA*

Correspondence should be addressed to Lorie D. Gottwald; lorie.gottwald@utoledo.edu

Academic Editor: Ravi Krishnan

Patients who suffer from rare skin diseases may try numerous therapies with many potential side effects before achieving remission. Livedoid vasculopathy (LV) is one such rare disease that lacks a definitive treatment as evidenced by randomized controlled trials. Although corticosteroids help reduce the pain flares associated with LV, they come at the risk of immunosuppression. We present a case of disseminated cutaneous infection of *M. chelonae/abscessus* arising in a diabetic patient on long-term corticosteroid therapy. This patient required an intensive antibiotic regimen and potentially lifelong antibiotic suppression pending improvement of her disseminated cutaneous infection. We report this case to increase awareness of the diagnostic consideration of atypical, rapidly growing mycobacterial (RGM) infection when encountering patients with a diffuse onset of ulcerative skin nodules amid a background of diabetes and long-term corticosteroid use.

1. Introduction

Livedoid vasculopathy (LV) is a chronic, painful condition that typically affects the cutaneous vasculature of the distal legs [1]. There is no standard or definitive treatment of livedoid vasculopathy as evidenced by a randomized controlled trial, perhaps due to its rare incidence at 1 : 100,000 [2]. Instead, case reports and series have demonstrated a multitude of therapeutic options with the most common being anticoagulants, antiplatelet drugs, systemic steroids, and intravenous immunoglobulins (IVIG) [3]. These therapies each have a wealth of adverse effects and contraindications that can make it difficult to treat a patient with comorbidities alongside a rare disease such as livedoid vasculopathy. Although the pathogenesis of LV is now thought to involve thrombotic occlusion, some patients may fail or have contraindications to the now commonly used anticoagulant/antiplatelet agents. These patients might then find relief with systemic corticosteroids, as some patients using corticosteroids have reported better healing and prompt resolution of pain flares associated with livedoid vasculopathy [4].

It is known that corticosteroids modulate the innate immune system and suppress cellular immunity [5]. Opportunistic infection is an unfortunate development of immunosuppression secondary to corticosteroids. A rare example of this is disseminated cutaneous infection with nontuberculous mycobacterial species such as the *Mycobacterium chelonae–abscessus complex*. These rapidly growing nontuberculous mycobacteria are ubiquitous in environmental soil and water [6] and can cause three different manifestations of disease—catheter infection, local infection of skin or bone, or a disseminated cutaneous infection; the latter being the most common clinical presentation of *M. chelonae* infection [7]. The morphology of disseminated cutaneous lesions include pustules, hyperkeratotic plaques, ulcers with sinus tracts, nodules which may suppurate, and finally a sporotrichoid appearance with proximal spread along lymphatic vessels [8]. In one study, 90% of these disseminated cutaneous infections occurred with corticosteroid therapy, with some underlying conditions including autoimmune disease, renal transplant, and rheumatoid arthritis [7]. Additionally, a retrospective study in 2016 suggested that soft-tissue infection with nontuberculous mycobacterial species were three times overrepresented in diabetic patients when compared to the general population [9].

We present a case of disseminated cutaneous infection of *M. chelonae/abscessus* occurring in a diabetic patient on long-term corticosteroid therapy for her rare livedoid vasculopathy.

2. Case Presentation

In July 2006, a 50-year-old female presented to the dermatology clinic with a complaint of painful skin changes in her bilateral lower extremities. She was employed as a dog groomer, and her past medical history was significant for type 2 diabetes mellitus with insulin requirements, gastritis, and severe valvular heart disease affecting the tricuspid, mitral, and aortic valves with surgical repair of the aortic valve. On physical examination, the patient was found to have linear, hyperpigmented macules on the bilateral lower legs with foci of scarring and ulceration. Two biopsies of the proximal and distal left lower leg suggested livedoid vasculopathy pending clinical correlation. She was additionally found to have an elevated antithrombin 3 activity of 124 (reference range 70.0–120.0), which is strongly suggestive of an underlying prothrombotic component to her condition [10]. At this time, therapeutic options for livedoid vasculopathy were considered and offered to the patient.

The patient's preferences and past medical history presented several obstacles to treatment of her LV. She repeatedly refused anticoagulant therapy because her husband had previously had issues with the diet restrictions and INR monitoring mandated by the use of warfarin. Antiplatelet agents were avoided due to her history of severe gastritis that was onset prior to our management of her LV. Intravenous immunoglobulin was considered; however, the patient could not afford the co-pay and her cardiologist recommended against IVIG due to the risk of these hyperosmolar preparations causing fluid overload in this patient with severe valvular heart disease. The patient was eventually started on an acceptable treatment regimen consisting of oral dapsone 100 mg once daily and prednisone 10 mg once daily, with the addition of doxepin or tramadol for intermittent pain control. With these medications, she achieved intermittent remission of her LV for several years.

In 2015, she began having intermittent, painful flares of her LV which were managed by increasing her dapsone to 150 mg once daily and increasing her prednisone to 20 mg. She sometimes required burst doses of 60 mg once daily. Attempts to wean her prednisone back down to 10 mg were rarely successful, and this dosing became an ongoing concern in 2018 when she began having severe hyperglycemic episodes which resulted in a brief hospitalization. Her insulin delivery was also switched to a pump system.

In the fall of 2018, she presented to dermatology during an acute LV pain flare and was coincidentally found to have an erythematous papule at the right dorsal forearm, which she attributed to a possible insect bite or a scratch from her dog. Three weeks later, she reported worsening of this right forearm lesion as well as new onset of two painful, ulcerative lesions on her right thigh and right forearm. On examination, the right dorsal forearm was now found to have two firm, tender erythematous papulonodules, one with central ulceration (Figure 1). The right lateral thigh was found to have a single purpuric patch with central ulceration and necrosis (Figure 2). The bilateral forearms additionally had a few scattered linear superficial abrasions consistent with animal scratches. No other new lesions were found on examination. She perceived these lesions as dissimilar from her typical LV, but at this time mycophenolate mofetil 500 mg twice daily was added for her ongoing LV flares. A 4 mm punch biopsy of a

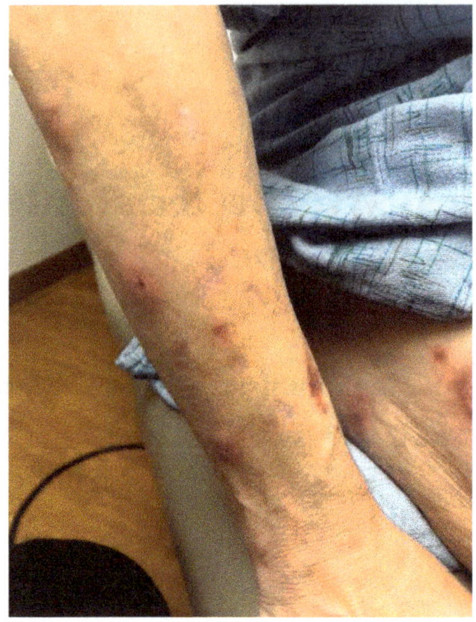

Figure 1: The right dorsal forearm was found to have two firm, tender erythematous papulonodules, one with central ulceration.

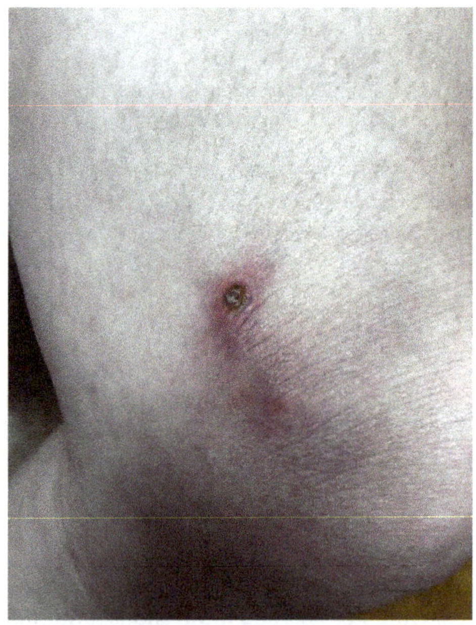

Figure 2: The right lateral thigh was found to have a purpuric patch with central ulceration and necrosis.

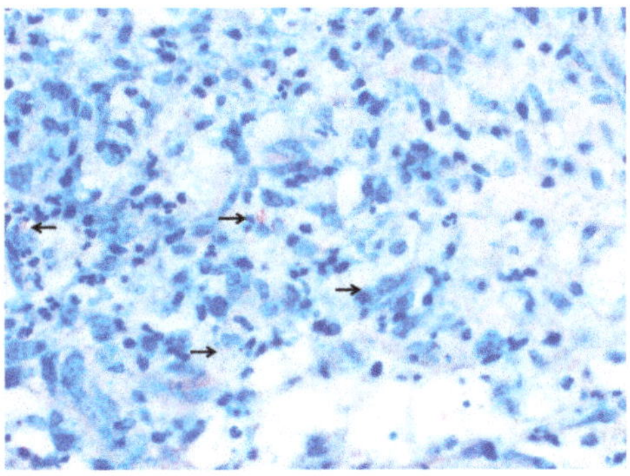

FIGURE 3: Kinyoun stain (40x). Acid fast bacilli (arrows) within the center of the suppurative granuloma.

right dorsal forearm lesion revealed suppurative, granulomatous inflammation in the deep reticular dermis with demonstration of acid-fast organisms on AFB stain (Figure 3).

The patient was subsequently evaluated for systemic mycobacterial disease. A chest X-ray showed no evidence of pulmonary mycobacterial disease. Laboratory testing was negative for HIV, AFB blood culture, and Tb QuantiFERON. Her CRP was elevated at 13.3, and the CBC revealed a mild leukocytosis of 13.00 with mild neutrophilia of 79.4%, elevated absolute neutrophils (10.3), and absolute immature granulocytes (0.4).

The state Department of Health identified rapidly growing *Mycobacterium abscessus/chelonae* on her right forearm tissue culture. Susceptibility testing and treatment guidance was subsequently provided by a national center specializing in mycobacterial consultation. Susceptibility results revealed resistance to cefoxitin, doxycycline, sulfamethoxazole-trimethoprim, and amoxicillin-clavulanic acid and sensitivity to clarithromycin, azithromycin, linezolid, imipenem, and amikacin. There was also intermediate sensitivity to ciprofloxacin and moxifloxacin.

The physicians of the Dermatology and Infectious Disease departments then coordinated management of her simultaneously flaring livedoid vasculopathy and disseminated cutaneous mycobacterial infection. The patient had a PICC line placed for her antimycobacterial regimen which consisted of oral azithromycin 250 mg once daily, intravenous imipenem 500 mg every 12 hours, and finally intravenous amikacin 12–15 mg/kg on Mondays, Wednesdays, and Fridays. Additional treatment with fluoroquinolones was not considered because she had a previously documented allergic reaction of a blistering skin eruption. This regimen was initially to be continued for a total of 8–12 weeks depending on her response, followed by oral azithromycin monotherapy for at least an additional 6 months. Lifelong suppression with oral monotherapy is also being considered pending her clinical response and tolerance to azithromycin.

At 10 weeks of treatment her physical exam revealed improvement of the ulcers of the right forearm, right thigh, and left foot. However, she also developed three new left knee ulcers consistent in appearance with her other mycobacterial lesions. For this reason, her current regimen is to be continued until her follow-up appointment for PICC line removal at 17 weeks of treatment. At that time, she will transition to daily maintenance therapy of oral azithromycin if she demonstrates adequate improvement in the existing lesions.

Meanwhile, the treatment of her livedoid vasculopathy was optimized by the dermatology team. Her prednisone was tapered down to 10 mg once daily, and both the dapsone and mycophenolate mofetil were discontinued. She has since been started on warfarin 1 mg once daily. This low dose was chosen due to reports of supratherapeutic INR from interaction of warfarin and azithromycin [11]. Her LV was found to be stable at her follow-up appointment 9 weeks after initiating and continuing the same dose of warfarin.

3. Discussion

Livedoid vasculopathy is a relatively rare condition with an incidence of 1 : 100,000 at a 3 : 1 ratio of women to men [2]. The clinical manifestations of early LV classically involve the bilateral distal legs and ankles with a reticular pattern of purple plaques and papules which intermittently flare into painful ulcers; late manifestations include stelliform, porcelain-white scarring known as "atrophie blanche" [1]. Because LV is not a true inflammatory vasculitis but rather a thrombotic vasculopathy, clinical suspicion must be confirmed with histopathologic evidence demonstrating dermal vascular changes such as segmental hyalinosis, thrombosis, and fibrin deposition [2].

This case exemplifies the struggles and complications that patients with rare skin diseases may encounter. There is no definitive treatment for livedoid vasculopathy, and in our case the preferred treatments were either contraindicated or deferred due to patient preference. This resulted in her being treated with dapsone and prednisone for years. The use of corticosteroids in LV is not unheard of, as steroids were the second-most prescribed drug for LV behind heparin in one pre-study population [10]. However, that same cohort study found approximately 12 patients with LV to have no better than a moderate response to steroids. On the other hand, Feng et al. described 22 patients with LV on combined regimens that included steroids, and they found that steroids were effective in hastening resolution of acute, ulcerative LV flares [12]. Our patient similarly responded well to increasing doses of prednisone during her acute LV flares. However, this treatment came with the well-known adverse effect of immunosuppression. Her diabetes and recent hospitalization for hyperglycemia were additional concerning factors in the management of this patient with corticosteroids.

This patient's development of a rapidly growing nontuberculous mycobacterial skin infection can be attributed to multiple factors including her corticosteroid therapy, ongoing poorly controlled diabetes mellitus, and a possible direct inoculation or environmental exposure. The most common presentation of disseminated RGM skin infections is with an underlying corticosteroid exposure or defective cellular immunity [8]. A case report in 2015 describes a patient who developed a disseminated cutaneous *M. chelonae* infection amid systemic corticosteroid and mycophenolate mofetil treatment for systemic lupus erythematosus [13]. Our patient did have a brief trial of mycophenolate mofetil for her LV flares. However, this was initiated after her initial right forearm lesion was first observed and it was discontinued when the patient began her antibiotic regimen for the confirmed RGM infection. Therefore, we do not believe mycophenolate mofetil played a role in the development of our patient's infection.

Diabetics have also been demonstrated to have increased tendency for developing RGM infections, and some case reports trace atypical mycobacterial infections to an inoculating event with unclean or improperly used insulin pens or syringes [14–16]. Other local inoculating events have been reported in the literature, including tattooing and surgical procedures such as liposuction and liposculpture [17, 18].

Our patient was interviewed regarding possible events surrounding the onset of her infection. Although one early lesion was on her right lateral thigh, she denied any known insulin injections at that site prior to onset of her infection. She denied recent falls, penetrating trauma, surgeries, cosmetic procedures, biopsies, tattoos, or injections besides the previous use of her insulin pens and glucometer. Of note, she was working as a part-time pet groomer and frequently bathed dogs in water. She also owned several dogs and cats and reported being frequently scratched on the forearms and legs by these animals.

The zoonotic potential of several mycobacterial species is well-documented, ranging from bovine tuberculosis to fish tank granuloma primarily caused by *Mycobacterium bovis* and *Mycobacterium marinum*, respectively [19, 20]. Zoonotic transmission of *Mycobacterium microti* infection by cats, racoon dogs, and mice has been suggested; however, like *M. bovis* and *M. marinum*, the *M. microti* species is a slow-growing mycobacterial species [21]. A search of medical and veterinary literature did not reveal any known cases of zoonosis involving the *M. chelonae* complex. Although our patient's profession as a dog groomer is intriguing, we suspect that she likely encountered her infection through a common environmental source of RGM such as water or soil.

Disseminated cutaneous infection with rapidly growing nontuberculous mycobacteria may result in significant morbidity due to the prolonged therapeutic timeline that typically lasts a minimum of 12 months [13]. The *M. abscessus* species is resistant to conventional antimycobacterial drugs and those that are usually effective against other RGM such as erythromycin and minocycline. The initial choice for local disease can be oral monotherapy with clarithromycin; however, disseminated cutaneous disease requires an oral agent (such as clarithromycin or azithromycin) with parental combination involving tobramycin, imipenem, and amikacin [16]. We consulted a national center for mycobacterial susceptibilities and treatment guidance, and we agreed upon a regimen with one oral agent and two parenteral agents administered via PICC line at home for a minimum of four months. This would be followed by potentially lifelong oral monotherapy with azithromycin. Her PICC line requirement has known risks including luminal occlusion, venous thrombosis, and local or systemic infection [22]. Our patient is now retired and has a good support system in place with her husband; however, she does require a visiting home nurse to aid with her PICC line.

Due to concerns of adverse effects of her antimicrobial regimen, our patient required weekly labs including complete blood count, basic metabolic panel, and serum amikacin levels. Of particular note was a time of 10 weeks into her treatment when amikacin was temporarily discontinued due to a concerning creatinine elevation of 1.62 compared to her baseline of 1.17 prior to initiating antibiotic therapy.

4. Conclusion

This case demonstrates the frustrations that both patients and dermatologists experience when treating a rare skin disease in a patient with multiple comorbidities. We report this case to increase awareness of the diagnostic consideration of atypical mycobacterial infection, especially when encountering patients with a diffuse onset of ulcerative skin nodules amid a background of immunosuppression secondary to long-term corticosteroid use and diabetes.

References

[1] N. Kerk and T. Goerge, "Livedoid vasculopathy—current aspects of diagnosis and treatment of cutaneous infarction," *Journal of the German Society of Dermatology*, vol. 11, no. 5, pp. 407–410, 2013.

[2] T. M. Gonzalez-Santiago and M. D. P. Davis, "Update of management of connective tissue diseases: livedoid vasculopathy," *Dermatologic Therapy*, vol. 25, no. 2, pp. 183–194, 2012.

[3] R. Micieli and A. Alavi, "Treatment for livedoid vasculopathy: a systematic review," *JAMA Dermatology*, vol. 154, no. 2, pp. 193–202, 2018.

[4] B. Vasudevan, S. Neema, and R. Verma, "Livedoid vasculopathy: a review of pathogenesis and principles of management," *Indian Journal of Dermatology, Venereology and Leprology*, vol. 82, no. 5, pp. 478–488, 2016.

[5] D. Franchimont, "Overview of the actions of glucocorticoids on the immune response: a good model to characterize new pathways of immunosuppression for new treatment strategies," *Annals of the New York Academy of Sciences*, vol. 1024, no. 1, pp. 124–137, 2004.

[6] M. A. De Groote and G. Huitt, "Infections due to rapidly growing mycobacteria," *Clinical Infectious Diseases*, vol. 42, no. 12, pp. 1756–1763, 2006.

[7] R. J. Wallace Jr., B. A. Brown, and G. O. Onyi , "Skin, soft tissue, and bone infections due to *Mycobacterium chelonae* chelonae: importance of prior corticosteroid therapy, frequency of disseminated infections, and resistance to oral antimicrobials other than clarithromycin," *The Journal of Infectious Diseases*, vol. 166, no. 2, pp. 405–412, 1992.

[8] P. Kullavanijaya, "Atypical mycobacterial cutaneous infection," *Clinics in Dermatology*, vol. 17, no. 2, pp. 153–158, 1999.

[9] T. Bridson, B. Govan, N. Ketheesan, and R. Norton, "Overrepresentation of diabetes in soft tissue nontuberculous mycobacterial infections," *The American Journal of Tropical Medicine and Hygiene*, vol. 95, no. 3, pp. 528–530, 2016.

[10] C. Weishaupt, A. Strolin, B. Kahle et al., "Characteristics, risk factors and treatment reality in livedoid vasculopathy—a multicentre analysis," *Journal of the European Academy of Dermatology and Venereology*, 2019.

[11] D. R. Foster and N. L. Milan, "Potential interaction between azithromycin and warfarin," *Pharmacotherapy*, vol. 19, no. 7, pp. 902–908, 1999.

[12] S. Feng, W. Su, P. Jin, and C. Shao, "Livedoid vasculopathy: clinical features and treatment in 24 chinese patients," *Advances in Dermatology and Venereology*, vol. 94, no. 5, pp. 574–578, 2014.

[13] S. Mankad, R. Karthik, P. Rupali, and J. S. Michael, "Fatal disseminated *Mycobacterium chelonae* infection in an immunocompromised host-a unique presentation," *The Journal of the Association of Physicians of India*, vol. 63, no. 1, pp. 49–52, 2015.

[14] K. Finucane, P. Ambrey, S. Narayan, C. B. Archer, and C. Dayan, "Insulin injection abscesses caused by *Mycobacterium chelonae*," *Diabetes Care*, vol. 26, no. 8, pp. 2483–2484, 2003.

[15] T. W. Yew, N. S. Chandran, K. B. Tan, and A. C. Thai, "Atypical mycobacterial infection in insulin injection sites," *QJM: An International Journal of Medicine*, vol. 108, no. 8, pp. 673–674, 2015.

[16] T. R. Bates, T. Keenher, L. C. O'Reilly, C. H. Heath, J. P. Flexman, and R. J. Murray, "Extensive cutaneous *Mycobacterium abscessus* infection due to contaminated insulin delivery system sites," *QJM: An International Journal of Medicine*, vol. 102, no. 12, pp. 881–884, 2009.

[17] B. S. Kennedy, B. Bedard, M. Younge et al., "Outbreak of *Mycobacterium chelonae* infection associated with tattoo ink," *The New England Journal of Medicine*, vol. 367, no. 11, pp. 1020–1024, 2012.

[18] J. Murillo, J. Torres, L. Bofill et al., "Skin and wound infection by rapidly growing mycobacteria: an unexpected complication of liposuction and liposculpture," *Archives of Dermatology*, vol. 136, no. 11, pp. 1347–1352, 2000.

[19] F. Olea-Popelka, A. Muwonge, A. Perera et al., "Zoonotic tuberculosis in human beings caused by *Mycobacterium bovis*—a call for action," *The Lancet Infectious Diseases*, vol. 17, no. 1, pp. e21–e25, 2017.

[20] M. Slany, P. Jezek, and M. Bodnarova, "Fish tank granuloma caused by *Mycobacterium marinum* in two aquarists: two case reports," *BioMed Research International*, vol. 2013, Article ID 161329, 4 pages, 2013.

[21] L. Michelet, K. de Cruz, G. Zanella et al., "Infection with *Mycobacterium microti* in animals in France," *Journal of Clinical Microbiology*, vol. 53, no. 3, pp. 981–985, 2015.

[22] D. Grau, B. Clarivet, A. Lotthé, S. Bommart, and S. Parer, "Complications with peripherally inserted central catheters (PICCs) used in hospitalized patients and outpatients: a prospective cohort study," *Antimicrobial Resistance and Infection Control*, vol. 6, no. 1, Article ID 18, 2017.

4

Treatment of Generalized Granuloma Annulare with Oral Griseofulvin

Chumsaeng Chumsaengsri and Jongjin Suwanthaweemeesuk

Institute of Dermatology, Bangkok, Thailand

Correspondence should be addressed to Jongjin Suwanthaweemeesuk; jsuwanthaw@gmail.com

Academic Editor: Alireza Firooz

Background. Granuloma annulare (GA) is a benign skin disease that has four clinical variants including localized, generalized, perforating, and subcutaneous GA. The most common type is localized GA, followed by generalized GA. Generalized GA was defined as at least 10 widespread annular plagues and frequently on the trunk, face, neck, and extremities. The diagnosis was made by clinical and histopathology. Generalized GA was difficult to treat. *Case Presentation.* We presented a Thai woman with nonscaly annular papules and plaques on the trunk and all extremities. A skin biopsy revealed a lesion that was compatible with granuloma annulare. She was partially resolved with 2-month course of oral griseofluvin 500 mg daily. *Discussion.* The regression of GA response to oral griseofulvin is consistent with the inflammatory nature, which identified IFN-gamma upregulated in GA. *Conclusion.* Griseofulvin is safe with few side effects and cost effectiveness. Further studies are needed to better understand the immunology and pathogenesis of GA.

1. Introduction

Granuloma annulare (GA) is an inflammatory granulomatous skin disease affecting all ages but most frequently during the fifth decade of life and more common in women [1]. Although the pathogenesis of GA is unclear, it represents a benign cutaneous reaction with a variety of trigger factors. Infectious agents including both viral and bacterial triggers, several vaccinations, medications, bee string, octopus bite, and red pigmented tattoo were leading to the development of GA [2]. Drug-induced granuloma annulare are typically resolved when discontinuing the culprit drug, and drug lists including angiotensin-converting enzyme inhibitors, anti-TNF agents (infliximab, adalimumab, etanercept, and lenalidomide), diuretics (furosemide), gold, methotrexate, and immunization (hepatitis B and anti-tetanus vaccination) [3]. Hyperlipidemia and hypothyroidism remained significantly associated with GA while type II diabetes mellitus was not a significant association [4].

A recent publication from New York reported the upregulation of T-helper cell type 1 (tumor necrosis factor (TNF)-alpha, interleukin (IL)-1beta, IL-12/23p40), and T-helper cell type 2 (IL4 and IL31) pathways in GA lesional skins compared with normal skin of healthy adults [5]. Furthermore, the significant upregulation of the Janus kinase signal transducer and activator of transcription (JAK-STAT) pathway in GA lesional skin [5]. Another recent publication reported JAK-STAT dependent cytokines, interferon (IFN)-gamma, and oncosatin M are upregulated in GA lesions, as well as IL-21 and IL-15 [6]. GA is T-cell-dependent disorder and the immune mechanism could be driving this disease [5, 6].

Currently, there are no effective treatments for GA due to lack of pathogenesis. The main purpose of treatment is to relieve pruritus and improve quality of life. Generalized GA is recalcitrant to therapy [5]. Multiple therapeutic options for generalized GA including hydroxychloroquine [7], PUVA [8], dapsone [9], methotrexate [10], TNF-alpha

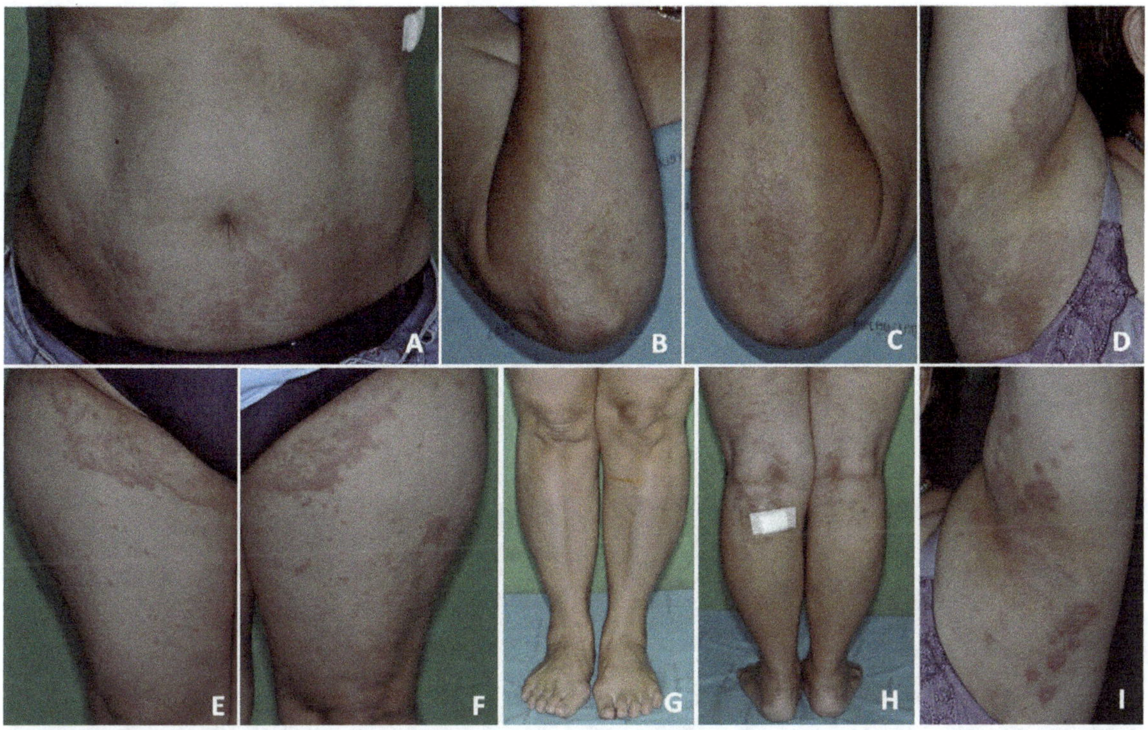

Figure 1: Clinical features: multiple well-defined nonscaly, erythematous annular papules, and plaques on the trunk, both axillar, both groin, and all extremities (a–i).

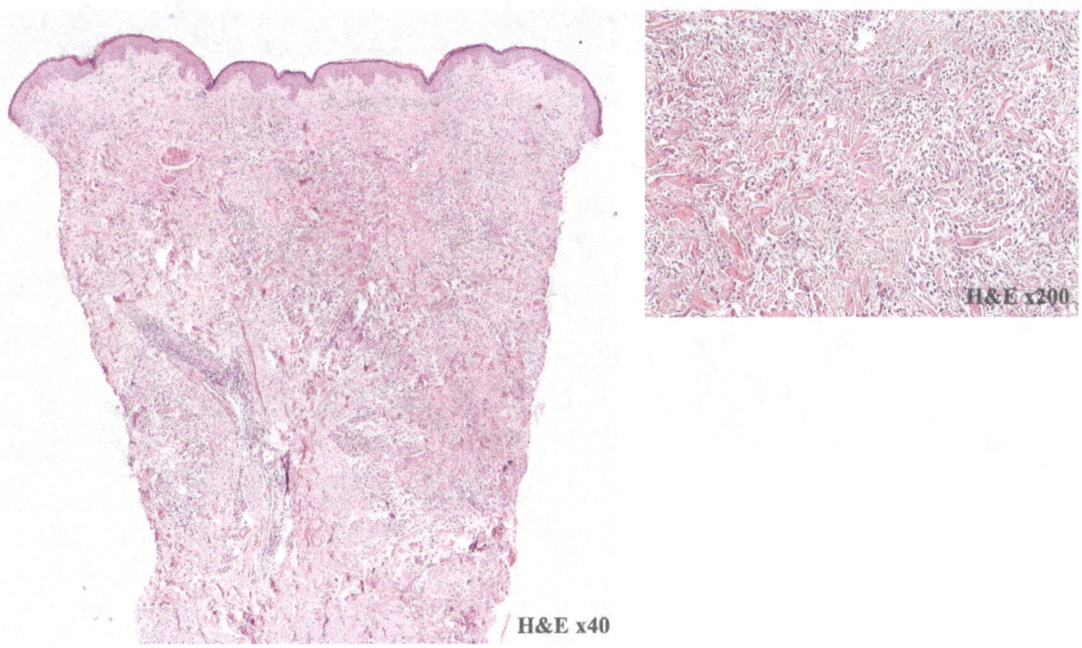

(a) (b)

Figure 2: Continued.

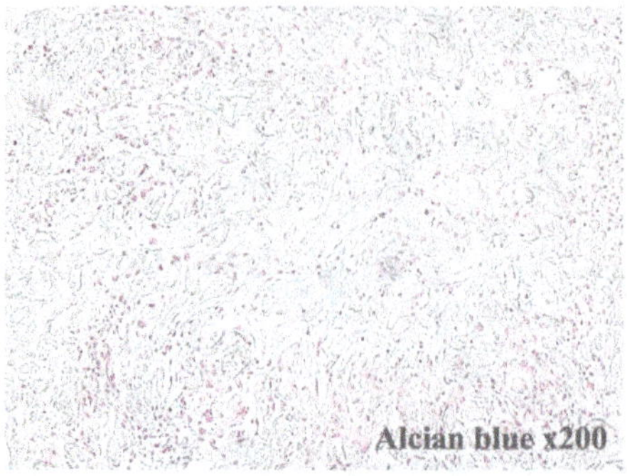

(c)

Figure 2: Histopathology showing palisading granuloma with mucin deposit (a and b). Alcian blue special stain is positive in the center of aggregate (c).

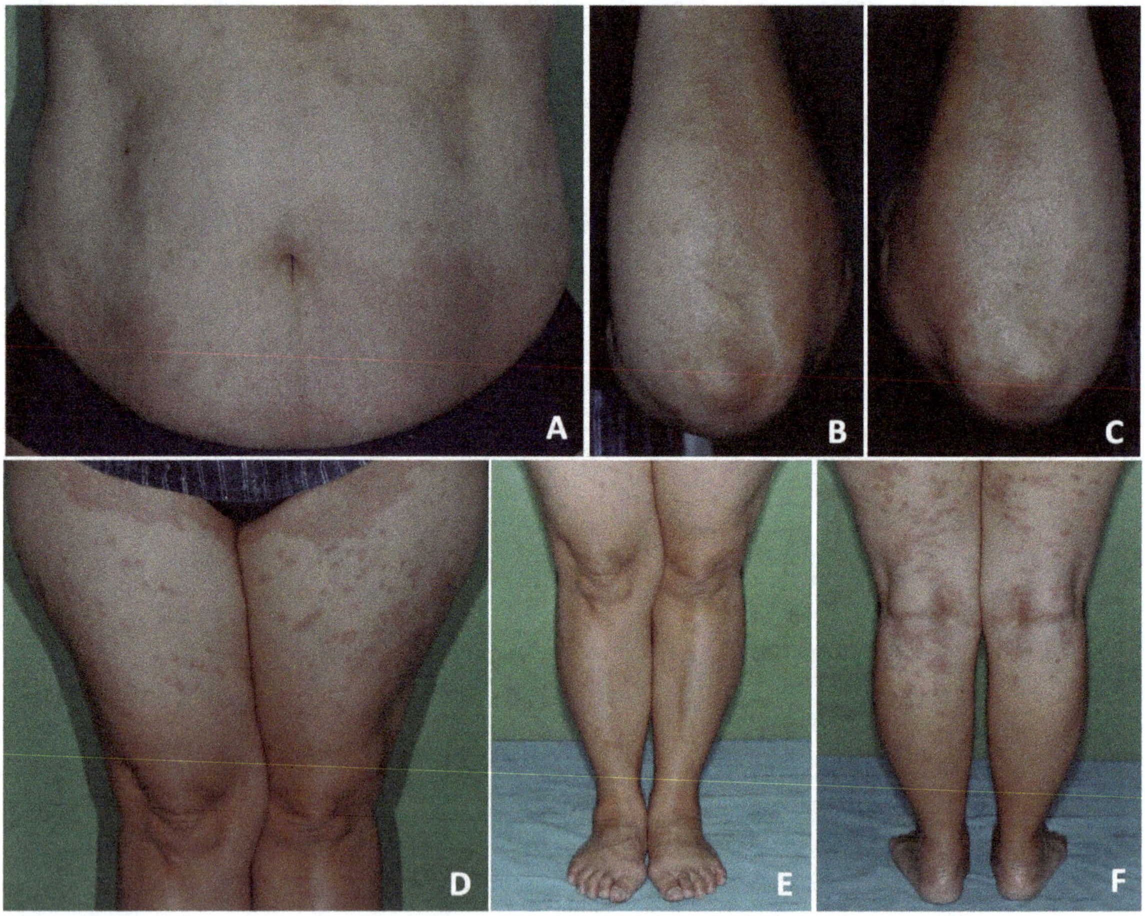

Figure 3: Clinical features of the improved patient: multiple well-defined nonscaly, erythematous annular papules, and plaques were faded in color (a–f).

inhibitor (adalimumab [11] and dupilumab [12]), apremilast [13], and JAK inhibitor (tofacitinib [14]) have been reported to be effective. Around 50% of patients spontaneously resolve within 2 years, and recurrence is also common [2].

2. Case Report

A 58-year-old Thai woman came to the outpatient clinic with pruritic, nonscaly erythematous annular papules and plaques on the trunk, both axillar, both groin, and all extremities for 3 months. At first, she had this clinical manifestation 2 years ago and treated with methotrexate and topical corticosteroids at the previous hospital, but the symptoms did not improve. She still had extremely pruritic, numerous nonscaly erythematous papules, and plaques on the same area so she went to another hospital. She had the same treatment with methotrexate, and her symptoms did not improve. No triggers were reported. She had well-controlled hypertension on losartan 50 mg per day. Dermatological examination revealed the same clinical manifestation as previously mentioned (Figures 1(a)–1(i)). Lymph nodes can not be palpated.

A potassium hydroxide preparation was negative. The skin biopsy of the trunk and left leg showed a focal aggregate of histiocytes reminiscing palisading granuloma and degeneration of collagen in the center is noted. No inflammatory cell is present. Alcian blue special stain is positive in the center of the aggregate (Figures 2(a)–2(c)). Her blood test showed normal fasting blood glucose (FBS 97 mg/dL) and normal lipid profile (cholesterol level 200 mg/dL, triglyceride level 72 mg/dL). She was diagnosed with generalized granuloma annulare. She was prescribed oral griseofulvin 500 mg per day and follow-up one month later, the rash was still present but had faded in color, so we prescribed our patient topical low potency corticosteroids (0.05% betamethasone valerate) applied twice daily on the trunk and all extremities. At follow-up two months later, her symptoms were improved and the rash had faded in color (Figures 3(a)–3(f)).

3. Discussion

Generalized GA can persist for a decade despite therapy [11]. In our case, the clinicopathological data supported the provisional diagnosis of granuloma annulare. Blood sampling for screening metabolic disease was normal. No precipitated factor was reported.

Griseofulvin is known as an antifungal drug for many years and has antibacterial activity [15]. In the previous study, Griseofulvin has potent immunomodulatory properties which its feature was a microtubule antagonist that caused rapid, reversible, and repeated dissociation of mitotic spindle compared to colchicine [16]. Furthermore, griseofulvin inhibited IFN-gamma-induced HLA-DR expression on human keratinocytes is similar to colchicine [16]. This drug has been reported to be a benefit in lichen planus [17, 18] and pigmented purpuric dermatosis [19]. Griseofulvin is safe with few side effects and cost effectiveness. We prescribed our patient oral griseofulvin 500 mg per day and followed up two months later, her symptoms were partially improved. The regression of GA response to oral griseofulvin is consistent with the recent study by Wang et al. [6], which performed single cell RNA sequencing to identified IFN-gamma target genes and has been upregulated by macrophages in GA.

To the best of our knowledge, this is the first case report of generalized GA being successfully treated with oral griseofulvin. Further studies are needed to understand the pathogenesis of GA, approach the new target therapy, and need to be done to corroborate our preliminary findings.

Acknowledgments

The authors would like to thank the Institute of Dermatology, Bangkok, for their assistance in this work.

References

[1] T. P. Joshi and M. Duvic, "Granuloma annulare: an updated review of epidemiology, pathogenesis, and treatment options," *American Journal of Clinical Dermatology*, vol. 23, pp. 37–50, 2021.

[2] E. W. Piette and M. Rosenbach, "Granuloma annulare: pathogenesis, disease associations and triggers, and therapeutic options," *Journal of the American Academy of Dermatology*, vol. 75, no. 3, pp. 467–479, 2016.

[3] N. Shah, M. Shah, A. M. Drucker, N. H. Shear, M. Ziv, and R. P. Dodiuk-Gad, "Granulomatous cutaneous drug eruptions: a systematic review," *American Journal of Clinical Dermatology*, vol. 22, no. 1, pp. 39–53, 2021.

[4] A. C. Leasure, W. Damsky, and J. M. Cohen, "Comorbidities associated with granuloma annulare: a case-control study in the all of Us research program," *Journal of the American Academy of Dermatology*, vol. 87, no. 1, pp. 197–199, 2022.

[5] M. S. Min, J. Wu, H. He et al., "Granuloma annulare skin profile shows activation of T-helper cell type 1, T-helper cell type 2, and Janus kinase pathways," *Journal of the American Academy of Dermatology*, vol. 83, no. 1, pp. 63–70, 2020.

[6] A. Wang, N.-T. Rahman, M. K. McGeary et al., "Treatment of granuloma annulare and suppression of proinflammatory cytokine activity with tofacitinib," *The Journal of Allergy and Clinical Immunology*, vol. 147, no. 5, pp. 1795–1809, 2021.

[7] M. Megna, A. Sidikov, A. Ruggiero et al., "A case of generalized granuloma annulare successfully treated by hydroxychloroquine," *Dermatologic Therapy*, vol. 33, no. 6, Article ID e13894, 2020.

[8] T. M. Nordmann, J.-R. Kim, R. Dummer, and F. Anzengruber, "A monocentric, retrospective analysis of 61 patients with generalized granuloma annulare," *Dermatology*, vol. 236, no. 4, pp. 369–374, 2020.

[9] M. L. Hrin, A. M. Bashyam, S. R. Feldman, and W. W. Huang, "Oral dapsone for the treatment of generalized granuloma annulare: a retrospective case series," *Journal of the American Academy of Dermatology*, vol. 86, no. 4, pp. 911–914, 2022.

[10] F. Naka and B. E. Strober, "Methotrexate treatment of generalized granuloma annulare: a retrospective case series," *Journal of Dermatological Treatment*, vol. 29, no. 7, pp. 720–724, 2018.

[11] M. Fässler and C. Schlapbach, "Granuloma annulare arising under systemic psoriasis therapy successfully treated with adalimumab," *JAAD case reports*, vol. 6, no. 9, pp. 832–834, 2020.

[12] E. J. Song, J. Bezecny, and S. Farrer, "Recalcitrant generalized granuloma annulare treated successfully with dupilumab," *JAAD Case Reports*, vol. 7, pp. 1-2, 2021.

[13] S. Blum and D. Altman, "Treatment of generalized granuloma annulare with apremilast: a report of 2 cases," *JAAD case reports*, vol. 5, no. 11, pp. 976–978, 2019.

[14] J. S. Durgin, B. E. Shields, and M. Rosenbach, "Generalized granuloma annulare: a widespread response to limited application of compounded 2% topical tofacitinib," *JAAD Case Reports*, vol. 6, no. 10, pp. 1113–1115, 2020.

[15] A. Geronikaki, V. Kartsev, A. Petrou et al., "Antibacterial activity of griseofulvin analogues as an example of drug

repurposing," *International Journal of Antimicrobial Agents*, vol. 55, no. 3, Article ID 105884, 2020.

[16] A. Asahina, Y. Tada, K. Nakamura, and K. Tamaki, "Griseofulvin has a potential to modulate the expression of cell adhesion molecules on leukocytes and vascular endothelial cells," *International Immunopharmacology*, vol. 1, no. 1, pp. 75–83, 2001.

[17] I. Bhuiyan, M. Wahab, A. Ali et al., "Comparative efficacy of hydroxychloroquine and griseofulvin in the treatment of lichen planus," *Journal of Pakistan Association of Dermatologists*, vol. 20, no. 2, pp. 79–83, 2010.

[18] K. Sen, R. Hira, A. Islam, S. Sarker, M. Sarker, and A. Biswas, "Effects of griseofulvin in the treatment of lichen planus-A study in BSMMU," *Faridpur Medical College Journal*, vol. 6, no. 2, pp. 86–88, 1970.

[19] I. Martínez Pallás, R. Conejero del Mazo, and V. Lezcano Biosca, "Pigmented purpuric dermatosis: a review of the literature," *Actas Dermo-Sifiliográficas*, vol. 111, no. 3, pp. 196–204, 2020.

5

Psoriasiform Dermatitis in a COVID-19 Patient

Marlyn Wu,[1] **Shereen Teymour**,[1] **Robin Ashinoff**,[1] **and Hira Ghani**[2]

[1]*Hackensack Meridian Palisades Medical Center, Palisades, NJ, USA*
[2]*Nassau University Medical Center, Long Island, NY, USA*

Correspondence should be addressed to Hira Ghani; hghani01@nyit.edu

Academic Editor: Ravi Krishnan

Psoriasis is a chronic inflammatory papulosquamous disorder which affects around 2% of the world's population. A peak exacerbation in psoriatic symptoms was noted during COVID-19 due to lack of access to dermatological care mixed with heightened emotional stress during the pandemic. This case report describes a 52-year-old admitted male patient who sustained a diffuse rash on multiple areas of his body a week prior to testing positive for COVID-19. We explore plausible causes for the occurrence of the rash, discuss our treatment plan, include relevant clinical pictures, and review published literature to examine conditions that present similarly to the rash seen in our patient. It is crucial for dermatologists to be able to discern various systemic manifestations associated with cutaneous lesions, such as the one seen in this patient, in order to make an accurate and prompt diagnosis. A better understanding of the association between COVID-19 infection and psoriasiform lesions is needed for improving the prognostic and therapeutic outcomes in patients.

1. Introduction

Psoriasis is a chronic inflammatory papulosquamous disorder which affects around 2% of the world's population [1, 2]. COVID-19 is a highly contagious respiratory infection caused by severe acute respiratory syndrome coronavirus 2 (SARS-CoV2) [3]. The World Health Organization officially declared COVID-19 a pandemic on March 2020 [3]. Psoriasis is noted to be a more common dermatological disease manifestation in patients with COVID-19. Lack of access to dermatologic care during the peak of COVID-19 pandemic and emotional stress resulting from the global disease outbreak significantly contributed to exacerbation of psoriatic symptoms in those suffering from this condition [4].

In this case report, we describe a patient who sustained a diffuse rash on his upper extremities, trunk, and groin one week prior to testing positive for COVID-19. We explore plausible causes for the occurrence of the rash, discuss our treatment plan, include relevant clinical pictures, and review published literature to examine conditions that present similarly to the rash seen in our patient.

2. Case

A 52-year-old admitted male with no significant past medical or surgical history was evaluated for a 2-week history of an intensely pruritic, diffuse rash starting on his upper extremities and extending to his trunk. Using over the counter topical steroids provided him with minimal symptomatic relief. There was no recent use of new medications. He was seen in the emergency department (ED) for gradual onset of fever, malaise, and shortness of breath, which prompted testing for COVID-19, human immunodeficiency virus (HIV), and syphilis. While his HIV and syphilis tests were negative, he tested positive for COVID-19. The patient was treated with IV fluids, acetaminophen, piperacillin-tazobactam, and vancomycin, and was admitted for further evaluation.

Upon physical exam in our dermatology clinic, diffuse salmon pink papules and plaques with overlying white scales were identified on the trunk, groin, and upper and lower extremities (Figures 1(a)–1(c)). In addition, punctate scaly papules with erythema on were noted on the palms and koebnerization was observed on the patient's old hernia repair surgical site on the abdomen. A 4 mm punch biopsy of

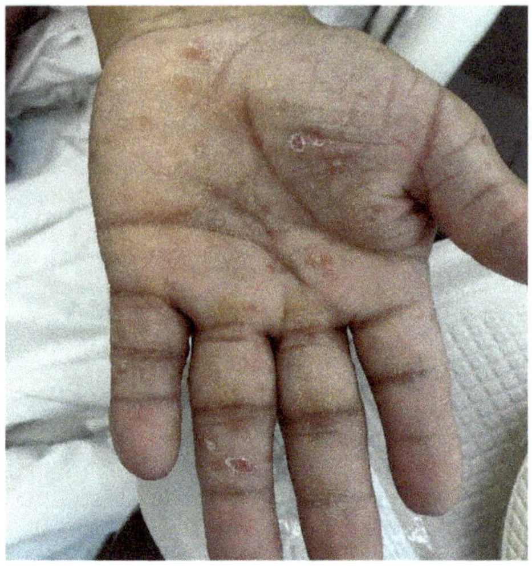

(a)

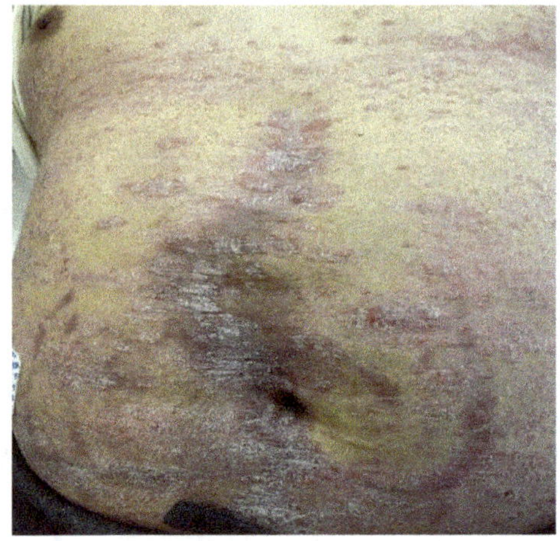

(b)

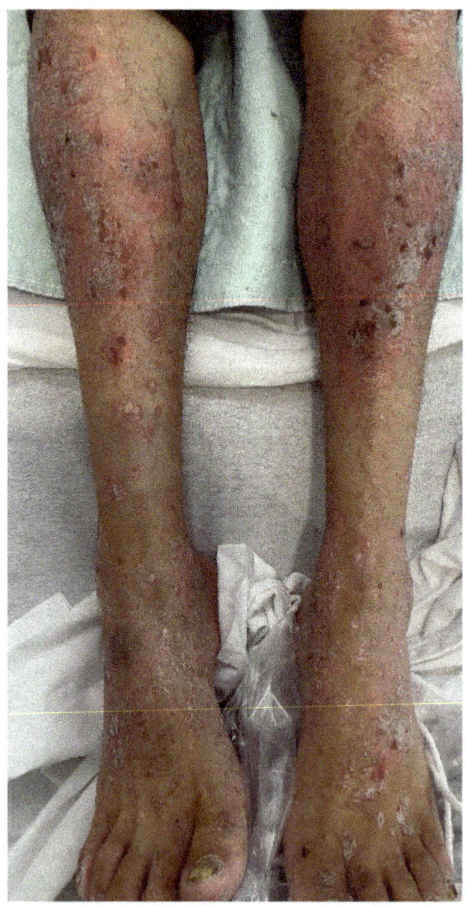

(c)

FIGURE 1: (a–c) Psoriasiform dermatitis. Clinical images depicting diffuse sharply demarcated pink plaques with white scale on the left palm, abdomen, and bilateral lower extremities.

left lower abdomen revealed psoriasiform epidermal hyperplasia, hypogranulosis, and areas of confluent parakeratosis. While intraepidermal neutrophils and eosinophils were not seen, a mild perivascular mononuclear inflammatory infiltrate was appreciated. Histopathological features were consistent with psoriasiform dermatitis and psoriasis vulgaris. A negative PAS silver stain confirmed against any fungal etiology. The absence of plasma cell infiltrates decreased the possibility of secondary syphilis as a differential diagnosis.

The patient was treated with triamcinolone 0.1% ointment twice a day to affected areas for 2 weeks. Upon follow-up, a complete resolution of lesions was noticed.

3. Discussion

Given the clinical findings of our patient, the most likely diagnosis appears to be psoriasiform dermatitis triggered by an underlying viral (COVID-19) etiology. Various factors can trigger psoriasis in genetically predisposed individuals or exacerbate the disease when it is in remission [5]. COVID-19 patients may exhibit features of a hyper-inflammatory state, such as significantly elevated biomarkers of inflammation (CRP, ferritin), cytokines, cardiac and muscle injury, liver and kidney dysfunction, and hyper-coagulation in patients with severe COVID19 [5].

It is postulated that psoriasis is a T lymphocyte-mediated disease in which activation of pathogenic T cells results in cutaneous inflammation by inducing hyperproliferation of keratinocytes. Dermal dendritic cells release certain cytokines, including interleukin-12 (IL-12) and interleukin-23 (IL-23), which results in T helper cell stimulation of epidermal hyperkeratosis and decreased apoptosis [6]. While a multitude of factors can cause psoriasis, there has been an increasing evidence suggesting the role of certain viruses such as hepatitis C, HIV, human papillomavirus (HPV), SARS-CoV2, and Zika in inducing or exacerbating psoriasis [7]. Kutlu and Metin reported a case of psoriasis exacerbation in a COVID-19 patient upon treatment with hydroxychloroquine and oseltamivir [7]. Although these drugs may worsen psoriasis, the onset of severe psoriasis within a short time frame may indicate that COVID-19 infection itself plays an crucial role in the pathogenesis of psoriasis. The presence of inflammatory cytokines, including IL-2, IL-7, and IL-10; granulocyte colony-stimulating factor; interferon-induced protein 10; monocyte chemokine 1; macrophage inflammatory protein 1; and tumor necrosis factor, have been reported to be potentially associated with the exacerbation of psoriasis in patients infected with SARS-CoV2 [7]. While we can positively identify the presence of some common cytokines mediating the underlying pathophysiology of both viral infections and psoriasis, more research is needed to better understand the pathogenesis of psoriasis induced by COVID-19 infection.

4. Conclusion

While many factors contribute to PSD, an underlying viral etiology such as COVID-19 or HIV infections may have a significant role in causing psoriasiform lesions in immunocompromised individuals. It is likely that the rash observed in our patient was secondary to COVID-19 infection, since no other underlying etiology could positively be identified. It is crucial for dermatologists to be able to discern various systemic manifestations associated with cutaneous lesions, such as the one seen in this patient, in order to make an accurate and prompt diagnosis. A better understanding of the association between COVID-19 infection and psoriasiform lesions is needed for improving the prognostic and therapeutic outcomes in patients.

References

[1] P. E. LeBoit, "Dermatopathologic findings in patients infected with HIV," *Dermatologic Clinics*, vol. 10, no. 1, pp. 59–71, 1992.

[2] M. R. Wick, "Psoriasiform dermatitides: a brief review," *Seminars in Diagnostic Pathology*, vol. 34, no. 3, pp. 220–225, 2017.

[3] ÖF. Elmas, A. Demirbaş, and Ö Kutlu, *Dermatologic Therapy*, vol. 33, no. 6, p. e13858, Article ID e13858, 2020.

[4] O. Kutlu and A. Metin, "Dermatological diseases presented before COVID-19: are patients with psoriasis and superficial fungal infections more vulnerable to the COVID-19?" *Dermatologic Therapy*, vol. 33, no. 4, p. e13509, Article ID e13509, 2020.

[5] B. M. Henry, M. H. S. de Oliveira, S. Benoit, M. Plebani, and G. Lippi, "Hematologic, biochemical and immune biomarker abnormalities associated with severe illness and mortality in coronavirus disease 2019 (COVID-19): a meta-analysis," *Clinical Chemistry and Laboratory Medicine*, vol. 58, no. 7, pp. 1021–1028, 2020.

[6] F. Grän, A. Kerstan, E. Serfling, M. Goebeler, and K. Muhammad, "Current developments in the immunology of psoriasis," *Yale J Biol Med*, vol. 93, no. 1, pp. 97–110, 2020.

[7] Y. Teng, W. Xie, X. Tao et al., "Infection-provoked psoriasis: induced or aggravated (review)," *Experimental and Therapeutic Medicine*, vol. 21, no. 6, p. 567, 2021.

6

Amelanotic Melanoma Treated as Fungal Infection for Years

Guilherme Kuceki[1] **Dekker C. Deacon**[2,3] **and Aaron M. Secrest**[2,4]

[1]*School of Medicine, University of Utah, Salt Lake, UT, USA*
[2]*Department of Dermatology, University of Utah, Salt Lake, UT, USA*
[3]*Huntsman Cancer Institute, University of Utah, Salt Lake, UT, USA*
[4]*Department of Population Health Sciences, University of Utah, Salt Lake, UT, USA*

Correspondence should be addressed to Aaron M. Secrest; aaron.secrest@hsc.utah.edu

Academic Editor: Ravi Krishnan

This study describes a case of amelanotic lentigo maligna melanoma in a 69-year-old female that had been growing for approximately 5 years. The asymptomatic lesion had been previously diagnosed and treated as a fungal skin infection, an inflammatory rash, and an actinic keratosis that did not respond to standard treatments. Biopsy revealed confluent and nested atypical melanocytes at the dermal-epidermal junction, consistent with melanoma in situ. Excisional biopsy revealed invasive lentigo maligna melanoma, Breslow depth 0.3 mm, with positive melanoma in situ at margins. She is now 3 years post-Mohs surgery without recurrence. When working up a patient with a hypopigmented or inflammatory lesion not responding to standard therapies, physicians should always consider biopsy to rule out unusual neoplastic etiologies, such as amelanotic melanomas.

1. Introduction

Melanoma can occur on any skin or mucosal surface. Despite melanoma accounting for only 4% of all skin cancers, it is responsible for approximately half of skin cancer-related deaths [1, 2]. Amelanotic melanoma occurs in up to 1–8% of all melanomas; however, the actual percentage might be lower as many hypopigmented melanomas are characterized as amelanotic [3]. These lesions are difficult to diagnose due to their ability to masquerade as other hypopigmented lesions [4]. Herein, we describe an amelanotic melanoma that was treated as tinea corporis, nummular dermatitis, and actinic keratosis for 5 years before biopsy established the diagnosis and led to appropriate treatment.

2. Case Report

A 69-year-old woman presented with an asymptomatic growth on her left arm that had consistently enlarged over the previous five years. Examination revealed a 5 cm ovoid pink-white, minimally scaly, thin plaque with intact sensation and without pain or itch (Figure 1(a), a′). This growth had been diagnosed clinically as tinea corporis and nummular dermatitis but did not respond to topical antifungals or steroids, respectively. The lesion had also been treated as an actinic keratosis with cryotherapy with subsequent growth. The patient denied a history of similar rashes and was growing increasingly frustrated with the lack of treatment response.

A shave biopsy was performed with additional clinical differential diagnoses, including lichen sclerosis and Bowen's disease. Pathology was consistent with a diagnosis of melanoma in situ, lentigo maligna-type (Figures 1(b) and 1(c)). The excision of the clinical residual was significant for invasive lentigo maligna melanoma, Breslow depth 0.3 mm (Figures 1(d) and 1(e)). Per our institutional protocol [5], she was treated with off-label imiquimod prior to Mohs surgery, three times weekly for 4 months, without perceptible improvement, though given the lack of pigmentation in this neoplasm, it was noted that response was challenging to assess. She subsequently underwent slow Mohs micrographic surgery with immunologic staining for Melan-A and Sox10, without residual melanoma being identified [5–8]. The defect was repaired linearly and healed well.

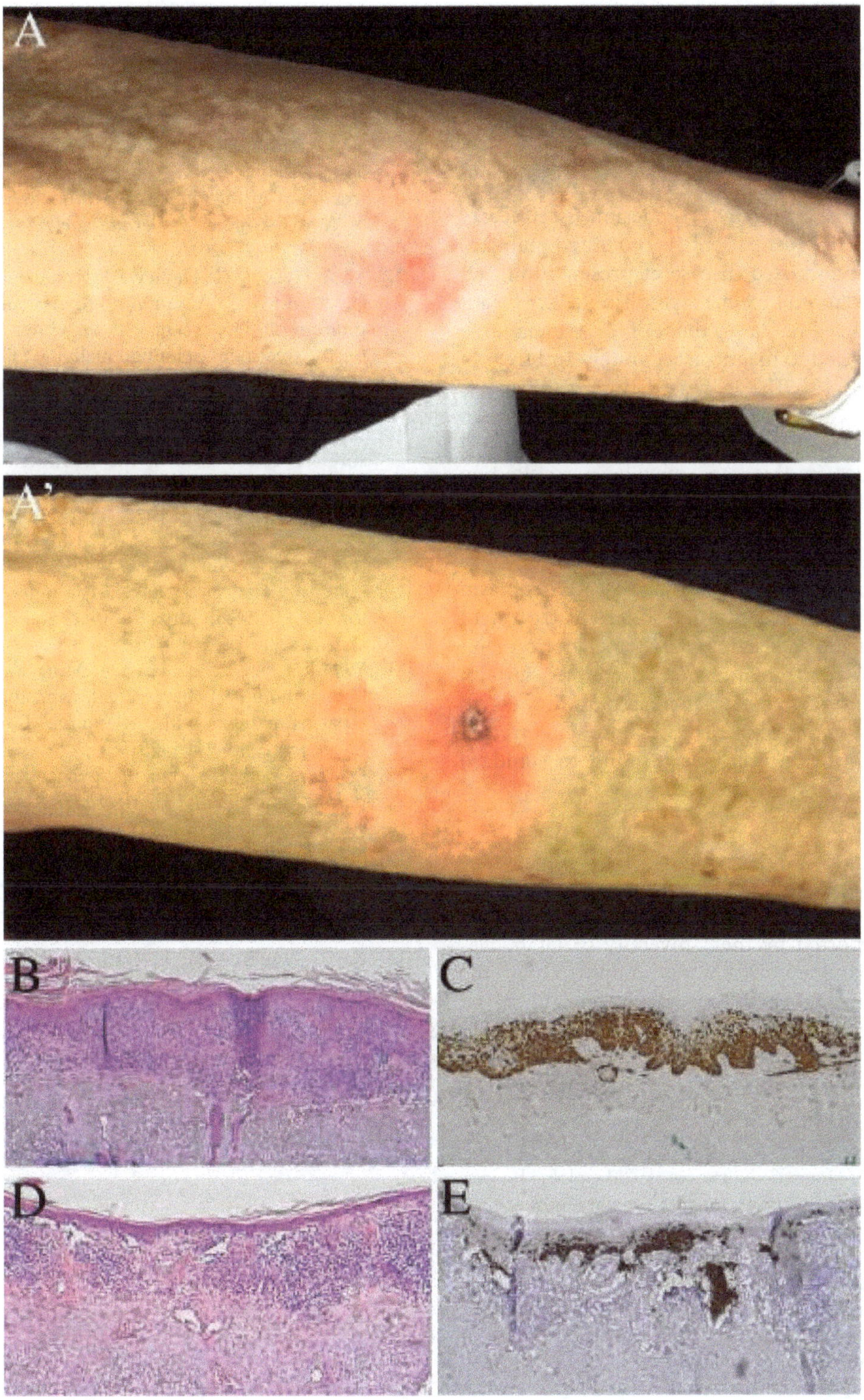

FIGURE 1: (a) A 5 cm ovoid, pink-white, minimally scaly, thin plaque on the arm of a 69-year-old female, Fitzpatrick skin type II. (a′) Postbiopsy. (b) H&E and (c) Melan-A immunohistochemistry revealing melanoma in situ, lentigo maligna type, on shave biopsy. (d) H&E and (e) Melan-A immunohistochemistry revealing invasive lentigo maligna melanoma, Breslow depth 0.3 mm. All microscopy is performed at 100x total magnification.

3. Discussion

Amelanotic melanoma arises from malignant melanocytes that do not produce mature melanin granules, with variable presentations, including amelanotic papules and nodules, desmoplastic plaques, subungual neoplasia with nail plate deformity, or secondary amelanotic growths that have metastasized from a primary pigmented melanoma [9]. The risk of developing a melanoma is modifiable, with the risk of melanoma doubling after 5 sunburns and halved with regular sunscreen use [10]. The ABCDE criteria recommended for patient evaluation of melanocytic neoplasia are not designed to help patients evaluate at-risk hypopigmented lesions [10]. However, as with other skin cancers, dermatoscopy and biopsy are indicated for all suspicious hypopigmented lesions, especially if the lesion is refractory to other treatments [3]. Most patients with lentigo maligna-type melanoma have localized disease at presentation, but once this type of melanoma reaches lymph node or distant metastasis, outcomes are similar to those of other melanoma subtypes, hence the need to diagnose accurately and treat in a timely manner [11, 12]. The increased time to diagnosis and definitive surgical treatment resulting from initial misdiagnosis and treatments for infectious and inflammatory etiologies in this case may have resulted in dermal invasion and increased risk for recurrence and metastasis [13, 14].

The key clinical features of this case presentation were the asymptomatic, slow-growing nature of this neoplasm and the failure to respond to multiple different treatment modalities for nonneoplastic etiologies. Amelanotic melanoma can be diagnostically challenging. Therefore, our aim with this case report is to bring increased awareness to clinicians of the need to biopsy a "rash" that does not present with classic symptoms (i.e., itch) or respond to standard topical treatments.

Acknowledgments

This work was supported by the University of Utah, Department of Dermatology. DCD was supported by the Melanoma Research Alliance, the American Cancer Society, and the Dermatology Foundation.

References

[1] C. Karimkhani, A. Green, T. Nijsten et al., "The global burden of melanoma: results from the Global Burden of Disease Study 2015," *British Journal of Dermatology*, vol. 177, no. 1, pp. 134–140, 2017.

[2] Gbd 2015 Mortality and Causes of Death Collaborators, "Global, regional, and national life expectancy, all-cause mortality, and cause-specific mortality for 249 causes of death, 1980-2015: a systematic analysis for the Global Burden of Disease Study 2015," *Lancet*, vol. 388, no. 10053, pp. 1459–1544, 2016.

[3] M. A. Pizzichetta, R. Talamini, I. Stanganelli et al., "Amelanotic/hypomelanotic melanoma: clinical and dermoscopic features," *British Journal of Dermatology*, vol. 150, no. 6, pp. 1117–1124, 2004.

[4] S. Kumar, V. Geethamani, M. Rehan, and A. Shetty, "Amelanotic melanoma masquerading as a superficial small round cell tumor: a diagnostic challenge," *Indian Journal of Dermatology*, vol. 59, no. 6, p. 631, 2014.

[5] J. M. Donigan, M. A. Hyde, D. E. Goldgar, M. L. Hadley, M. Bowling, and G. M. Bowen, "Rate of recurrence of lentigo maligna treated with off-label neoadjuvant topical imiquimod, 5%, cream prior to conservatively staged excision," *JAMA Dermatol*, vol. 154, no. 8, pp. 885–889, 2018.

[6] S. M. Siscos, B. C. Neill, E. W. Seger, T. A. Hooton, and T. L. H. Hocker, "The current state of Mohs surgery for the treatment of melanoma: a nationwide cross-sectional survey of Mohs surgeons," *Dermatologic Surgery*, vol. 46, no. 10, pp. 1267–1271, 2020.

[7] M. A. Hyde, M. L. Hadley, P. Tristani-Firouzi, D. Goldgar, and G. M. Bowen, "A randomized trial of the off-label use of imiquimod, 5%, cream with vs without tazarotene, 0.1%, gel for the treatment of lentigo maligna, followed by conservative staged excisions," *Archives of Dermatology*, vol. 148, no. 5, pp. 592–596, 2012.

[8] B. P. Sampson and G. M. Bowen, "Strategies for reducing final surgical defect sizes in the treatment of lentigo maligna," *Dermatologic Surgery*, vol. 46, no. 4, pp. 537–545, 2020.

[9] S. E. Koch and J. R. Lange, "Amelanotic melanoma: the great masquerader," *Journal of the American Academy of Dermatology*, vol. 42, no. 5, pp. 731–734, 2000.

[10] American Cancer Society, "Melanoma Skin Cancer Statistics for 2016," 2016, https://www.cancer.org/cancer/melanoma-skin-cancer.html.

[11] Y. Fujisawa, S. Yoshikawa, A. Minagawa et al., "Clinical and histopathological characteristics and survival analysis of 4594 Japanese patients with melanoma," *Cancer Medicine*, vol. 8, no. 5, pp. 2146–2156, 2019.

[12] L. M. Cohen, "Lentigo maligna and lentigo maligna melanoma," *Journal of the American Academy of Dermatology*, vol. 33, no. 6, pp. 923–936, 1995.

[13] S. M. Swetter, H. Tsao, C. K. Bichakjian et al., "Guidelines of care for the management of primary cutaneous melanoma," *Journal of the American Academy of Dermatology*, vol. 80, no. 1, pp. 208–250, 2019.

[14] Z. H. Hopkins, R. P. Carlisle, Z. E. Frost, J. A. Curtis, L. K. Ferris, and A. M. Secrest, "Risk factors and predictors of survival among patients with amelanotic melanoma compared to melanotic melanoma in the national cancer database," *J Clin Aesthet Dermatol*, vol. 14, no. 12, pp. 36–43, 2021.

7

Piperacillin/Tazobactam as Cause of Acute Generalized Exanthematous Pustulosis

Aikaterini Kyriakou,[1] **Sofia-Chrysovalantou Zagalioti**,[2] **Aikaterini Patsatsi**,[1] **Nikiforos Galanis**,[3] **and Elizabeth Lazaridou**[1]

[1] *Second Department of Dermatology and Venereology, Medical School, Aristotle University of Thessaloniki, Greece*
[2] *Papageorgiou Hospital, Thessaloniki, Greece*
[3] *Department of Orthopedics, Medical School, Aristotle University of Thessaloniki, Greece*

Correspondence should be addressed to Aikaterini Kyriakou; docmouli@gmail.com

Academic Editor: Ioannis D. Bassukas

Acute generalized exanthematous pustulosis (AGEP) is a rare cutaneous adverse reaction mainly attributed to antibiotics. It is characterized by numerous, nonfollicular, sterile pustules, arising on an exanthematous and edematous base. It is a serious adverse reaction accompanied by fever and leukocytosis. Piperacillin/tazobactam is indicated for the treatment of patients with moderate to severe infections. Herein is reported a case of AGEP caused by piperacillin/tazobactam. A 78-year-old woman with metastatic breast cancer was presented to the emergency department reporting fever and groin pain. The laboratory analysis and more specifically urine cultivation showed a urinary tract infection by *E. coli* with sensitivity to piperacillin/tazobactam. She had no known allergies. She was started on intravenous piperacillin/tazobactam; she improved clinically on the second day, but on the fourth day of intravenous therapy, she developed extensive pustular rash on the folds and anterior proximal thighs, accompanied by fever and neutrophilia. Piperacillin/tazobactam administration was interrupted and she was given prednisolone for ten days. The patient improved clinically and her laboratory tests returned to normal after two weeks. AGEP is an uncommon side effect of piperacillin/tazobactam treatment and there are few cases reported.

1. Introduction

Acute generalized exanthematous pustulosis (AGEP) is a rare and severe cutaneous adverse reaction. Its incidence is estimated to be one to five cases per million people per year [1]. The vast majority of the cases reported in the literature are attributed to antibiotics, mainly penicillin and macrolide [2]. However, viral infection, UV radiation, and hypersensitivity reaction to mercury have also been reported as uncommon causes of AGEP [3]. It is presented with an abrupt onset of numerous, nonfollicular, sterile pustules, arising on an erythematous and edematous base [4–6]. The lesions are preferentially located either on the face or on the intertriginous areas; then they spread to the trunk and limbs within a few hours [3]. Latency time for antibiotics is generally short, while for other drugs it is longer [1], and rash is accompanied by fever and leukocytosis with neutrophilia [2, 5, 6]. Piperacillin/tazobactam is an antibiotic indicated for the treatment of patients with moderate to severe infections [7]. A case of a patient who developed this rare condition with the use of piperacillin/tazobactam is presented and discussed.

2. Case Presentation

A 78-year-old, Caucasian female patient with metastatic breast cancer under chemotherapy was presented to the emergency department reporting fever, groin pain, vomiting (over 10 times per day) and being unable to get up of the bed for the past four days after the last chemotherapy. The initial laboratory workup revealed increased serum creatinine level of 3.20 mg/dl (GFR=14.89 mL/min/1.73m2, baseline= 0.57-1.11). Moreover, the urine analysis showed increased pyocytes (>100), while the urine cultivation highlighted *E. coli* with sensitivity to piperacillin/tazobactam.

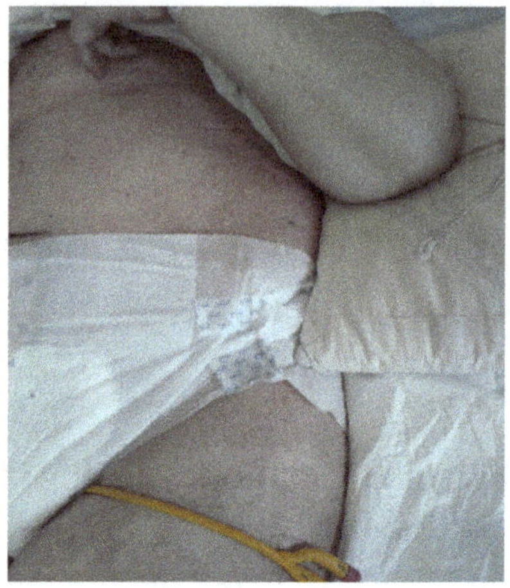

FIGURE 1: Extensive pustular rash located on the folds and proximal limp sessions.

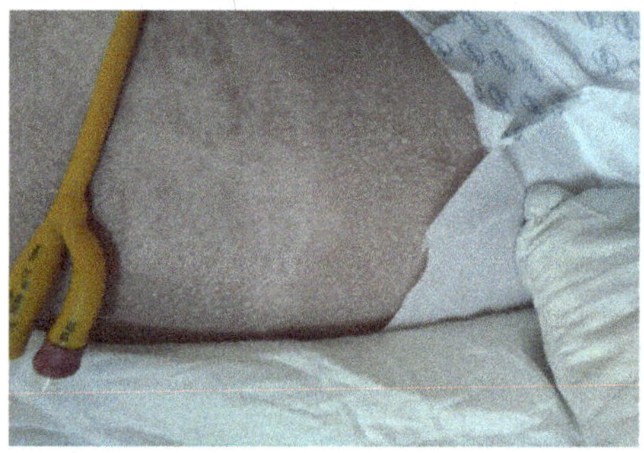

FIGURE 2: Numerous, pinhead-sized, nonfollicular, sterile pustules, arising on an erythematous and edematous base.

She was started on intravenous piperacillin/tazobactam (4.5g x 4, due to the impairment of renal function serum creatinine= 1.44 mg/dl) for urinary tract infection and at the same time she was kept hydrated. She had no known drug allergies and no history of psoriasis. She was clinically improved after two days of antibiotic therapy. On the fourth day of the intravenous piperacillin/tazobactam administration protocol, she abruptly developed extensive erythema and pustules that were located predominantly on the folds and anterior proximal thighs (Figures 1 and 2). The Nikolsky sign was negative and there was no mucosal involvement. The rash was accompanied by fever (38.5°C) and mild pruritus. The blood tests showed significant leukocytosis neutrophilia. Impressively, the white blood cells increased from 5.26 K/μl (with neutrophils 3.5 K/μl) to 39.6 x 10^3 K/μl (with neutrophils 27.7 K/μl) within two days of developing the rash. The patient refused to undergo a skin biopsy. However, Tzanck smear showed mainly neutrophils accompanied by the presence of eosinophils and lymphocytes, without any bacterial cocci. Moreover, bacterial culture from pustule content was negative.

Based on the clinical and laboratory results, it was concluded that the patient presented AGEP. Moreover, based on the AGEP validation score of the EuroSCAR study group [1], our patient's score was 9, which is compatible with a definite diagnosis of AGEP. Piperacillin/tazobactam administration was interrupted (Day 4) and the patient was given 30 mg of prednisolone intravenously once a day, which was tapered and stopped within 10 days. Both the skin rash resolved, followed by postpustular desquamation, and the white blood cells returned to their normal levels two weeks after the discontinuation of the drug. Based on the WHO-UMC causality categories, association of the described side effect to the culprit drug could be characterized as "probable/likely." The limitation of this work was the fact that there was no systemic rechallenge.

3. Discussion

AGEP was first described by Beylot et al. in 1980 [8], while in 1991 Roujeau et al. characterized the disease as a drug-induced, severe reaction and differentiated it from pustular psoriasis [3].

Until 2000, AGEP was characterized by the diagnostic triad nonfollicular, intraepidermal, or subcorneal pustules, fever greater than 38C, and neutrophil count above 7000 cells/mL [9]. Since 2001, the diagnosis of AGEP is based on morphology, course, and histology [1]. The mucous membranes are not frequently affected.

Overlap of AGEP and toxic epidermal necrolysis is a nonexisting diagnosis [10]. Cases of AGEP and drug-related rash with eosinophilia and systemic symptoms syndrome have previously been reported [11]. Biopsy should be performed, whenever is possible, since histopathology is part of the validation score of AGEP [1]. Moreover, there are histopathological, diagnostic clues in favor of AGEP in patients with a pustular eruption [12].

AGEP is suggested to be type IV hypersensitivity reaction which is mediated by T cells [13]. Recently, Pinho et al. reported that patch testing is a safe and useful tool for confirming the culprit drug involvement in most nonimmediate cutaneous adverse drug reactions from antibiotics [14]. Based on their findings, in AGEP cases, patch tests were mainly useful in detecting reactivity to fluoroquinolones. Moreover, a negative patch test result cannot be used to exclude drug imputability, since overall reactivity was relatively low [14]. In our case, no patch test was performed, which places a limitation.

The necessity of steroids in the treatment of AGEP is still a matter of debate [1]. However, except for cessation of the causative agent, close monitoring based on the immune status of the patient is indicated, since AGEP is not always easily controlled [12].

AGEP is a rarely reported severe cutaneous adverse drug reaction [11, 15]. In general, AGEP has a self-limited course lasting ≤ 15 days and its treatment lies mainly in withdrawing the offending drug. However, systematically administered corticosteroids may be necessary in refractory or severe cases.

References

[1] A. Sidoroff, S. Halevy, J. N. B. Bavinck, L. Vaillant, and J.-C. Roujeau, "Acute generalized exanthematous pustulosis (AGEP)—a clinical reaction pattern," *Journal of Cutaneous Pathology*, vol. 28, no. 3, pp. 113–119, 2001.

[2] A. De, S. Das, A. Sarda, D. Pal, and P. Biswas, "Acute generalised exanthematous pustulosis: An update," *Indian Journal of Dermatology*, vol. 63, no. 1, pp. 22–29, 2018.

[3] J.-C. Roujeau, P. Bioulac-Sage, C. Bourseau et al., "Acute generalized exanthematous pustulosis: analysis of 63 cases," *JAMA Dermatology*, vol. 127, no. 9, pp. 1333–1338, 1991.

[4] C. Thienvibul, V. Vachiramon, and K. Chanprapaph, "Five-year retrospective review of acute generalized exanthematous pustulosis," *Dermatology Research and Practice*, vol. 2015, Article ID 260928, 2015.

[5] Y. Lin, C. Yang, H. Sindy et al., "Severe cutaneous adverse reactions related to systemic antibiotics," *Clinical Infectious Diseases*, vol. 58, no. 10, pp. 1377–1385, 2014.

[6] M. J. Choi, H. S. Kim, H. J. Park et al., "Clinicopathologic manifestations of 36 Korean patients with acute generalized exanthematous pustulosis: a case series and review of the literature," *Annals of Dermatology*, vol. 22, no. 2, pp. 163–169, 2010.

[7] H. McCormick, N. Tomaka, S. Baggett et al., "Comparison of acute renal injury associated with intermittent and extended infusion piperacillin/tazobactam," *American journal of health-system pharmacy : AJHP : official journal of the American Society of Health-System Pharmacists*, vol. 72, no. 11, pp. S25–S30, 2015.

[8] C. Beylot, P. Bioulac, and M. S. Doutre, "Acute generalized exanthematic pustuloses (four cases) (author's transl)]," *Ann Dermatol Venereol*, vol. 107, no. 1-2, pp. 37–48, 1980.

[9] J.-C. Roujeau, "Neutrophilic drug eruptions," *Clinics in Dermatology*, vol. 18, no. 3, pp. 331–337, 2000.

[10] S. Van Hattem, G. I. Beerthuizen, and S. H. Kardaun, "Severe flucloxacillin-induced acute generalized exanthematous pustulosis (AGEP), with toxic epidermal necrolysis (TEN)-like features: Does overlap between AGEP and TEN exist? Clinical report and review of the literature," *British Journal of Dermatology*, vol. 171, no. 6, pp. 1539–1545, 2014.

[11] T. I. Kim, K. H. Jeong, M. K. Shin, and N. I. Kim, "Piperacillin/tazobactam-associated hypersensitivity syndrome with overlapping features of acute generalized exanthematous pustulosis and drug-related rash with eosinophilia and systemic symptoms syndrome," *Annals of Dermatology*, vol. 28, no. 1, pp. 98–101, 2016.

[12] S. Halevy, S. H. Kardaun, B. Davidovici, and J. Wechsler, "The spectrum of histopathological features in acute generalized exanthematous pustulosis: A study of 102 cases," *British Journal of Dermatology*, vol. 163, no. 6, pp. 1245–1252, 2010.

[13] W. J. Pichler, "Delayed Drug Hypersensitivity Reactions," *Annals of Internal Medicine*, vol. 139, no. 8, pp. 683–146, 2003.

[14] A. Pinho, I. Coutinho, A. Gameiro, M. Gouveia, and M. Gonçalo, "Patch testing – a valuable tool for investigating non-immediate cutaneous adverse drug reactions to antibiotics," *Journal of the European Academy of Dermatology and Venereology*, vol. 31, no. 2, pp. 280–287, 2017.

[15] S. Talati, M. Lala, H. Kapupara, and Z. Thet, "Acute generalized exanthematous pustulosis: A rare clinical entity with use of piperacillin/tazobactam," *American Journal of Therapeutics*, vol. 16, no. 6, pp. 591-592, 2009.

8

Interstitial Granulomatous Drug Reaction to Ustekinumab

A. Walker,[1] J. S. Westerdahl,[1] J. Zussman,[2] and J. Mathis[2]

[1]*University of Utah School of Medicine, Salt Lake City, Utah 84132, USA*
[2]*University of Utah, Department of Dermatology, Salt Lake City, Utah 84111, USA*

Correspondence should be addressed to A. Walker; amanda.walker@hsc.utah.edu

Academic Editor: Ioannis D. Bassukas

Interstitial granulomatous drug reaction (IGDR) is a distinct inflammatory process that often presents as annular, violaceous plaques distributed on the extremities, proximal trunk, and intertriginous areas. The list of drugs implicated for inciting IGDR is growing, but most prominently includes ACE inhibitors, antihistamines, beta-blockers, antidepressants, and anticonvulsants. Ustekinumab is a human monoclonal antibody that targets inflammatory cytokines IL-12 and IL-23 and has been have shown to be effective in treating IGDR. However, we present a case that suggests ustekinumab can also act as an inciting agent for IGDR.

1. Introduction

Interstitial granulomatous drug reaction (IGDR) is a distinct inflammatory process characterized histologically by interstitial histiocytes distributed between reticular collagen bundles, prominent eosinophils, and lymphoid atypia [1]. It often presents as annular, violaceous plaques distributed on the extremities, proximal trunk, and intertriginous areas [2].

The list of drugs implicated for inciting IGDR is growing and currently includes ACE inhibitors, antihistamines, beta-blockers, antidepressants, and anticonvulsants alongside many others [1, 2]. Some biologics have been shown to be effective in the treatment of similar granulomatous processes including granuloma annulare and interstitial granulomatous dermatitis [3, 4]. Ustekinumab (Stelara), a human monoclonal antibody that targets inflammatory cytokines IL-12 and IL-23, is currently an effective treatment option for many chronic inflammatory conditions including ulcerative colitis (UC), Crohn's disease, psoriatic arthritis, and psoriasis, and case reports have suggested that it may also be effective in treating IGDR [3, 4]. However, we present a novel case that suggests ustekinumab can also act as an inciting agent for IGDR.

2. Case

A 33-year-old male presented to our dermatology clinic for a pruritic rash. The rash was limited to his arms, but the pruritis involved his entire body. His medical history was significant for extensive biologic, steroid, and immunomodulatory therapy for the management of his UC. Three months prior, he switched from to facitinib to ustekinumab due to refractory symptoms. According to the patient, the rash presented shortly after the initiation of ustekinumab. Exam at that time revealed pruritic pink papules coalescing into plaques on bilateral forearms (Figure 1). Beyond that, he had been treated in the past with prednisone, budesonide, allopurinol, azathioprine, sulfasalazine, adalimumab, vedolizumab, and finally tofacitinib.

A lesional punch biopsy was performed, which demonstrated spongiosis of the *epidermis*, perivascular lymphohistiocytic inflammation with scattered eosinophils, and interstitial histiocytes between superficial reticular collagen bundles (Figure 2). After biopsy, the patient did not improve with topical steroids and antihistamines. Instead, he elected to discontinue ustekinumab and restart vedolizumab with resolution of his symptoms. Excluding UC, the patient had no signs or symptoms of other autoimmune conditions, so further immunologic workup was not deemed necessary

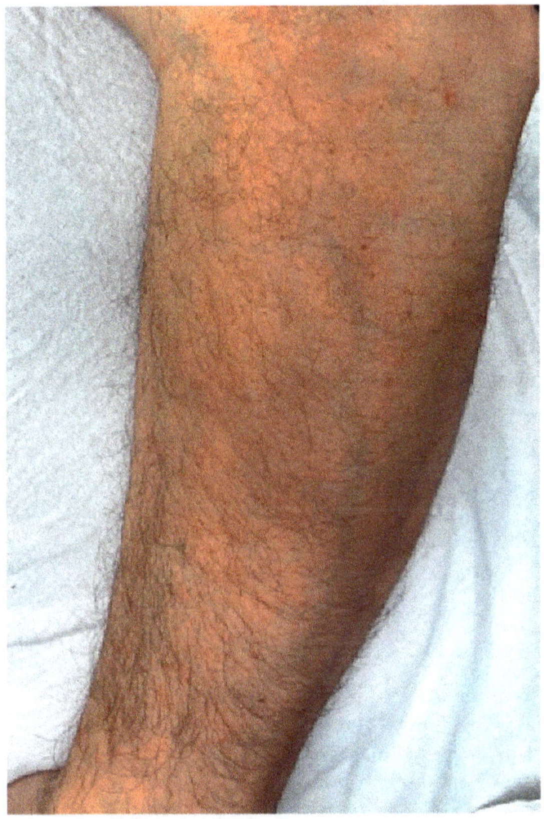

FIGURE 1: Pink papules coalescing into plaques on the left forearm. The rash extends into the posterior arm and is present bilaterally.

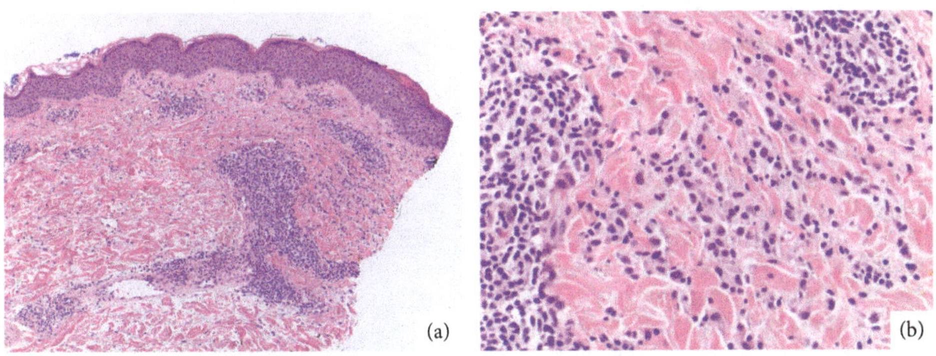

FIGURE 2: Histopathology with H&E demonstrating (a) epidermal acanthosis and mild spongiosis at 100X. There is dense perivascular inflammation, and interstitial histiocytes are noted at the edge of the specimen. (b) Histiocytes are seen between collagen bundles as well as scattered eosinophils, 400X.

after cessation of ustekinumab resolved the patient's presenting complaint.

3. Discussion

We present a novel case of IGDR arising in a patient with ulcerative colitis after treatment initiation with ustekinumab. Based upon the clinical and histological findings, the patient was diagnosed as a probable case of drug reaction associated with ustekinumab, with a score of 5 (probable adverse drug reaction (ADR)) by the ADR Probability Scale [5]. No single clinical or histological feature is specific of drug reactions, and findings like spongiosis is common [6]. But the perivascular lymphohistiocytic inflammation and eosinophilia are consistent with interstitial granulomatous dermatitis and cannot otherwise be explained, particularly in the context of his medication history.

It is also possible for a granulomatous reaction to manifest as a part of the natural disease process of chronic inflammatory bowel disease (IBD) [7]. However, given the excellent control of underlying IBD on ustekinumab, onset after initiation of ustekinumab, resolution with its cessation, and lack of other possible etiologies at the time of onset, we believe ustekinumab to be the most likely culprit. Furthermore, interstitial granulomatous reactions caused by inflammatory bowel disease often have a neutrophilic component, which was not seen here.

The itching was bothersome enough that the patient wished to discontinue a medication that had improved his IBD significantly. Whether it could be "treated through" or would progress on the medication is not clear. Paradoxical adverse events (PAEs) related to biologic use are increasing in the literature and may complicate effective treatment of disabling diseases. PAEs include psoriasis, hidradenitis suppurativa, and other granulomatous disease processes linked to biologics, particularly anti-TNF inhibitor therapy [8]. We believe we have identified the first known case implicating ustekinumab as an inciting agent for IGDR.

Acknowledgments

Funding for submission was provided by the University of Utah Department of Dermatology.

References

[1] C. M. Magro, A. N. Crowson, and B. L. Schapiro, "The interstitial granulomatous drug reaction: a distinctive clinical and pathological entity," *Journal of Cutaneous Pathology*, vol. 25, no. 2, pp. 72–78, 1998.

[2] M. Rosenbach and J. C. English, "Reactive granulomatous dermatitis," *Dermatologic Clinics*, vol. 33, no. 3, pp. 373–387, 2015.

[3] A. Chen, A. K. Truong, and S. Worswick, "The role of biologics in the treatment of chronic granuloma annulare," *International Journal of Dermatology*, vol. 58, no. 5, pp. 622–626, 2019.

[4] H. Cornillier, T. Kervarrec, F. Tabareau-Delalande, S. Mammou, A.-P. Jonville Bera, and L. Machet, "Interstitial granulomatous dermatitis occurring in a patient with SAPHO syndrome one month after starting leflunomide, and subsequently disappearing with ustekinumab," *European Journal of Dermatology*, vol. 26, no. 6, pp. 614-615, 2016.

[5] C. A. Naranjo, U. Busto, E. M. Sellers et al., "A method for estimating the probability of adverse drug reactions," *Clinical Pharmacology and Therapeutics*, vol. 30, no. 2, pp. 239–245, 1981.

[6] W. Weyers and D. Metze, "Histopathology of drug eruptions-general criteria, common patterns, and differential diagnosis," *Dermatology Practical & Conceptual*, vol. 1, no. 1, p. 9, 2001.

[7] K. M. Stiff and P. R. Cohen, "Palisaded granulomatous dermatitis associated with ulcerative colitis: a comprehensive literature review," *Cureus*, vol. 6, 2017.

[8] É. Toussirot and F. Aubin, "Paradoxical reactions under TNF-α blocking agents and other biological agents given for chronic immune-mediated diseases: an analytical and comprehensive overview," *RMD Open*, vol. 2, no. 2, Article ID e000239, 2016.

9

An Atypical Presentation of Lichen Planus-Like Reaction from Pembrolizumab

Matthew Lee[1] **and Nagashree Seetharamu**[2]

[1]*Department of Medicine, North Shore University Hospital-Long Island Jewish Medical Center, 300 Community Dr, Manhasset, NY 11030, USA*
[2]*Department of Oncology, Donald and Barbara Zucker School of Medicine at Hofstra/Northwell, 500 Hofstra Blvd, Hempstead, NY 11549, USA*

Correspondence should be addressed to Matthew Lee; mlee37@northwell.edu

Academic Editor: Soner Uzun

Introduction. With the advent of immunotherapy, a new subtype of side effects called IRAEs or immune related adverse effects have become more common. They may present in various organ systems as colitis, pneumonitis, hypophysitis, and thyroiditis and commonly as dermatological reactions. *Case.* This is a case report of a lung cancer patient that was started on Pembrolizumab and developed shortly after what appeared to be clinically at first pustular psoriasis but on biopsy was confirmed to be lichen planus. She was discontinued on the Pembrolizumab and treated with both systemic and topical steroids and improved. *Conclusion.* This case highlights a cutaneous reaction from Pembrolizumab and the subsequent management that helped resolve her condition but also weighing the benefits against the risk of treatments and potential prognostic implications of having cutaneous side effects.

1. Introduction

Cancer growth has long been linked to the ability of malignant cells to avoid detection by the patient's own immune system and leads to uninhibited growth. With increased understanding of tumor immunity, new medications have been developed to selectively target checkpoints in the cell cycle known as checkpoint inhibitors. Some of the most common targets include programed cell death protein and ligand-1 (PD-1/PD-L1) and cytotoxic T lymphocyte associated protein-4 (CTLA-4) now utilized in metastatic melanoma, lung cancer, and renal, gastric, and hepatocellular carcinomas management [1, 2]. Activating and improving the patient's own innate immune system to recognize and to act against cancer cells have led to improved outcomes with less toxicity than traditional chemotherapy. However, this has also led to nonspecific activation that causes a new class of side effects known as immune-related adverse side effects (IRAEs). Examples of the most common side effects related to checkpoint inhibitors are colitis, diarrhea, thyroiditis, and hypothyroidism with autoantibodies against thyroid peroxidase or thyroid stimulating hormone receptors, hypophysitis, pneumonitis, autoimmune hepatitis, and polyarthralgia. Of these IRAEs, dermatological reactions are the most common including pruritus, maculopapular rashes, vitiligo, lichenoid skin reactions, psoriasis, and rarely life threatening effects like bullous pemphigoid, Stevens-Johnson syndrome, and drug rash with eosinophilia and systemic symptoms (DRESS) [3, 4]. In this case report, the patient was on Pembrolizumab and developed lichen planus and we will discuss further its presentation, management, and potential prognostic implications if patients have cutaneous side effects from immunotherapy.

2. Case

This is a case of a 60-year-old female with stage IV T3N3M1 lung adenocarcinoma metastatic to adrenals and bone was found to have EGF, ROS, ALK WT, and KRAS mutation and lymphangitic disease. She initially received six cycles of carboplatin and pemetrexed and then switched to maintenance Alimta after three cycles. However, CT scans showed progression of disease and she was switched to Nivolumab. For dosing convenience for the patient, she was then switched

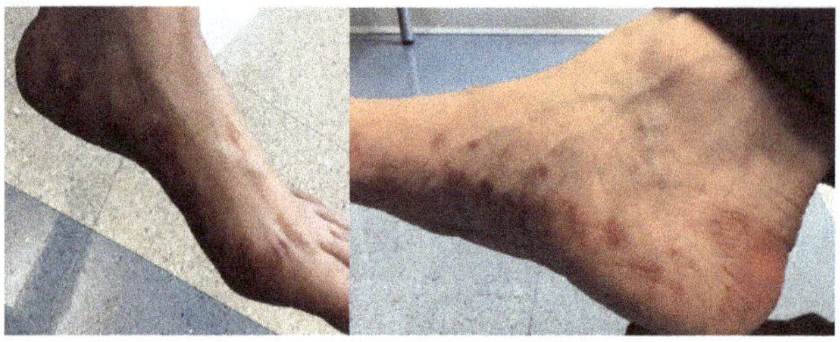

FIGURE 1: Photograph of lichen planus lesions on the patient's feet.

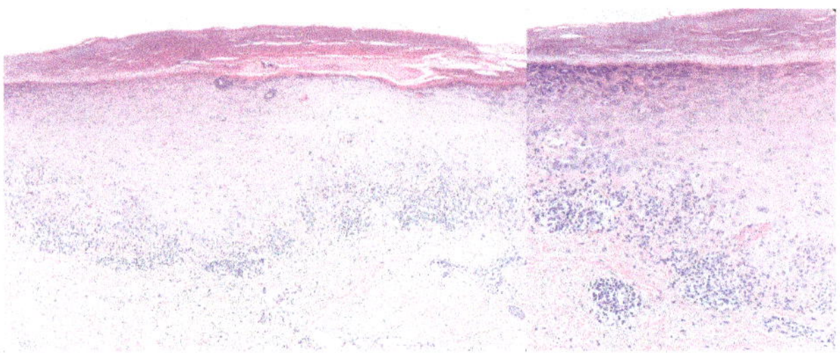

FIGURE 2: Skin biopsy shows a lichenoid lymphocytic infiltrate with acanthosis, hyperkeratosis, hypergranulosis, and civatte bodies (apoptotic basal keratinocytes).

to Pembrolizumab for every 3 weeks. Five months since starting Pembrolizumab, the patient then developed a pruritic rash on her wrists, feet, and buttocks and oral mucosal lesions. She was given clobetasol ointment and benadryl but on a follow-up visit a month afterwards she had developed a worsening rash. It became more difficult to walk and on physical exam the lesions appeared to be fluid filled and weeping bilaterally on feet and hands with psoriasiform papules, patches on back and buttocks, indurated pustules, and plaques on palms and sole. It was initially diagnosed by her dermatologist on clinical exam to be possibly pustular psoriasis and the patient was then started on oral prednisone 20 mg once a day and urea cream 40% twice a day and her Pembrolizumab was held. She improved within the next week but still had persistent maculopapular lesions on her feet (Figure 1) and then a punch biopsy of a left thigh lesion showed a diagnosis of palmoplantar lichen planus reaction (Figure 2). After five months of stopping the Pembrolizumab the rash started to decrease and her oral mucosal lesions disappeared. One year after the first cycle of Pembrolizumab, the patient now has healing hyperpigmented lesions with residual pain where the prior lesions were with Nystatin-Triamcinolone 10000-0.1 unit/gm external cream three times a day and Pembrolizumab is still being held. Furthermore, her lung adenocarcinoma is currently well maintained and has not progressed despite having Pembrolizumab being held and no further treatment.

3. Discussion

Although there is a wide variety of IRAEs, cutaneous side effects are the most commonly associated with checkpoint inhibitors. In a study by Hofman et al. it has been reported that 8.7% of melanoma patients treated with anti-PD1 therapy developed primary adverse dermatological events [5]. Specifically, Pembrolizumab, an IgG4 antagonist antibody to PD-1, was associated with cutaneous adverse events in 42% of its patients and 8 months from onset on average [6–9].

Lichen planus and lichenoid reactions are chronic inflammatory, T cell mediated reactions to an unknown antigen seen in various medications including beta-blockers, antimalarials, antihypertensive and proton pump inhibitors. Clinically, lichenoid reactions have different subtypes based on the sites it is involved with and morphology. Classically, it presents as papular/plaques, purple, pruritic, polygonal, and planar. Other types include hypertrophic that is common on extremities, vesiculobullous with blisters on lower extremities, and palmoplantar lesions that are scaly, bilateral, and symmetrical on malleoli and internal plantar arch. Other locations lichen planus can affect other than cutaneous locations are mucous membranes including oral, vulvovaginal, conjunctival, and laryngeal/esophageal [10–15]. As in our case, the patient presented with bullous vesicular lesions originally thought to be pustular psoriasis due to the clinical picture but found on biopsy to be ultimately lichen planus. Moreover, the lesions were also found on her oral mucosa along with flat papular polygonal lesions bilaterally on the plantar arch and malleoli areas.

The mechanism of how this occurs is still unknown but is thought to be T cell mediated. PD-1 itself is an inhibitory molecule on T cells that have immune tolerance to self-antigens and malignant tumors can express PD-L1 in order to evade immune responses [10]. PD-1 is also involved in epidermal preservation during inflammatory reactions and, by blocking PD-L1, there is not only an increase in the immune function of tumor-specific T cells but also an unmasking effect of self-immunity or prior antigen immune response. This leads to a widespread nonspecific T cell activation with an increase in T cell and TCR binding resulting in IRAEs in multiple organ systems and cutaneous reactions. In lichenoid reactions, they specifically affect keratinocytes expressing PD-L1 with lymphocyte infiltration in subepithelium and necrosis of keratinocytes, dense CD4 positive and CD8 positive T cells, spongiotic dermatitis, acanthosis, lymphocytic infiltrate of basal membrane, and hypergranulosis [10–15]. Interestingly, lichenoid reactions are not seen in other targeted therapies such as Ipilimumab, Epidermal Growth Factor Receptor (EGFR) inhibitors like Erlotinib and Bevacizumab or chemotherapies [9]. This may indicate that cutaneous reactions are a target effect on PD-1/PD-L1 pathway than nonspecific hypersensitivity reaction.

Treatment for cutaneous IRAEs in general is based primarily on grade severity which is referred most commonly by The National Cancer Institute's Common Terminology Criteria for Adverse Events (CTCAE) [16] (Table 1). However, psoriasis and lichenoid lesions were not specifically mentioned in CTCAE version 5.0 [16]. Furthermore, there is no standardized treatment for many IRAEs and management is based on case reports, case series, and expert consensus and opinions. Generally, Grade 1 and 2 cutaneous reactions and events are treated with topical corticosteroids and an oral antipruritic or antihistamine. For Grade 3-4 a skin biopsy is

TABLE 1: Skin and subcutaneous tissue disorders management of different gradings based on CTCAE (Common Terminology Criteria for Adverse Events) [16].

Grading (CTCAE)	General Cutaneous Features	Steroids	Immunosuppressives	Management of Immunotherapy	Outpatient or Inpatient care
1	Covers <10% BSA, limited, asymptomatic	Not recommended	Not recommended	Continue	Outpatient
2	Covers 10-30% BSA, minimal to moderate symptoms	Topical or systemic steroids oral 0.5-1 mg/kg/d	Not recommended	Continue	Outpatient
3	Covers >30% BSA, moderate or severe symptoms, limiting self-care ADLs	Systemic steroids oral or IV 1-2 mg/kg/d for 3 days then to 1mg/kg/d	Can consider if unresolved after 3-5 days of steroids	Suspend, discuss risk/benefit with patient	Outpatient or Inpatient for IV steroids
4	>30% BSA and fluid/electrolyte abnormalities	Systemic IV methylprednisolone 1-2mg/kg/d for 3 days	Can consider if unresolved after 3-5 days of steroids	Discontinue permanently	Inpatient and possible ICU or burn unit

BSA: body surface area.

needed for classification and systemic steroids are needed for at least 2-4 weeks. Steroids can be gradually reduced over 1 month if there is a response with most IRAEs resolving within 6-12 weeks [17]. Furthermore, cessation of immunotherapy (temporary or permanent) is needed with these high-grade reactions [5, 18, 19]. Lastly is the case of being refractory to steroids, immunomodulatory or immunosuppressive agents such as TNF-alpha (tumour necrosis factor) antagonists, azathioprine, and MMF (mycophenolate mofetil) [20, 21].

In terms of specifically for lichenoid reactions the main management includes topical and systemic corticosteroids [22]. The majority are able to be maintained on their anti-PD1 therapy (81%) and it was concluded that treatment can still be continued [23]. Furthermore, it has been reported that the majority respond well to topical steroids and holding immunotherapy may not be needed in contrast to more severe immunobullous toxicities [24]. Evidence of reduced efficacy of immunotherapy with immunosuppressive medications is mixed and no definitive conclusions [25, 26] and it is preferred still especially in high-grade cutaneous toxicity as it can enable reinitiation of immunotherapy [25]. In this atypical case of lichen planus, the lesions were initially severe enough to cause our patient substantial clinical effects and concerning features of bullous lesions that were resistant to topical steroids that oral steroids were needed and cessation of therapy in order for it to finally resolve.

Many of the cutaneous lichenoid side effects resolve within 6 months to 1 year. However, it can also reoccur and have periods of waxing and waning depending on different subtypes including erosive lichen planus or hypertrophic variants [27]. In terms of prognosis, cutaneous side effects have also been shown as potential positive prognostic factors. A study by Sanlorenzo et al. had examined a sample of patients treated with Pembrolizumab who had cutaneous adverse effects and their survival analysis showed that those who had cutaneous adverse effects had longer progression free intervals irregardless of treatment regimens [6]. Another study by Freeman et al. involved Nivolumab and metastatic melanoma patients and also showing a longer progression free survival compared to those who did not experience cutaneous toxicity [28]. Furthermore, adverse cutaneous effects such as hypopigmentation and vitiligo have been shown to be possible positive prognostic factors but mainly in melanoma patients [29–31]. However, what could potentially affect these findings is that patients who progress with immunotherapies like pembrolizumab or nivolumab would not have the same cumulative amount compared to those who do not progress and continue taking it. Thus, those that stay on treatment have a higher chance of developing a cutaneous adverse effect and may have a longer progression-free survival.

Lastly, there is controversy over whether oral lichen planus is a potential risk factor for oral squamous cell carcinoma (SCC). It has been debated that since oral lichen planus has been shown to have had a loss of heterozygosity and microsatellite instability and possible risk of malignant transformation [32]. Further, it was shown that 2.4% of oral lichen planus patients developed oral SCC in previously treated areas [33] with transformation ratios ranging from 1% to 5% [34, 35]. However, there is a need to have larger prospective cohort studies and further studies.

4. Conclusion

As for this patient in this case report she had developed a lichen planus eruption after 3 months of an anti-PD-L1 treatment, Pembrolizumab. Management for her case included topical treatment that initially failed and then systemic treatment with steroids and cessation of Pembrolizumab which eventually led to the resolution of the rashes and cutaneous lesions. This case highlights how different ways cutaneous side effects can be managed and present as and the subsequent difficulties based on clinical exam alone. Recognizing toxicities from immune checkpoint therapies becomes increasingly important as the number of patients on these treatments continues to grow and decisions on whether to stop or continue immunotherapies continue to be based on clinical experience as the field advances. Side effects such as vitiligo and hypopigmentation have been shown to be potentially prognostic and future studies should examine if other cutaneous findings can be also.

Abbreviations

PD-1/PD-L1: Programed cell death protein-1 and programed cell death ligand-1
CTLA-4: Cytotoxic T lymphocyte associated protein-4
IRAEs: Immune-related adverse side effects
TSH: Thyroid stimulating hormone
DRESS: Drug rash with eosinophilia and systemic symptoms
EGF: Epidermal growth factor
ROS: Protooncogene tyrosine protein kinase
ALK WT: Anaplastic Lymphoma Kinase
KRAS: Oncogene Kristen Rat Sarcoma
CTCAE: Common Terminology Criteria for Adverse Events
AE: Adverse events.

Consent

In accordance with the Declaration of Helsinki, informed written and verbal consent to participate and share publication of this case report and any potentially-identifying information/images was obtained by the patient.

Authors' Contributions

Matthew Lee and Nagashree Seetharamu prepared the paper and analysis. All authors read and approved the final paper.

Acknowledgments

The authors would like to thank all members of the study team, the patient's family, and Northwell Health System for their support.

References

[1] S. L. Topalian, F. S. Hodi, J. R. Brahmer et al., "Safety, activity, and immune correlates of anti-PD-1 antibody in cancer," *The New England Journal of Medicine*, vol. 366, no. 26, pp. 2443–2454, 2012.

[2] D. M. Pardoll, "The blockade of immune checkpoints in cancer immunotherapy," *Nature Reviews Cancer*, vol. 12, no. 4, pp. 252–264, 2012.

[3] L. K. Collins, M. S. Chapman, J. B. Carter, and F. H. Samie, "Cutaneous adverse effects of immune checkpoint inhibitors," *Current Problems in Cancer*, vol. 41, no. 2, pp. 125–128, 2017.

[4] L. Spain, S. Diem, and J. Larkin, "Management of toxicities of immune checkpoint inhibitors," *Cancer Treatment Reviews*, vol. 44, pp. 51–60, 2016.

[5] L. Hofmann, A. Forschner, and C. Loquai, "Cutaneous, gastrointestinal, hepatic, endocrine, and renal side-effects of anti-PD-1 therapy," *European Journal of Cancer*, vol. 60, pp. 190–199, 2016.

[6] M. Sanlorenzo, I. Vujic, A. Daud et al., "Pembrolizumab cutaneous adverse events and their association with disease progression," *JAMA Dermatology*, vol. 151, no. 11, p. 1206, 2015.

[7] S. Hwang, G. Carlos, and D. Wakade, "Cutaneous adverse events (AEs) of anti-programmed cell death(PD)-1 therapy in patients with metastatic melanoma:a single-institution cohort," *Journal of the American Academy of Dermatology*, vol. 74, no. 4, pp. 455–461, 2016.

[8] M. Maarouf, C. Alexander, and V. Y. Shi, "Nivolumab reactivation of hypertrophic lichen planus, a case report and review of published literature," *Dermatology Online Journal*, vol. 24, no. 1, p. 9, 2018.

[9] V. J. Shi, N. Rodic, S. Gettinger et al., "Clinical and histologic features of lichenoid mucocutaneous eruptions due to anti-programmed cell death 1 and anti-programmed cell death ligand 1 immunotherapy," *JAMA Dermatology*, vol. 152, no. 10, pp. 1128–1136, 2016.

[10] G. J. Freeman, A. J. Long, Y. Iwai et al., "Engagement of the PD-1 immunoinhibitory receptor by a novel B7 family member leads to negative regulation of lymphocyte activation," *The Journal of Experimental Medicine*, vol. 192, no. 7, pp. 1027–1034, 2000.

[11] V. Belum, B. Benhuri, M. Postow et al., "Characterisation and management of dermatologic adverse events to agents targeting the PD-1 receptor," *European Journal of Cancer*, vol. 60, pp. 12–25, 2016.

[12] S. M. Goldinger, P. Stieger, B. Meier et al., "Cytotoxic cutaneous adverse drug reactions during anti-PD-1 therapy," *Clinical Cancer Research*, vol. 22, no. 16, pp. 4023–4029, 2016.

[13] T. Komori, T. Honda, H. Irie, A. Otsuka, and K. Kabashima, "Lichen planus in irradiated skin during nivolumab treatment," *Acta Dermato-Venereologica*, vol. 97, no. 3, pp. 391-392, 2017.

[14] R. D. Sontheimer, "Lichenoid tissue reaction/interface dermatitis: Clinical and histological perspectives," *Journal of Investigative Dermatology*, vol. 129, no. 5, pp. 1088–1099, 2009.

[15] M. R. Roopashree, R. V. Gondhalekar, M. C. Shashikanth, J. George, S. H. Thippeswamy, and A. Shukla, "Pathogenesis of oral lichen planus—a review," *Journal of Oral Pathology & Medicine*, vol. 39, no. 10, pp. 729–734, 2010.

[16] National Institutes of Health, National Cancer Institute. Common Terminology Criteria for Adverse Events (CTCAE), Version 5.0, November 2017. https://ctep.cancer.gov/protocolDevelopment/electronic_applications/docs/CTCAE_v5_Quick_Reference_8.5x11.pdf.

[17] J. S. Weber, R. Dummer, V. de Pril, C. Lebbé, and F. S. Hodi, "Patterns of onset and resolution of immune-related

adverse events of special interest with ipilimumab: detailed safety analysis from a phase 3 trial in patients with advanced melanoma," *Cancer*, vol. 119, no. 9, pp. 1675–1682, 2013.

[18] I. Puzanov, A. Diab, K. Abdallah et al., "Managing toxicities associated with immune checkpoint inhibitors: consensus recommendations from the Society for Immunotherapy of Cancer (SITC) Toxicity Management Working Group," *Journal for ImmunoTherapy of Cancer*, vol. 5, no. 1, p. 95, 2017.

[19] V. Sibaud, "Dermatologic reactions to immune checkpoint inhibitors: skin toxicities and immunotherapy," *American Journal of Clinical Dermatology*, vol. 19, no. 3, pp. 345–361, 2018.

[20] Merck. Highlights of prescribing information for Keytruda. 2015.

[21] Squibb Bristol-Myers, *Yervoy (Ipilimumab), Immune-Mediated Adverse Reaction Management Guide*, 2011.

[22] P. R. Massey, K. M. Jones, and M. C. Fox, "New yellow plaques in a patient taking pembrolizumab," *JAMA Oncology*, vol. 3, no. 1, pp. 119-120, 2017.

[23] J. Bonigen, C. Raynaud-Donzel, J. Hureaux et al., "Anti-PD1-induced psoriasis: a study of 21 patients," *Journal of the European Academy of Dermatology and Venereology*, vol. 31, no. 5, pp. e254–e257, 2017.

[24] M. T. Tetzlaff, P. Nagarajan, S. Chon et al., "Lichenoid dermatologic toxicity from immune checkpoint blockade therapy," *American Journal of Dermatopathology*, vol. 39, no. 2, pp. 121–129, 2017.

[25] A. Garant, C. Guilbault, T. Ekmekjian, Z. Greenwald, P. Murgoi, and T. Vuong, "Concomitant use of corticosteroids and immune checkpoint inhibitors in patients with hematologic or solid neoplasms: A systematic review," *Critical Review in Oncology/Hematology*, vol. 120, pp. 86–92, 2017.

[26] T. Z. Horvat, N. G. Adel, T.-O. Dang et al., "Immune-related adverse events, need for systemic immunosuppression, and effects on survival and time to treatment failure in patients with melanoma treated with ipilimumab at memorial sloan kettering cancer center," *Journal of Clinical Oncology*, vol. 33, no. 28, pp. 3193–3198, 2015.

[27] Farzam Gorouhi, Parastoo Davari, and Nasim Fazel, "Cutaneous and mucosal lichen planus: a comprehensive review of clinical subtypes, risk factors, diagnosis, and prognosis," *The Scientific World Journal*, vol. 2014, Article ID 742826, 22 pages, 2014.

[28] M. Freeman-Keller, Y. Kim, H. Cronin, A. Richards, G. Gibney, and J. S. Weber, "Nivolumab in resected and unresectable metastatic melanoma: Characteristics of immune-related adverse events and association with outcomes," *Clinical Cancer Research*, vol. 22, no. 4, pp. 886–894, 2016.

[29] J. J. Nordlund, J. M. Kirkwood, B. M. Forget, G. Milton, D. M. Albert, and A. B. Lerner, "Vitiligo in patients with metastatic melanoma: a good prognostic sign," *Journal of the American Academy of Dermatology*, vol. 9, no. 5, pp. 689–696, 1983.

[30] P. Quaglino, F. Marenco, S. Osella-Abate et al., "Vitiligo is an independent favourable prognostic factor in stage III and IV metastatic melanoma patients: Results from a single-institution hospital-based observational cohort study," *Annals of Oncology*, vol. 21, no. 2, pp. 409–414, 2010.

[31] J.-C. Bystryn, D. Rigel, R. J. Friedman, and A. Kopf, "Prognostic significance of hypopigmentation in malignant melanoma," *JAMA Dermatology*, vol. 123, no. 8, pp. 1053–1055, 1987.

[32] B. T. Accurso, B. M. Warner, T. J. Knobloch et al., "Allelic imbalance in oral lichen planus and assessment of its classification as a premalignant condition," *Oral Surgery, Oral Medicine, Oral Pathology, Oral Radiology, and Endodontology*, vol. 112, no. 3, pp. 359–366, 2011.

[33] G. P. Bombeccari, G. Guzzi, M. Tettamanti et al., "Oral lichen planus and malignant transformation: A longitudinal cohort study," *Oral Surgery, Oral Medicine, Oral Pathology, Oral Radiology, and Endodontology*, vol. 112, no. 3, pp. 328–334, 2011.

[34] L. Lo Muzio, M. D. Mignogna, G. Favia, M. Procaccini, N. F. Testa, and E. Bucci, "The possible association between oral lichen planus and oral squamous cell carcinoma: A clinical evaluation on 14 cases and a review of the literature," *Oral Oncology*, vol. 34, no. 4, pp. 239–246, 1998.

[35] D. Eisen, "The clinical features, malignant potential, and systemic associations of oral lichen planus: A study of 723 patients," *Journal of the American Academy of Dermatology*, vol. 46, no. 2, pp. 207–214, 2002.

10

Inflammatory Nasal Swelling due to *Leishmania tropica*

Hajiba Fellah,[1,2] Maryam Hakkour,[1,2] Bouchra Delouane,[2] Asmae Hmamouch,[3] Abdelhakim Bouyahya,[4] Faiza Sebti,[2] and Abderrahim Sadak[1]

[1]*Laboratory of Biodiversity, Ecology and Genome, Faculty of Sciences, Mohammed V University in Rabat, Rabat, Morocco*
[2]*National Reference Laboratory of Leishmaniasis, National Institute of Hygiene, Rabat, Morocco*
[3]*Laboratory of Microbial Biotechnology, Sciences and Techniques Faculty, Sidi Mohammed Ben Abdellah University, Fez, Morocco*
[4]*Laboratory of Human Pathologies Biology, Department of Biology, Faculty of Sciences, and Genomic Center of Human Pathologies, Faculty of Medicine and Pharmacy, Mohammed V University in Rabat, Rabat, Morocco*

Correspondence should be addressed to Abdelhakim Bouyahya; boyahyaa-90@hotmail.fr

Academic Editor: Alireza Firooz

Since its discovery in the 19th century, cutaneous leishmaniasis has been a major public health problem, especially with the appearance of more and more unusual cases of cutaneous lesions due to this parasite. Indeed, the present study joins the previous studies and describes a typical case of a nasal lesion due to *Leishmania* infection. This is a 20-year-old young man, with no particular pathological history, from an epidemic focus who presented with inflammatory nasal swelling similar to a mucocutaneous form. However, the X-ray data showed that no lysis of the bones proper to the nose was detected and no damage to the underlying mucosa was observed. Nevertheless, the parasitological diagnosis confirmed the presence of amastigotes, and the results of the molecular study showed that the electrophoretic profile was comparable to that of *L. tropica*. After diagnosis and confirmation, treatment with meglumine antimonate at the rate of two ampoules/injection (one ampoule = 5 ml) of antimony salt for one month was administered intramuscularly with favorable outcome. Atypical forms of cutaneous leishmaniasis constitute a rare and unusual entity often leading to diagnostic delay. For this, the clinical examination must take into account both exceptional presentations of *Leishmania* infection, in particular in subjects living or having stayed in an endemic area, in order to ensure appropriate and early treatment.

1. Introduction

Leishmaniases include several clinical forms depending on the pathogen, ranging from skin ulcers and nodules to mucosal disorders with more serious lesions, up to visceral infections that damage internal organs [1]. This multiplicity of clinical pictures results both from a wide variety of species and from the variation in the immune response of the infected host.

In Morocco, cutaneous-mucous leishmaniasis has never been declared. However, cutaneous leishmaniasis (CL) constitutes a major national public health problem. It is caused by three *Leishmania* species, namely, *Leishmania major* (*L. major*), *Leishmania tropica* (*L. tropica*), and *Leishmania infantum* (*L. infantum*) [2]. Nevertheless, each species is characterized by a different clinical polymorphism [3].

In order to examine the epidemiological and clinical particularities of CL, a rare form of facial lesion has been studied and described. Thus, a molecular study was developed to determine the species responsible for this unusual lesion.

2. Case Description

This is a case of a 20-year-old patient with no particular pathological history, originally from the province of Taounate and moving between this province and the province of

Meknes. However, he was infected in the province of Taounate, especially in the rural sector of Ghafsai where he carries out his agricultural activities. He consulted for a skin lesion in the nose. The disease started around May 2018 with a small localized lesion (Figure 1). Four months later, the lesion has spread over the entire lobe of the nose and appeared erythematous (Figure 2).

In front of all these clinical elements, the patient had received antibiotic treatment without improvement. After that, several diagnoses were suggested, namely, sarcoidosis and leishmaniasis, and the observational clinical examination had suspected cutaneous mucosal leishmaniasis. The pathological anatomy results performed in a private center showed an inflammatory reaction composed of mononuclear cells, sometimes epithelioid with a vaguely granulomatous arrangement without caseous necrosis. However, these same results showed the absence of a formal argument for sarcoidosis as well as the absence of an obvious *Leishmania* body. As for the X-ray results, no lysis of the specific bones of the nose was detected and no damage to the underlying mucosa was observed (Figure 3). One month later, the patient was presented to the national leishmaniasis reference laboratory at the national institute of hygiene in order to confirm the diagnosis of CL. Clinical examination revealed an ulcerative, infiltrated, and poorly limited erythematous placard (Figure 4).

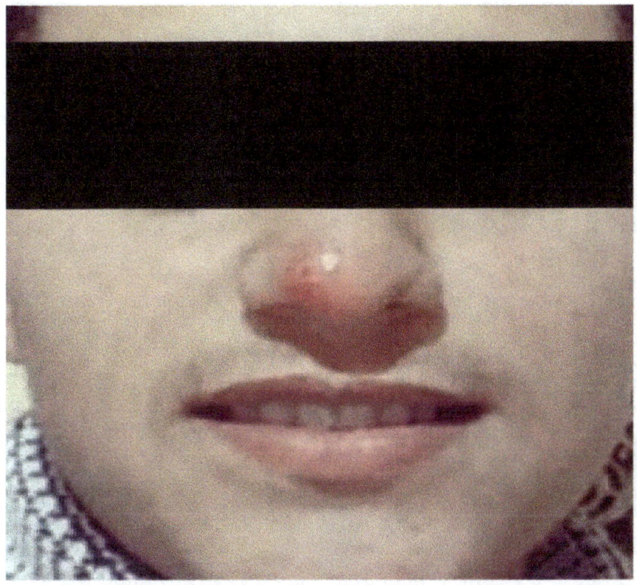

Figure 1: Onset lesion of the nasal infection.

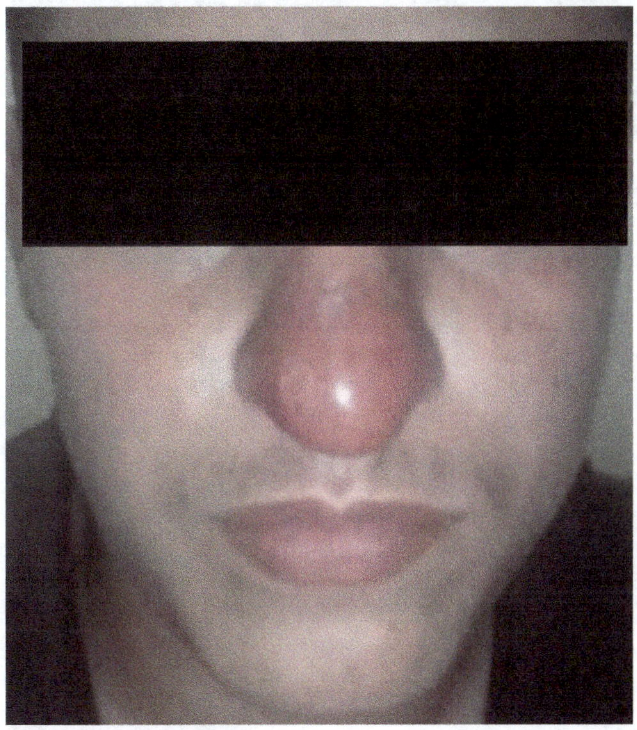

Figure 2: Erythematous appearance covering the entire lobe of the nose.

The microscopic diagnosis from skin samples showed the presence of *Leishmania* amastigotes within the macrophages. These results were confirmed by molecular diagnosis using the ITS1 PCR-RFLP technique. In addition, the enzymatic digestion carried out by MN1-I enzyme made it possible to compare the sample received and the three *Leishmania* species circulating in Morocco, namely, *L. tropica*, *L. major*, and *L. infantum*. However, the results showed that the electrophoretic profile was comparable to that of *L. tropica* (Figure 5).

Lane 1-2: patient smears and lane WM: weight marker 100 bp. Positive controls: Lt, *L. tropica*; Li: *L. infantum*; Lm: *L. major*; and NTC: negative control. The electrophoretic profile of the strain isolated in the patient was comparable to the *L. tropica* profile.

Immediately after laboratory confirmation and after an X-ray of the healthy liver and lungs, treatment with meglumine antimonate (Glucantime®) was initiated according to the protocol described by the Ministry of Health, generally 20 mg of SB5+/kg, without exceeding 2 ampoules, for 3 weeks. For our patient, two ampoules/injection (one ampoule = 5 ml) of antimony salt were administered intramuscularly. Due to the extent and location of the lesion, the duration of treatment was one month.

The initiation of treatment had shown good tolerance and satisfactory results (Figure 6). A week later, a clear clinical improvement was noticed and the skin lesion healed completely without relapse (Figure 7). Nevertheless, the patient still retains partial healing of the lesion (Figure 8). However, cosmetic surgery was subsequently mandatory to remove the residue from the lesion. This was the consequence of late treatment because the patient did not come to the leishmaniasis reference center (INH) until after having consulted quite a few private centers.

3. Discussion

Leishmaniases are caused by a heterogeneous group of protozoan parasites belonging to the *Leishmania* genus which are responsible for many clinical presentations.

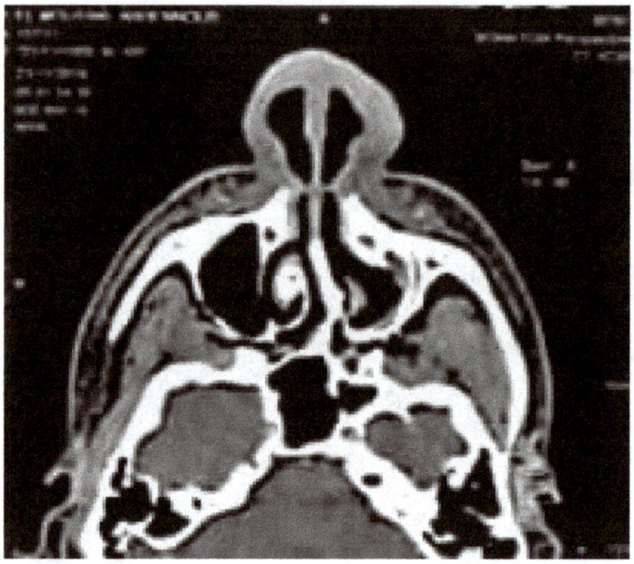

FIGURE 3: CT scan of the facial mass: no destruction of the nasal septum.

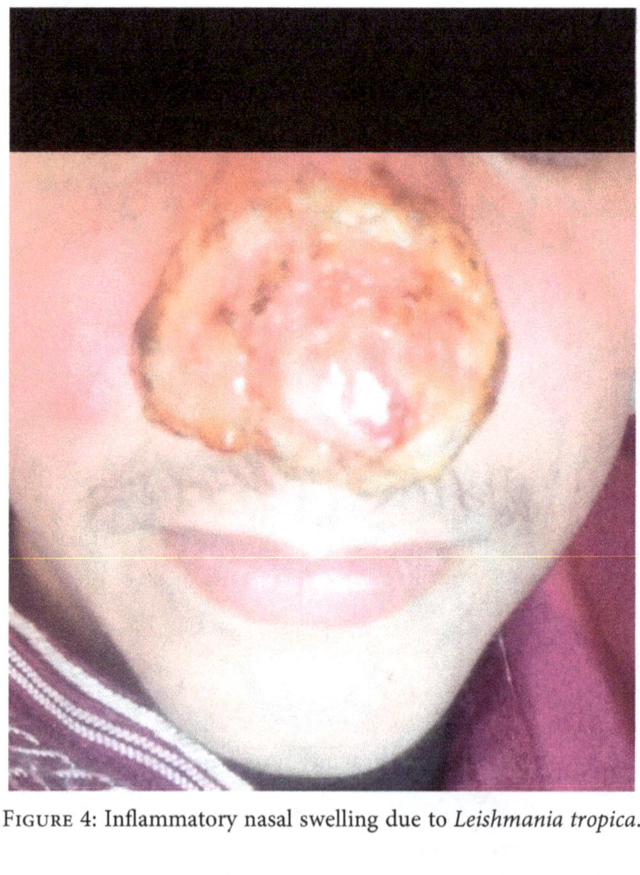

FIGURE 4: Inflammatory nasal swelling due to *Leishmania tropica*.

The epidemiology of the cutaneous form is complex due to intra- and interspecific variations in transmission cycles, reservoir hosts, sandfly vectors, and clinical manifestations, as well as the presence of multiple *Leishmania* species in the same geographical area which are phylogenetically distinct [4].

Mucocutaneous leishmaniasis is the most severe form of the disease, and it is mainly caused by the *L. braziliensis* complex. About diffuse cutaneous leishmaniasis, it is caused by *L. aethiopica*, and the Daman constitutes the main reservoir of the parasite.

In Morocco, neither of these two integumentary forms has been described so far, giving way to localized cutaneous leishmaniasis, which constitutes a major public health problem.

The study is the subject of a rare clinical appearance of a lesion caused by the *L. tropica* species. Indeed, this species has the largest geographical distribution in Morocco compared to the Maghreb countries. Its transmission can be both urban and rural [5–7]. In Morocco, leishmaniasis is a real public health problem. To deal with this pathology, a National Leishmaniasis Control Program has been established since 1997 [8]. The control measures for this program are as follows:

(i) Earlier detection and treatment of leishmaniasis cases (screening in schools and localities)

(ii) Vector control action: chemical action (intradomiciliary insect control or in stables, caves, household refuse, and manure dumps); physical action (sanitation and hygienic disposal of household waste and collective hygiene); and individual protection (by impregnated mosquito nets)

(iii) Action to control the reservoir through the fight against stray dogs and rodents through intersectoral collaboration

(iv) Information, education, and communication (training and information of staff; awareness of the population; and associations)

(v) Intersectoral collaboration: the Ministry of the Interior (environmental sanitation and hygiene and fight against stray dogs); Ministry of Agriculture (rodent control and fight against stray dogs as part of the fight against zoonoses); and Ministry of Health (patient care)

Unusual lesions due to *L. tropica* or other *Leishmania* species are no longer surprising in both reservoirs and humans. The usual clinicopathological picture of human CL varies from erythematous papules to noduloulcerative forms. However, in various endemic countries, unusual forms of CL have been described including erysipeloid, lupoid, annular, mucocutaneous, chancriforms, acute paronychic, palmoplantar, fissure leishmaniasis, zosteriform, submaxillary subcutaneous nodule, leishmaniasis scarring, whiteness, discoid lupus erythematosus-like, eczematous, squamous cell carcinoma-like, verrucous, and panniculiticvariants [9–14].

The clinical picture of leishmaniasis depends not only on the infecting leishmaniasis species but also on the host's immune response, which is largely mediated by cellular immunity. This immunity actually leads to a wide variety of presentations in a geographically restricted area. The response may be associated with the resistance of the *Leishmania* strain to macrophages, defective macrophage function, decreased production of interferon, imbalance between TH1 and TH2 cells, decreased chemotaxis, or increased delayed hypersensitivity [11].

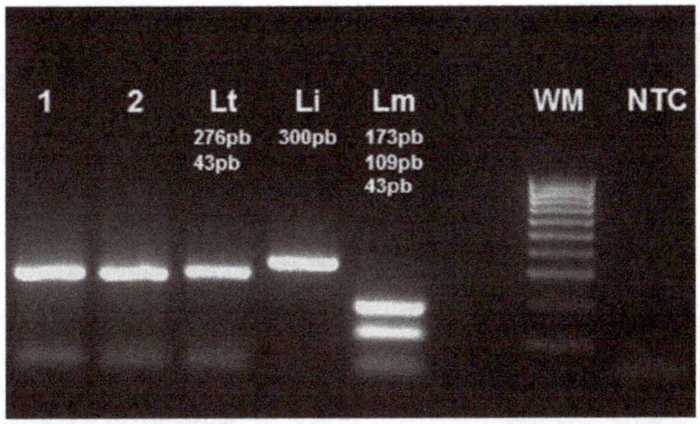

Figure 5: PCR-RFLP technique used for identification of *Leishmania* species (enzymatic digestion of PCR fragments by Mn1-I).

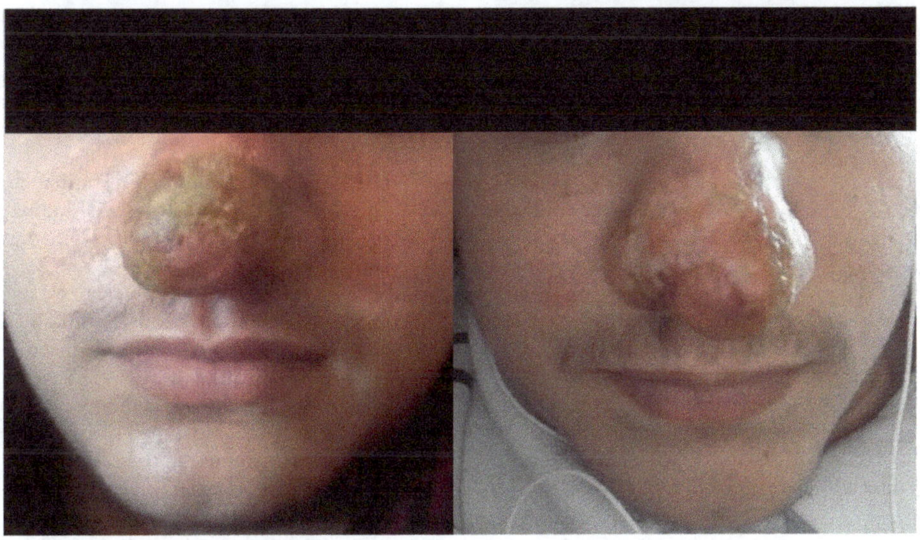

Figure 6: Response of the lesion to meglumine antimoniate treatment: one week after beginning of treatment.

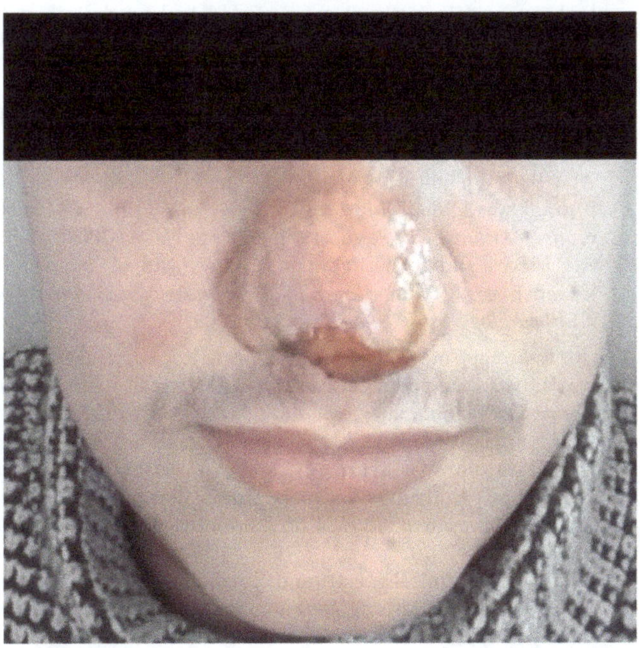

Figure 7: Response of the lesion to meglumine antimoniate treatment: 2 weeks after beginning of treatment.

In addition to the immune status, other factors can affect the clinical picture including the number of parasites inoculated, the site of inoculation, the nutritional status of the host, old age, menopause with its hormonal changes, and use of oral steroids and even wound contamination with inorganic materials.

Coinfection with human immunodeficiency virus (HIV) can also alter the clinical picture of CL. Indeed, HIV infection has led to the development of atypical forms of VL with an increased incidence of skin involvement. Several forms of the skin lesions have been reported worldwide including papulonodular lesions, psoriasiform-like and dermatomyositis-like eruption, erythroderma, and polymyositis-like syndrome [15].

Our patient is male and younger than the described cases, which works against senile immune impairment. In addition, he does not suffer from any disease of the immune system, and no trauma has been described. However, he resides in a province known for its history of leishmaniasis, both the cutaneous and visceral form.

Usually lesions are seen on the exposed parts of the body. Several studies have described isolated cases of nasal involvement following CL. However, nasal leishmaniasis was

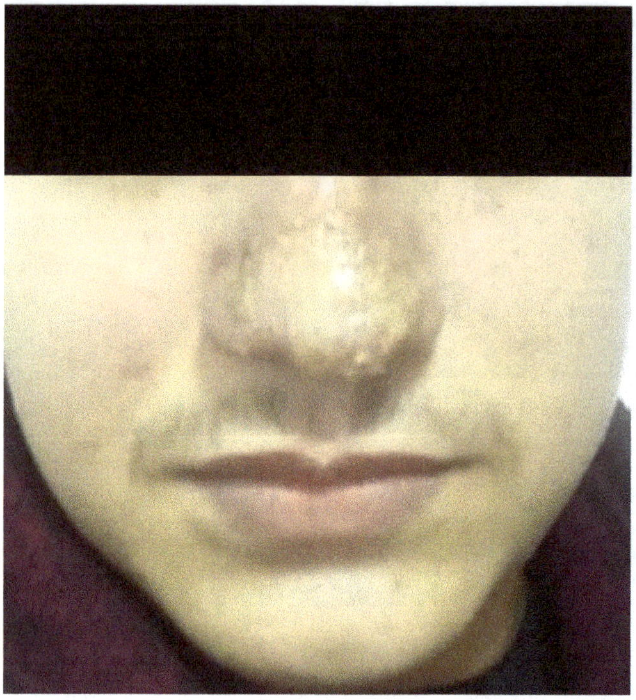

Figure 8: Response of the lesion to meglumine antimoniate treatment: stopping treatment.

considered infrequent. On the other hand, a study showed that 29% of cases of CL had a nasal infection and that young people, adolescents, and young adults were the most affected [11]. This nasal infection may be due to the fact that the nose is the most projected part of the face and its inability to avoid sandfly bites by pushing it away. However, this is the first time that such an aspect of lesion has been observed in the nose, whether at the institute level or at the provincial level.

Finally, due to the wide spectrum of nasal CL diseases in endemic areas, practitioner training is essential taking into account all lesions resulting from *Leishmania* infection which do not respond to appropriate conventional therapies.

4. Conclusions

Our observation shows an *L. tropica* infection with an unusual lesion in a young man with no particular pathological history. However, he resides in a province known for its history of being foci of cutaneous and visceral forms of leishmaniasis. Given these facts, the clinical examination must always take into account the unusual lesions resulting from infection with *Leishmania*, especially in subjects living or having stayed in the endemic area, in order to ensure appropriate and early treatment.

Authors' Contributions

Hajiba Fellah and Maryam Hakkour contributed equally to this work.

Acknowledgments

The authors would like to thank the technician Ms. Ouahdi Fouzia for the good skin sample. Also, they send big thanks to the patient A.E.M for agreeing to publish his experience with leishmaniasis.

References

[1] WHO, "Leishmaniasis," 2021, https://www.who.int/westernpacific/health-topics/leishmaniasis.

[2] M. Rhajaoui, F. Sebti, H. Fellah et al., "Identification of the causative agent of cutaneous leishmaniasis in Chichaoua province, Morocco," *Parasite: Journal de la Société Française de Parasitologie*.vol. 19, no. 1, p. 81, 2012.

[3] A. Masmoudi, N. Ayadi, S. Boudaya et al., "Clinical polymorphism of cutaneous leishmaniasis in centre and south of Tunisia," *Bulletin de la Société de Pathologie Exotique*, vol. 100, no. 1, pp. 36–40, 2007.

[4] E. Handman, "Leishmaniasis: current status of vaccine development," *Clinical Microbiology Reviews*, vol. 14, no. 2, pp. 229–243, 2001.

[5] H. Asmae, A. Fatima, F. Hajiba et al., "Coexistence of Leishmania tropica and Leishmania infantum in sefrou province, Morocco," *Acta Tropica*, vol. 130, pp. 94–99, 2014.

[6] S. Faiza, H. Asmae, A. Fatima et al., "Molecular epidemiological study of cutaneous leishmaniasis in beni mellal and fquih ben saleh provinces in Morocco," *Acta Tropica*, vol. 149, pp. 106–112, 2015.

[7] M. M. M. El Alem, M. Hakkour, A. Hmamouch et al., "Risk factors and prediction analysis of cutaneous leishmaniasis due to Leishmania tropica in Southwestern Morocco," *Infection, Genetics and Evolution*, vol. 61, pp. 84–91, 2018.

[8] "Leishmaniose_guide_national_2010_Maroc.pdf," 2010, https://www.who.int/leishmaniasis/burden/Leishmaniose_guide_national_2010_Maroc.pdf.

[9] A.-G. Kibbi, P. G. Karam, and A. K. Kurban, "Sporotrichoid leishmaniasis in patients from Saudi Arabia: clinical and histologic features," *Journal of the American Academy of Dermatology*, vol. 17, no. 5, pp. 759–764, 1987.

[10] K. M. Raja and B. Rahman, "Unusual clinical variants of cutaneous leishmaniasis in Pakistan," *British Journal of Dermatology*, vol. 139, no. 1, pp. 111–113, 1998.

[11] AU Bari, "Clinical spectrum of nasal leishmaniasis in Muzaffarabad," *Journal of the College of Physicians and Surgeons-Pakistan: JCPSP*, vol. 19, no. 3, pp. 146–9, 2009.

[12] A. U. Bari and S. B. Rahman, "Many faces of cutaneous leishmaniasis," *Indian Journal of Dermatology Venereology and Leprology*, vol. 74, no. 1, p. 23, 2008.

[13] M. R. Bongiorno, G. Pistone, and M. Aricò, "Unusual clinical variants of cutaneous leishmaniasis in Sicily," *International Journal of Dermatology*, vol. 48, no. 3, pp. 286–289, 2009.

[14] A. Eryılmaz, M. Durdu, M. Baba, N. Bal, and F. Yiğit, "A case with two unusual findings: cutaneous leishmaniasis presenting as panniculitis and pericarditis after antimony therapy," *International Journal of Dermatology*, vol. 49, no. 3, pp. 295–297, 2010.

[15] A. U. Bari, "Clinical spectrum of cutaneous leishmaniasis: an overview from Pakistan," *Dermatology Online Journal*, vol. 18, no. 2, p. 4, 2012.

11

Polypoid Basal Cell Carcinoma on the Nose Tip

Mutsuki Hirakawa, Yuki Ishikura, Taketoshi Futatsuya, Reimon Yamaguchi, and Akira Shimizu

Department of Dermatology, Kanazawa Medical University, Uchinada, Ishikawa, Japan

Correspondence should be addressed to Akira Shimizu; ashimizu@kanazawa-med.ac.jp

Academic Editor: Ioannis D. Bassukas

Basal cell carcinoma (BCC) is usually seen on the face as a pigmented nodule. We herein report a patient who presented with a polypoid BCC on the nose tip. Clinically, we suspected adnexal tumor; however, the findings of dermoscopy were consistent with that of BCC. Although the tumor was excised at the stalk, it was completely resected. Since the clinical manifestation was characteristic, we reviewed previously reported polypoid BCCs and found that this tumor can occur at any site, including the trunk and inguinal region, which are not preferential sites for ordinary BCC. There have been no reports of polypoid BCC on the nasal tip. The initial diagnoses varied, including adnexal tumors, and dermoscopic examinations proved useful for suspecting polypoid BCC. Histopathologically, the tumor cells in the resected specimens were within the polypoid area. Although BCC is a common tumor, polypoid BCC has distinct clinical features, and we should keep this rare subtype in mind.

1. Introduction

Basal cell carcinoma (BCC) is one of the most common cancers of the skin. It is seen on skin that is frequently exposed to sunlight. BCC has various clinical appearances and histological features. Some forms of common BCC, such as superficial, nodular, morphoeic, and ulcerated, are clinically recognized [1]. BCC rarely shows a pedunculated form, except for fibroepithelioma, which presents with a fibroma-like manifestation and is located on the back. In addition, polypoid BCC, which differs from fibroepithelioma, was reported by Megahed [2].

We herein report a patient with polypoid BCC presenting with a cystic and pedunculated nodule on the nose tip.

2. Case Report

A 104-year-old male patient was referred to us with a tumor on the nose tip. The nodule had been noted for decades but had rapidly grown over the past two months. An elastic, hard, $40 \times 25 \times 15$-mm, pedunculated red-black nodule with a smooth surface was found on the nose (Figures 1(a) and 1(b)). At first, we suspected an adnexal tumor rather than BCC based on its clinical appearance. However, a dermoscopy examination clearly showed arborizing vessels and black dots on its lower surface (Figure 1(c)), and a biopsy specimen revealed the nodular and cystic structure of basaloid cells, which was consistent with BCC.

The tumor was resected at the base of the stem, and the defect was cauterized with monopolar cautery. Histopathologically, there were two parts to this lesion, and a nodular and adenoid structure of basaloid cells was observed in the dermis (Figure 1(d)). The nuclei of the peripheral cell layer of the tumor masses were arranged in a palisade pattern. A cleft between the tumor and stroma was observed (Figure 1(e)). Cystic spaces containing mucinous and hyalinized tissues were also observed. There were some areas of adenoid differentiation and pseudocyst formation due to tumor necrosis (Figure 1(f)). Comparing the shallow lesions with the deep lesions, the deep lesions were marked by edema and myxomatous changes between tumor cells. Furthermore, immunohistochemical Ber-EP4 staining which is a useful marker for the diagnosis of neoplasms with follicular germinative differentiation was positive. The staining was more strongly positive in shallow lesions than in deep lesions

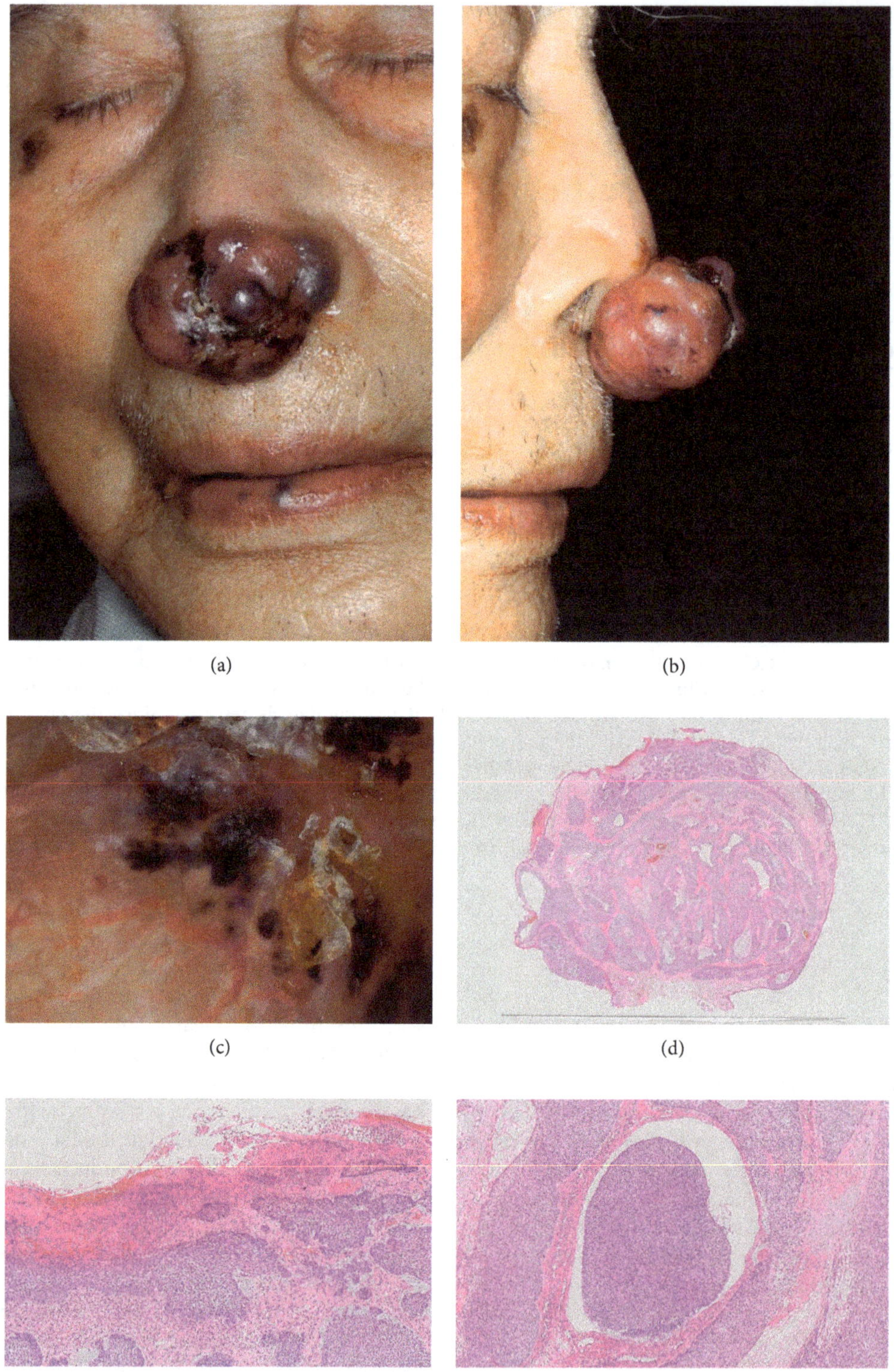

(a) (b) (c) (d) (e) (f)

FIGURE 1: Continued.

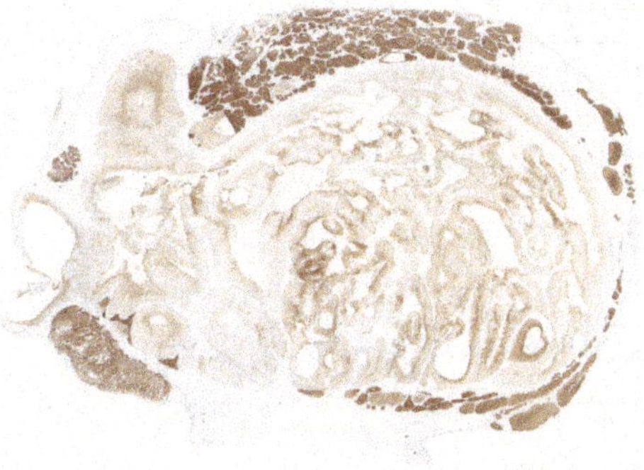

(g)

FIGURE 1: Clinical manifestation and histopathology. (a) A polypoid nodule was seen on the nose tip. (b) The lateral view shows a stalk on the nose. (c) Dermoscopy shows arborizing vessels and pigmented ovoid nests. (d) A low-power view showed basophilic nests in the dermis (hematoxylin and eosin staining, ×20). (e) A high-power view of the upper square showed basaloid cells with palisading (hematoxylin and eosin staining, ×200). (f) A high-power view of the lower square showed cystic spaces (hematoxylin and eosin staining, ×200). (g) Immunostaining with Ber-EP4 is more strongly positive in shallow lesions.

TABLE 1: Clinical and pathological summary of PBCC.

No	Year	Author	Age	Sex	Location	Size (mm)	Initial diagnosis	DS	Histopathology	TR	Others
1	1969	Gaughan[3]	68	F	forearm	50 × 40 × 25	ND	ND	ND	ND	Arising from burn scar
2	1985	Love[16]	64	M	Back	50 × 20	ND	ND	Adenoid	Yes	
3	1996	McElroy[17]	56	M	Shoulder	70 × 40	ND	ND	Nodular/ Adenoid	ND	
4	1985	Morimoto[18]	69	M	Buttock	10 × 15	Pedunculated nevus, soft fibroma, neurofibroma	ND	Nodular/ Adenoid	Yes	Deep margin positive
5	1995	Foley[19]	62	F	Eyelid	ND	ND	ND	ND	ND	Keratotic lesion
6	1999	Megahed[2]	87	F	ear	10 × 8	BCC, adnexal tumor, amelanotic melanoma	ND	Nodular	Yes	
7	1999	Megahed	76	F	Scalp	20 × 10	Adnexal tumor, verruca seborrheic,	ND	ND	Yes	
8	1999	Megahed	52	F	Scalp	15 × 10	Adnexal tumor, pedunculated dermal nevus	ND	ND	Yes	
9	1999	Megahed	20	F	Scalp	13 × 8	BCC, syringocystadenoma papilliferum, angioma developing on a nevus sebaceous	ND	Nodular	Yes	
10	2001	Morita[7]	33	F	Scalp	15 × 17	Pigmented nevus, fibroma	ND	Nodular/cystic	Yes	
11	2003	Sahin[5]	56	F	Inguinal region	40 × 30 × 25	Adnexal neoplasm	ND	Nodular	ND	Keratotic lesion
12	2004	Misago[8]	88	F	Buttock	35 × 20	PBCC, melanoma, adnexal neoplasm	ND	Nodular	Yes	
13	2006	Wang[6]	56	M	Perineum	21 × 15	PBCC, acrochordon, nevus	ND	Nodular	Yes	Multiple lesions, BCNS
14	2007	Sakai[9]	70	M	Eyelid	7	Neurofibroma, pigmented nevus	ND	Nodular	Yes	
15	2007	Choi[10]	56	F	Inguinal region	25 × 20	Pyogenic granuloma	ND	ND	Yes	
16	2007	Choi	69	F	calf	20 × 20	Melanoma, seborrheic keratosis	ND	Nodular	Yes	
17	2007	Choi	28	M	Scalp	15 × 10	Pyogenic granuloma	ND	ND	Yes	

Table 1: Continued.

No	Year	Author	Age	Sex	Location	Size (mm)	Initial diagnosis	DS	Histopathology	TR	Others
18	2008	Feito-Rodriguez[11]	7	M	face, neck	2 (mean)	BCC	done	Nodular	Yes	Multiple lesions, BCNS
19	2008	Ouchi[12]	54	M	Scrotum	17	ND	ND	Nodular/cystic	Yes	
20	2008	Yadav[13]	57	F	Cheek	30×20	BCC, pyogenic granuloma,	ND	Nodular/ Adenoid	ND	
21	2010	Kim[14]	61	M	Lower back	$86\times52\times10$	ND	ND	Nodular/Death	Yes	Metastasis
22	2017	Yildiz[15]	60	F	Postauricular region	7×5	BCC	done	Nodular	Yes	
23	2021	Present report	104	M	Nose tip	$40\times25\times15$	BCC, adnexal tumor	done	Nodular/ Adenoid	Yes	

BCC, basal cell carcinoma; PBCC, polypoid BCC; DS, dermoscopy; TR, tumor restriction within the polypoid area; ND, not described; BCNS, basal cell nevus syndrome.

(Figure 1(g)). ki67-positive cells were not clearly different between shallow and deep lesions, and EMA was negative (data not shown).

We finally diagnosed the patient with polypoid BCC on the nose tip. Two months later, the ulcer was epithelized by topical treatment. No recurrence has been seen for three months since excision.

3. Discussion

Megahed [2] proposed polypoid BCC as a new clinicopathological variant of nodular BCC in 1999 based on a few case reports. The author characterized BCC as follows: polypoid appearance, female predominance, and tumor restriction within the polypoid area. Our search identified 22 previously reported cases of polypoid BCC described in the English literature (Table 1) [2–18]. In our search, Gaughan [3] reported a giant pedunculated BCC on the forearm which arose from burn scar. Following that report, four more cases had been reported before Megahed's publication [2]; however, the characteristics of polypoid BCC were not fully described (Table 1). Among the 22 patients, there were 9 men and 13 women. The mean age was 58 years old (20–88, median 57 years old) which was younger than seen with ordinary BCC. The average size of the polyps was 28 mm. Despite the large size, most of the lesions displayed well-circumscribed nodules without any aggressive infiltrative pattern. The anatomic distribution of these polypoid BCC was distinctive: 5 (21%) on the scalp; 6 (25%) in the genital/perianal/buttock region; 3 (13%) on the trunk; 4 (17%) on the face; 2 (8%) in the periotic region; and 3 (13%) on the extremities. Typically, BCCs are commonly found on sun-exposed areas; however, polypoid BCC preferentially occurs on the scalp, genital areas, and back or buttock area. Polypoid BCC on the nose tip, as in our case, has never been reported. Adachi et al. [19] reviewed nine cases of Japanese polypoid BCC from their institution and noted that the polypoid BCC tumor was larger than other nodular BCCs, and the tumor site varied, including sites at the upper extremities, lower extremities, and genital area.

The manifestation is characteristic, and it is sometimes difficult to suspect BCC clinically. Seven cases of the reports stated that the initial clinical diagnosis was adnexal tumor or neurofibroma rather than BCC (Table 1). Our case clinically resembled adnexal tumor, but the findings of dermoscopy were consistent with BCC. Dermoscopy can be a valuable technique for distinguishing polypoid BCC from other pedunculated tumors. Some cases have demonstrated additional characteristics of polypoid BCC. Sahin et al. [4] described a case of keratotic BCC with polypoid manifestation. Wang et al. [5] reported multiple polypoid BCCs in a patient with basal cell nevus syndrome.

Histopathologically, 15 cases of polypoid BCC have shown the nodular type. Some cases also showed an adenoid/cystic structure histopathologically. The tumor nest was restricted to the polyp, which is important information for surgical excision. However, Kim et al. [13] described a case of polypoid BCC in the lower back, which progressed to pulmonary metastasis and death. Notably, in that case, the tumor was restricted to the polyp; however, it was the largest among the reported polyploid BCCs (Table 1).

The mechanism underlying the formation of polypoid BCC is unclear. Clothing-associated stimuli may be a cause, or there may be anatomical reasons, such as a rare fat condition. As Morita et al. [6] speculated, there are two patterns: preexisting lesions, such as fibroma and sebaceous nevus, and de novo lesions.

In our case, the positivity of the Ber-EP4 immunocytochemistry was stronger in shallow lesions than in deep lesions, suggesting that BCC is composed of two distinct tumour components. In our case, therefore, it was assumed that the shallow lesions developed first and that the rapid growth of the deeper mucinous lesions pushed the shallow lesions upwards. In addition, since the nose tip is located just above the bone, the rapid increase of the mucinous lesion may have resulted in this characteristic polypoid shape.

More cases of polypoid BCC need to be collected to clarify the characteristics.

Consent

The patient provided written informed consent to publication of the case details and photographs.

Acknowledgments

The authors thank Dr. Kazushi Anzawa and Ms. Yumi Okada for their technical assistance.

References

[1] K. Peris, M. C. Fargnoli, C. Garbe et al., "Diagnosis and treatment of basal cell carcinoma: European consensus-based interdisciplinary guidelines," *European Journal of Cancer*, vol. 118, pp. 10–34, 2019.

[2] M. Megahed, "Polypoid basal cell carcinoma: a new clinicopathological variant," *British Journal of Dermatology*, vol. 140, no. 4, pp. 701–703, 1999.

[3] L. J. Gaughan, J. R. Bergeron, and J. F. Mullins, "Giant basal cell epithelioma developing in acute burn site," *Archives of Dermatology*, vol. 99, no. 5, pp. 594-595, 1969.

[4] M. T. Sahin, M. A. Demir, Y. Kaya, M. Can, I. Inanir, and S. Ozturkcan, "Inguinal keratotic Basal cell carcinoma mimicking giant solitary trichoepithelioma," *The Journal of Dermatology*, vol. 30, no. 5, pp. 395–399, 2003.

[5] S. Q. Wang and L. H. Goldberg, "Multiple polypoid basal cell carcinomas on the perineum of a patient with basal cell nevus syndrome," *Journal of the American Academy of Dermatology*, vol. 57, no. 2, pp. S36–S37, 2007.

[6] K. Morita, A. Ikoma, and K. Takagaki, "Pedunculated basal cell epithelioma which is not Pinkus tumor," *The Journal of Dermatology*, vol. 28, no. 2, pp. 103–105, 2001.

[7] N. Misago, Y. Suzuki, Y. Miura, and Y. Narisawa, "Giant polypoid basal cell carcinoma with features of fibroepithelioma of Pinkus and extensive cornification," *European Journal of Dermatology*, vol. 14, no. 4, pp. 272–275, 2004.

[8] N. Sakai, K. Kurihara, and S. Kawana, "Polypoid basal cell carcinoma on the face," *Journal of Dermatology*, vol. 34, no. 8, pp. 588-589, 2007.

[9] J. E. Choi, N. Y. Ko, S. H. Seo, S. N. Kim, Y. C. Kye, and H. H. Ahn, "Polypoid basal cell carcinoma as a new variant of basal cell carcinoma: three Korean cases," *Acta Derm Venereol*, vol. 87, pp. 282-283, 2007.

[10] M. Feito-Rodriguez, E. Sendagorta-Cudos, M. Moratinos-Martinez, M. J. Gonzalez-Beato, R. de Lucas-Laguna, and A. Pizarro, "Dermatoscopic characteristics of acrochordon-like basal cell carcinomas in Gorlin-Goltz syndrome," *Journal of the American Academy of Dermatology*, vol. 60, no. 5, pp. 857–861, 2009.

[11] T. Ouchi and M. Sugiura, "Polypoid basal cell carcinoma on the scrotum," *The Journal of Dermatology*, vol. 35, no. 12, pp. 804-805, 2008.

[12] S. Yadav, G. P. Thami, A. Bhatnagar, S. Gill, and A. BhAtnAgAr, "Polypoid Basal cell carcinoma masquerading as pyogenic granuloma," *Indian Journal of Dermatology*, vol. 55, no. 3, p. 296, 2010.

[13] J. R. Kim, N. H. Lee, Y. S. Kim, J. H. Park, and S. K. Yun, "Pulmonary metastasis from a giant polypoid basal cell carcinoma in the lumbosacral area," *Dermatologic Surgery*, vol. 36, no. 1, pp. 128–132, 2010.

[14] S. Yildiz, I. Karaarsian, B. Yaman, and F. Ozdemir, "Dermoscopy and reflectance confocal microscopy in pedunculated basal cell carcinoma," *Dermatology Practical & Conceptual*, vol. 7, pp. 51-52, 2017.

[15] C. L. Love and D. P. Sarma, "Giant polypoid basal cell carcinoma," *Journal of Surgical Oncology*, vol. 28, no. 3, pp. 230-231, 1985.

[16] J. McElroy, T. E. Knight, and L. Chang-Stroman, "Giant polypoid basal cell carcinoma," *Cutis*, vol. 58, no. 4, pp. 289–292, 1996.

[17] S. S. Morimoto and A. W. Gurevitch, "Residents' corner: pedunculated pigmented basal-cell carcinoma on the buttock of a black man," *The Journal of Dermatologic Surgery and Oncology*, vol. 11, no. 2, pp. 115–117, 1985.

[18] P. Foley and G. Mason, "Keratotic basal cell carcinoma of the upper eyelid," *Australasian Journal of Dermatology*, vol. 36, no. 2, pp. 95-96, 1995.

[19] K. Adachi, Y. Yoshida, H. Goto, H. Noma, and O. Yamamoto, "Clinicopathological features of polypoid basal cell carcinoma: the first study in Japan," *European Journal of Dermatology*, vol. 30, no. 4, pp. 433–435, 2020.

12

The Management of Erythrodermic Psoriasis Complicated by Cyclosporine

Suman Rao, Michelle Bernshteyn, Raman Sohal, Rachael Proumen, Alexandra Goodman, and Zachary Shepherd

SUNY Upstate Medical University Hospital, 750 E Adams St., Syracuse, NY 13210, USA

Correspondence should be addressed to Suman Rao; raosu@upstate.edu

Academic Editor: Sergio A. Cuevas Covarrubias

We present a 64-year-old woman with past medical history of psoriasis and alcoholic liver cirrhosis who presented with a diffuse, erythematous, and scaly rash. Pertinent medications included topical triamcinolone 0.1% cream. She was started on oral prednisone 40 milligrams (mg) and oral cyclosporine 150 mg daily and was continued on topical triamcinolone. After the administration of two doses of this regimen, the serum creatinine increased to 1.76 mg/dL, and serum potassium increased to 6.7 mEq/L. The serum creatinine continued to uptrend to 2.42 mg/dL, and the glomerular filtration rate (GFR) decreased to 20 mL/min. The patient was emergently hemodialyzed. The patient was placed on an extended steroid taper, alleviating the psoriatic rash. However, the patient needed to be placed on a steroid-sparing regimen. Because of its rarity and ensuing complications, erythrodermic psoriasis must be identified and managed promptly. Cyclosporine is currently the first-line treatment. However, initiation of this therapy in our patient resulted in an acute kidney injury (AKI). Even though a steroid taper assisted in alleviating erythroderma, a steroid-sparing regimen needed to be started. This led to the consideration of alternate methods of therapy for further management of erythrodermic psoriasis with renal impairment.

1. Introduction

Psoriasis affects 3% of the adult population in the US. However, erythrodermic psoriasis is the rarest subtype, manifesting in less than 3% of patients with psoriasis [1]. Because of its rarity and capability to become life-threatening, the identification and appropriate treatment of erythrodermic psoriasis is essential. Erythrodermic psoriasis typically presents with erythema encompassing more than 75% of the skin surface [2]. It can be associated with pustules, scaling, or exfoliation. Although there is a scarcity of epidemiologically relevant data, erythrodermic psoriasis has a preference for manifestation in men and an average age of presentation at 48. Even though the immunopathogenesis of erythrodermic psoriasis is not fully understood, studies have shown it to be similar to that of plaque psoriasis, related to differential expression of the interleukin 17A signaling pathway [3]. Risk factors for the development of erythrodermic psoriasis include the administration of systemic glucocorticoids, abrupt withdrawal of either methotrexate/cyclosporine, treatment with topical retinoids, overuse of topical steroids, or TNF alpha inhibitors [2]. Complications of erythrodermic psoriasis include increased frequency of infections, including sepsis, due to breakdown of the skin defense barrier, and electrolyte abnormalities due to loss of fluid [4].

Cyclosporine is the treatment of choice for patients with erythrodermic psoriasis, even though the efficacy of this medication is limited [5]. The adverse side effects of this medication, specifically nephrotoxicity, have mainly been studied in patients undergoing kidney, liver, or heart transplants [6]. Chronic cyclosporine-induced nephrotoxicity can be seen in the form of chronic kidney disease and electrolyte/acid-base disturbances such as hyperkalemia, hyperuricemia, or gout [7, 8]. The pathogenesis of chronic nephropathy is secondary to renal insufficiency due to glomerular and vascular disease, tubular function abnormalities, and hypertension. Acute cyclosporine-induced nephrotoxicity can be characterized by AKI secondary to vasoconstriction of the afferent and efferent arterioles and a subsequent decrease in renal blood flow and GFR [8].

2. Case Presentation

We present a 64-year-old woman with past medical history of poorly controlled psoriasis and alcoholic liver cirrhosis who presented with a diffuse, erythematous, and scaly rash and desquamation for three weeks, worsening over the past week. She also complained of progressive weakness, subjective fevers, dyspnea at rest, and bilateral lower extremity swelling. She was in excruciating pain, tearful, and had intense pruritus. This patient had a diffuse, erythematous, and scaly rash and large plaques on her scalp, chest, abdomen, arms, and legs, which are the clinical presenting signs of erythrodermic psoriasis. She had a previous skin biopsy which confirmed her diagnosis of psoriasis as well.

Physical examination was remarkable for tachycardia at 115 beats per minute and new-onset hypoxia requiring 4 liters of oxygen by nasal cannula. Skin examination revealed large psoriatic plaques on her scalp, chest, abdomen, arms, and legs, along with diffuse erythroderma. The skin was dry, thin, and tender to palpation. The dorsal aspect of the left leg showed a weeping ulceration with serosanguinous discharge. 3+ bilateral lower extremity pitting edema was also present. Labs on admission showed a white blood cell count of 11,600 cell/mm^3, hemoglobin of 12.1 g/dL, hematocrit of 36.5%, sodium of 122 mEq/L, potassium of 5.8 mEq/L, chloride of 89 mEq/L, bicarbonate of 21 mEq/L, blood urea nitrogen of 22 mEq/L, and creatinine of 1.95 mg/dL (with a baseline creatinine 0.9 mg/dL). GFR was 26 mL/min. Chest X-ray on admission showed atelectasis of the left lower lobe, and electrocardiogram showed sinus tachycardia.

Past surgical history and family history were noncontributory. Social history included former smoking at one pack per day, which she quit ten years prior to admission, and her last alcoholic drink was three months prior to admission. She did not qualify for the liver transplant list due to extent of alcohol use and relapses. Pertinent medication history included topical triamcinolone 0.1% ointment, without any systemic steroidal therapy. Other medication history included diuretics (furosemide and spironolactone), naproxen, lactulose, baclofen, ranitidine, and potassium supplements. She was treated with apremilast two years prior with significant improvement in psoriatic plaques. However, due to worsening hepatic function and underlying cirrhosis, apremilast was discontinued a year prior to presentation.

The patient denied chest pain, cough, vomiting, or diarrhea. She denied having chills, night sweats, or weight loss. The patient did not have signs of onycholysis or arthritis. She has no prior history of chronic kidney disease or recent history of infections.

After admission, the electrolyte abnormalities and AKI were the first two problems that were managed. Hyperkalemia was treated with insulin, furosemide, Kayexalate, and lactulose. Asymptomatic hyponatremia and AKI were treated with normal saline. After this regimen, the serum creatinine began trending down toward normal at 1.67 mg/dL a day after admission. GFR began to uptrend to 31 mL/min.

Dermatology was consulted and recommended starting oral prednisone 40 mg daily and oral cyclosporine 150 mg daily. They also recommended oral antihistamines for pruritus, topical emollients for moisturization, and continuing topical triamcinolone.

After the administration of two doses of this regimen, the serum creatinine began to uptrend to 1.76 mg/dL, and the potassium level increased to 6.7 mEq/L. Cyclosporine was discontinued at this time. The serum creatinine continued to uptrend to 2.42 mg/dL on the following day. GFR continued decreasing to 20 mL/min. The patient was sent for vascular catheter placement and emergent hemodialysis, after a serum potassium level of 6.7 mEq/L.

After completing hemodialysis, her lab work showed serum sodium of 126 mEq/L, potassium of 4.4 mEq/L, chloride of 91 mEq/L, bicarbonate of 22 mEq/L, blood urea nitrogen of 16 mEq/L, creatinine of 1.58 mg/dL, and GFR of 34 mL/min. On the sixth day after admission, her lab work showed serum sodium of 128 mEq/L, potassium of 4.0 mEq/L, chloride of 95 mEq/L, bicarbonate of 24 mEq/L, blood urea nitrogen of 19 mEq/L, creatinine of 0.73 mg/dL, and GFR of 89 mL/min.

The patient was continued exclusively on extended steroid taper. The generalized psoriatic rash appeared significantly decreased. However, the patient needed to be placed on a steroid-sparing regimen.

3. Discussion

3.1. Approach to the Initial Management of Erythrodermic Psoriasis. This patient was previously diagnosed with psoriasis confirmed on skin biopsy, presenting with the tell-tale signs of this disease. The progression toward erythrodermic psoriasis in this patient was likely the result of poorly managed psoriasis. Her only treatment on admission was topical triamcinolone 0.1% cream. Studies have shown that excessive use of topical triamcinolone alone can trigger the manifestations of erythrodermic psoriasis. In addition, this patient was not on any systemic antipsoriatic medications after the discontinuation of apremilast two years ago, which could have contributed to her current presentation. During her admission, a decision was made against restarting apremilast due to underlying cirrhosis.

Cyclosporine is currently the first-line treatment for erythrodermic psoriasis, even though data on the efficacy of this drug for this specific disease subtype are lacking [5].

3.2. Acute Cyclosporine-Induced Nephropathy. After the initiation of cyclosporine, the patient experienced AKI, with the serum creatinine trending upward to 1.76 mg/dL and the potassium level to 6.7 mEq/L. After discontinuation of cyclosporine, the serum creatinine continued to trend upward to 2.42 mg/dL on the following day, attributable to cyclosporine's half-life of 8.4 hours. Observably, the only two medications started prior to the AKI were the steroid taper and the cyclosporine. Since steroids do not have any documentation of causing nephrotoxic symptoms, we propose that the cyclosporine was the cause of her ensuing AKI.

Although there have been several studies that demonstrate the nature of cyclosporine-induced nephropathy, there are distinct aspects of this presentation that are intriguing. More commonly, the nephropathy secondary to cyclosporine occurs after a prolonged exposure with chronic use. The onset of this patient's nephrotoxicity was within a couple of hours after the administration of cyclosporine and persisted until the completion of emergent hemodialysis. Although acute nephrotoxicity secondary to cyclosporine has been studied, most of these studies have been in post-kidney transplant patients [6].

3.3. Alternative Methods of Therapy. After the discontinuation of cyclosporine, the patient was continued on an extended steroid taper. She seemed to experience alleviation of her symptoms and a decrease in her psoriatic rash. However, she needed to be placed on a steroid-sparing regimen, and alternative methods of therapy were explored.

Studies have shown that infliximab is another first-line of therapy for erythrodermic psoriasis [9]. Other alternative therapies such as acitretin and methotrexate are less studied but are known to have a slower onset of action. Adalimumab and ustekinumab have also been useful in treating patients with moderate to severe plaque psoriasis [10].

In patients with acute renal failure or chronic kidney disease, alternative pharmacological agents must be considered in order to ensure an efficacious treatment, with minimal side effects. Studies have shown that methotrexate as well as apremilast should be avoided in patients with psoriasis [11]. In patients with decreased renal function, etanercept has been shown to be tolerated well in the management of psoriasis. Leflunomide has also been an appropriate alternative [12]. Other studies have shown that adalimumab can be safely used in patients presenting with end-stage renal disease, requiring hemodialysis [13].

4. Conclusion

Erythrodermic psoriasis manifests in less than 3% of all patients with psoriasis, presenting with scaly, erythematous rash, desquamation, and exfoliation involving more than three-fourths of the skin surface area. Because of its rarity and the ensuing complications, identifying and managing erythrodermic psoriasis is highly important. Cyclosporine is currently considered the first-line treatment for erythrodermic psoriasis. However, initiation of this therapy in our patient resulted in acute presentation of AKI. Although discontinuation of cyclosporine and initiation of a steroid taper assisted in resolving her AKI and alleviating the erythroderma, a steroid-sparing regimen that was compatible with her renal issues needed to be added to the management of this patient.

References

[1] T. D. Rachakonda, C. W. Schupp, and A. W. Armstrong, "Psoriasis prevalence among adults in the United States," *Journal of the American Academy of Dermatology*, vol. 70, no. 3, pp. 512–516, 2014.

[2] A. S. Boyd and A. Menter, "Erythrodermic psoriasis," *Journal of the American Academy of Dermatology*, vol. 21, no. 5, pp. 985–991, 1989.

[3] P. Zhang, H.-X. Chen, Y.-Q. Duan et al., "Analysis of Th1/Th2 response pattern for erythrodermic psoriasis," *Journal of Huazhong University of Science and Technology (Medical Sciences)*, vol. 34, no. 4, pp. 596–601, 2014.

[4] M. S. Green, J. H. Prystowsky, S. R. Cohen, J. I. Cohen, and M. G. Lebwohl, "Infectious complications of erythrodermic psoriasis," *Journal of the American Academy of Dermatology*, vol. 34, no. 5, pp. 911–914, 1996.

[5] B. Giannotti, P. Carli, and C. Veller-Fornasa, "Management of erythrodermic psoriasis with low-dose cyclosporin," *Dermatology*, vol. 187, no. 1, pp. 30–37, 1993.

[6] E. A. Burdmann, T. F. Andoh, L. Yu, and W. M. Bennett, "Cyclosporine nephrotoxicity," *Seminars in Nephrology*, vol. 23, no. 5, pp. 465–476, 2003.

[7] A. O. Ojo, P. J. Held, F. K. Port et al., "Chronic renal failure after transplantation of a nonrenal organ," *New England Journal of Medicine*, vol. 349, no. 10, pp. 931–940, 2003.

[8] J. A. Oates, J. J. W. Alastair, and B. D. Kahan, "Cyclosporine," *New England Journal of Medicine*, vol. 321, no. 25, pp. 1725–1738, 1989.

[9] F. Rongioletti, M. Borenstein, R. Kirsner, and F. Kerdel, "Erythrodermic, recalcitrant psoriasis: clinical resolution with infliximab," *Journal of Dermatological Treatment*, vol. 14, no. 4, pp. 222–225, 2003.

[10] T. Tsakok, N. Wilson, N. Dand et al., "Association of serum ustekinumab levels with clinical response in psoriasis," *Journal of the American Medical Association Dermatology*, vol. 155, no. 11, pp. 1235–1243, 2019.

[11] C. A. Elmets, C. L. Leonardi, D. M. R. Davis et al., "Joint AAD-NPF guidelines of care for the management and treatment of psoriasis with awareness and attention to comorbidities," *Journal of the American Academy of Dermatology*, vol. 80, no. 4, pp. 1073–1113, 2019.

[12] A. Ogdie, S. Schwartzman, L. Eder et al., "Comprehensive treatment of psoriatic arthritis: managing comorbidities and extraarticular manifestations," *The Journal of Rheumatology*, vol. 41, no. 11, pp. 2315–2322, 2014.

[13] Y. Kusakari, K. Yamasaki, T. Takahashi et al., "Successful adalimumab treatment of a psoriasis vulgaris patient with hemodialysis for renal failure: a case report and a review of the previous reports on biologic treatments for psoriasis patients with hemodialysis for renal failure," *The Journal of Dermatology*, vol. 42, no. 7, pp. 727–730, 2015.

13

Oral Isotretinoin Therapy in Recalcitrant Molluscum Contagiosum in an Immunocompromised Patient

Vikash Paudel[1] **and Deepa Chudal**[2]

[1]*Department of Dermatology and Venereology, National Medical College, Birgunj, Nepal*
[2]*Nepal Police Hospital, Kathmandu, Nepal*

Correspondence should be addressed to Vikash Paudel; vikashpoudel@iom.edu.np

Academic Editor: Ioannis D. Bassukas

Molluscum contagiosum is a viral infection caused by the Poxvirus characterized by multiple umbilicated papules. It is common in children and can be present at any body site. Severe molluscum is common in immunocompromised patients. We report a 20-year-old HIV-positive individual with widespread molluscum contagiosum, recalcitrant to topical therapy, under antiretroviral therapy, who was treated with oral isotretinoin and had a dramatic outcome. Although studies are needed to confirm the effectiveness of oral isotretinoin therapy in molluscum contagiosum, its easy availability, cost, and excellent safety profile appear to offer a promising therapeutic option.

1. Introduction

Molluscum contagiosum (MC) is a viral infection caused by a DNA virus, and the transmission is by direct contact. It is common in children and immunosuppressed adults [1]. Although topical retinoids have been used in the treatment of MC, their systemic use in MC is not reported in the literature. Thus, we report a rare case of recalcitrant MC where the efficacy of oral isotretinoin for the treatment of severe and recalcitrant MC in an HIV patient is demonstrated.

2. Case Report

A 20-year-old male patient presented to the outpatient clinic with an eruption of widespread skin-colored, dome-shaped lesions over his face and neck for one year. The lesions were asymptomatic but gradually increasing in size and number. A routine history revealed that the patient was HIV positive along with both of his parents. His CD4 + count was 82 cells/mm3 (normal > 500/mm3). He had the signs and symptoms of neither HIV nor the opportunistic infections. Besides, his medical and surgical history was also insignificant. He was taking standard antiretroviral therapy (ART) regimen regularly for the last five years, according to the national guidelines of Nepal. The ART used was tenofovir (300 mg), lamivudine (300 mg), and efavirenz (600 mg). For those eruptions, he was prescribed multiple topical medications (salicylic acid 5%, retinoic acid 0.05%, and other local remedies made from plant extract) and oral medications (not documented). However, there was no significant improvement of the lesions. No systemic modalities of retinoid or other antiviral medication were used previously.

On examination, several lesions were widespread over the eyelids, forehead, cheeks, nose, and neck, sparing the trunk and extremities (Figures 1(a) and 1(b)). They were pearly in color, umbilicated, dome-shaped papules which were discrete to coalescing, with a size ranging from a few millimeters to one centimeter. We made our clinical diagnosis as molluscum contagiosum in an immunocompromised patient and confirmed it after extirpation with a needle to find molluscae bodies in some of the skin lesions. Skin biopsy was not considered an option for diagnosis as a clinical diagnosis was sufficient in such cases. Dermoscopy might have assisted us with the confirmative diagnosis but was not performed due to its unavailability. Due to the

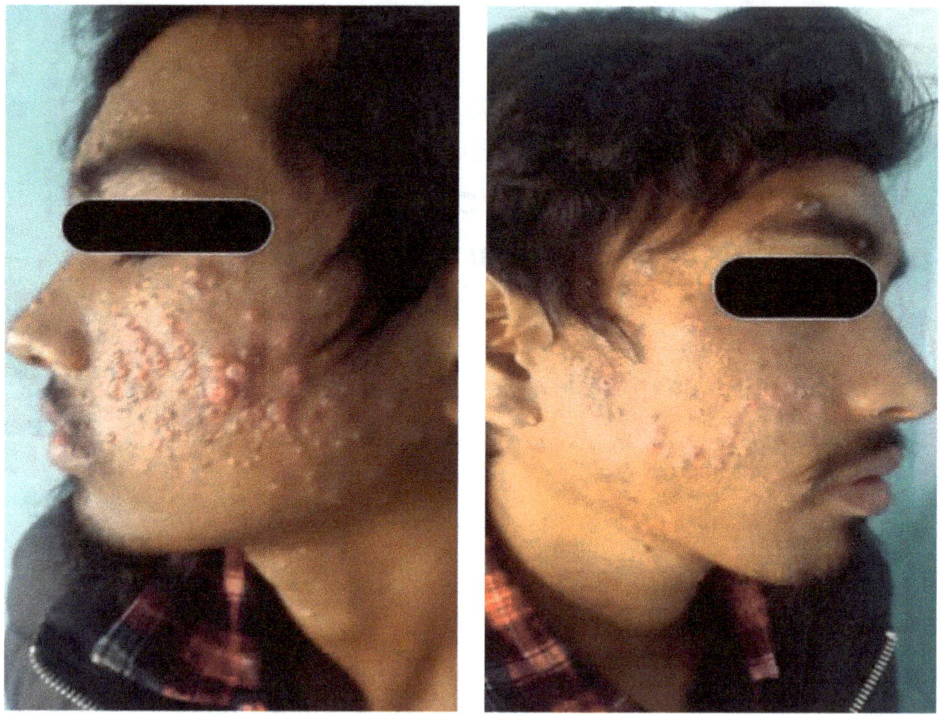

(a) (b)

FIGURE 1: (a, b) MC lesions before oral isotretinoin.

widespread location in the face and neck, recalcitrant nature, unavailability of other proven therapies (imiquimod gel, ingnelol gel, interferon, and cidopovir), and possibilities of side effects associated with systemic drugs, we decided to treat the patient with retinoid derivatives but systemically, i.e., oral isotretinoin 0.5 mg/kg. Isotretinoin was used as an option because of its property of being a systemic retinoid with intracellular conversion into tretinoin and its effects on cellular proliferation and differentiation. After discussing its possible side effects and measures to prevent them, isotretinoin (20 mg twice daily) was prescribed for a month to see the possible outcome. After one month of follow-up, there was subjective (both the patient and physician) and objective improvement in the appearance and count of the lesions with almost no lesions in the right half of the face and few lesions in the left half of the face (Figures 2(a) and 2(b)). The patient had no adverse effects of oral isotretinoin use except dry lips which were managed using petrolatum jelly. The remission was maintained even after two months of follow-up.

3. Discussion

Molluscum contagiosum is a cutaneous viral infection that is caused by a DNA virus that replicates only in human epidermal keratinocytes [1]. The virus is assumed to be the only existing poxvirus that specifically affects human beings. MC virus has 4 different genotypes: MCV 1, MCV 2, MCV 3, and MCV 4. It is transmitted by direct contact with infected skin, sexual, nonsexual, or by autoinoculation. Additionally, it can be transmitted by contaminated fomites.[2]. It usually presents as single or multiple, spherical, shiny, pearly white papules that classically have a central dimple. In immunocompetent patients, infection is self-limited with spontaneous resolution. Risk factors for infection in adult patients include sexual transmission and severe immunosuppression. Extragenital molluscum contagiosum in adults occurs almost exclusively in HIV-infected or immunocompromised ones. People with HIV infection are more prone to molluscum contagiosum; prevalence in this population has been reported up to 20% [3].

In immunocompetent individuals, MC is self-limiting with spontaneous resolution. Resolution of the lesions could be accelerated by its destruction and production of inflammatory responses. Many treatment options such as doing nothing (natural resolution), physical destruction (i.e., cryotherapy, extraction, and curettage and pricking with a needle), and topical agents (tretinoin, tazarotene, salicylic acid, imiquimod, potassium hydroxide, podophyllin, phenol, and contact immunotherapies) are discussed in the literature. Few systemic treatment modalities such as antivirals (cidofovir and interferon) or cimetidine have been suggested as a possible treatment for their antiviral and systemic immunomodulatory effects. Besides, interferon alfa is a proinflammatory cytokine that is used in the treatment of MC in immunosuppressed patients with severe or refractory disease and can be administered subcutaneously or intralesionally [4]. No therapy is universally effective in MC in HIV patients except the initiation of ART therapy [5]. Because the unavailability of such systemic therapies and the patient being already on an ART regimen, oral isotretinoin

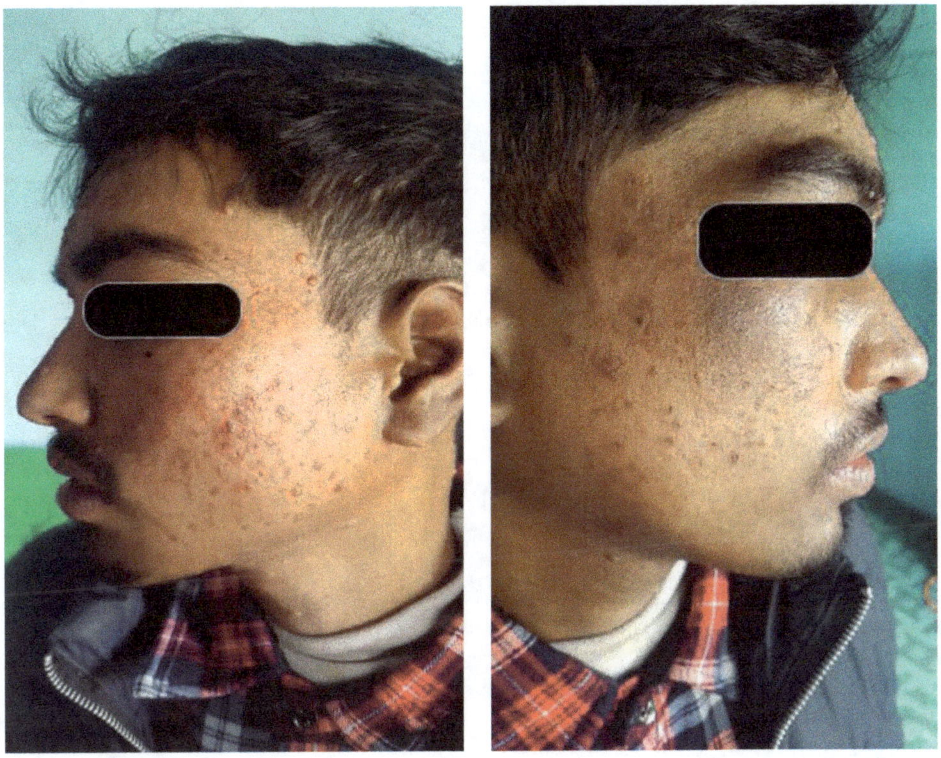

(a) (b)

FIGURE 2: (a, b) Resolution of MC after one month of therapy with oral isotretinoin.

was tried as an alternative due to its effects in the keratinocytes microenvironment.

Retinoids have been used in dermatology for many decades; indications for their use include psoriasis, acne, and disorders of keratinization. Their mechanism is attributed to the ability to control abnormal growth and differentiation of keratinocytes. Isotretinoin has remarkable efficacy on keratinocytes by influencing cell cycle progression, cellular differentiation, cell survival, and apoptosis [6]. It results in a significant reduction in sebum production and has anti-inflammatory properties. Study data suggest that all-trans-retinoic acid may be the active intracellular form of isotretinoin after isomerization which induces apoptosis in cells cultured from different human cells. Although oral isotretinoin has no direct antimicrobial action, it alters the microenvironment of keratinocytes leading to an unfavorable milieu for the poxvirus to survive which could be one possible mechanism of its efficacy in MC [7]. The role of isotretinoin in our condition might also be explained by its efficacy from the Fox O1 hypothesis leading to apoptosis of virally infected cells and resolution of MC [8].

When evaluating the response rate of any treatment modality, the possibility of spontaneous resolution should be considered as in other cases of MC. Notably, the patient had exhibited long durations of MC and had failed to respond to the known treatment modalities. Hence, the results were less likely to be influenced by the effect of spontaneous remission, and isotretinoin could be a newer modality of treatment in recalcitrant MC.

4. Conclusions

Although topical retinoic acids have been used in the treatment of molluscum, oral isotretinoin could be promising in widespread and recalcitrant MC. Indeed, randomized controlled studies are needed to confirm the effectiveness of this treatment, but its excellent safety profile appears to offer an attractive therapeutic option.

Consent

Consent was obtained from the patient for publication of this case report.

Authors' Contributions

All authors read and approved the final manuscript.

References

[1] A. K. C. Leung, B. Barankin, and K. L. E. Hon, "Molluscum contagiosum: an update," *Recent Patents on Inflammation & Allergy Drug Discovery*, vol. 11, no. 1, pp. 22-31, 2017.

[2] R. Meza-Romero, C. Navarrete-Dechent, and C. Downey, "Molluscum contagiosum: an update and review of new perspectives in etiology, diagnosis, and treatment," *Clinical, Cosmetic and Investigational Dermatology*, vol. 12, pp. 373–381, 2019.

[3] A. Czelusta, A. Yen-Moore, M. Van der Straten, D. Carrasco, and S. K. Tyring, "An overview of sexually transmitted diseases. Part III. Sexually transmitted diseases in HIV-infected patients," *Journal of the American Academy of Dermatology*, vol. 43, no. 3, pp. 409–436, 2000.

[4] J. C. Van der Wouden, R. Van der Sande, E. J. Kruithof, A. Sollie, L. W. Van Suijlekom-Smit, and S. Koning, "Interventions for cutaneous molluscum contagiosum," *Cochrane Database of Systematic Reviews*, vol. 5, no. 5, Article ID CD004767, 2017.

[5] P. Martin, "Interventions for molluscum contagiosum in people infected with human immunodeficiency virus: a systematic review," *International Journal of Dermatology*, vol. 55, no. 9, pp. 956–966, 2016.

[6] A. Layton, "The use of isotretinoin in acne," *Dermato-Endocrinology*, vol. 1, no. 3, pp. 162–169, 2009.

[7] M. Tsukada, M. Schröder, C. E. Orfanos et al., "13-cis retinoic acid exerts its specific activity on human sebocytes through selective intracellular isomerization to all-trans retinoic acid and binding to retinoid acid receptors," *Journal of Investigative Dermatology*, vol. 115, no. 2, pp. 321–327, 2000.

[8] B. Melnik, "Isotretinoin and FoxO1," *Dermato-Endocrinology*, vol. 3, no. 3, pp. 141–165, 2011.

14

Ultra-Low-Dose Radiotherapy for Palliation of Mycosis Fungoides

İpek Pınar Aral,[1] **Neşe Göçer Gürok**,[2] **Aykut Oğuz Konuk**,[3] **and Özlem Üçer**[4]

[1]*Nevsehir Public Hospital, Radiation Oncology Department, Göreme, Turkey*
[2]*Elazığ Fethi Sekin City Hospital, Dermatology Department, Elazig, Turkey*
[3]*Elazığ Fethi Sekin City Hospital, Radiation Oncology Department, Elazig, Turkey*
[4]*Fırat Univercity, Pathology Department, Elazig, Turkey*

Correspondence should be addressed to İpek Pınar Aral; ipekpt@hotmail.com

Academic Editor: Soner Uzun

Introduction. Mycosis fungoides (MF) is a form of primary cutaneous T-cell lymphomas, and radiotherapy (RT) has been used to treat localized/limited lesions of MF. In this case report, the results of low-dose RT applied for palliative purpose are shared. *Case Report.* A 70-year-old male patient was admitted to the outpatient clinic 7 months ago with a generalized itchy rash. The result of the biopsy was reported as mycosis fungoides. Systemic treatment was not performed due to comorbid diseases. The hemibody RT was applied. 2 Gy was given per fraction, with a total dose of 6 Gy. The significant clinical relief was observed with 6 Gy RT. The patient died due to multiorgan failure 2 months later, and no recurrence was observed. *Conclusion.* The palliation was achieved in the advanced MF patient with fractionated 6 Gy hemibody RT for the remaining 2 months of life.

1. Introduction

Mycosis fungoides (MF) is the most common form of primary cutaneous T-cell lymphomas [1]. Radiotherapy (RT) has been used to treat localized/limited lesions of MF since 1902. However, large-area skin irradiations using low-energy X-rays or electrons cannot be applied frequently due to equipment, experience, and technical deficiencies [2]. Total skin electron irradiation (TSEI) or total skin irradiation that uses photons (TSI) is performed in a limited number of experienced clinics, especially in MF patients with extensive involvement [3]. TSEI is a method used in the treatment of several dermatological malignant diseases, not only in MF but also in Sézary syndrome or Kaposi's sarcoma; successful results were seen [3–5]. Despite the successful results of RT, the clinician's awareness of this treatment remains low because of concern about side effects [4, 5]. In this case report, the results of ultra-low-dose RT applied for palliative purpose are shared.

2. The Case Report

A 70-year-old male patient was admitted to the outpatient clinic 7 months ago with a generalized itchy rash. A punch biopsy was taken from the thigh region in Firat University Hospital. Epidermis showed significant spongiosis and mild irregular acanthosis. Also, lymphocytes and infrequent neutrophil infiltration were observed in the epidermis. Significant vacuolization was observed in the basal layer. Lymphocytes with irregular hyperchromatic nuclei were detected in the basal layer. Inflammation of mixed cells in the superficial dermis has been reported. Immunohistochemical staining was performed, or CD3, CD4, and CD8 staining was observed. The result of the biopsy was reported as mycosis fungoides. Systemic treatments were not performed due to comorbid diseases (coronary Artery disease (CAD), chronic obstructive pulmonary disease (COPD), paraplegia due to stroke, and hypertension (HT)). The patient also had not started any palliative or symptomatic treatment. He had hypothermia attacks in the last month before admitted to our clinic. On examination, plaques with erythematous, slightly hyperpigmented, widespread flooding were observed throughout the body (Figure 1). The patient was hospitalized in our clinic. The patient was consulted by the dermatology department. The clobetasol propionate, diphenhydramine hydrochloride, and undermine were administered by the dermatologist. This

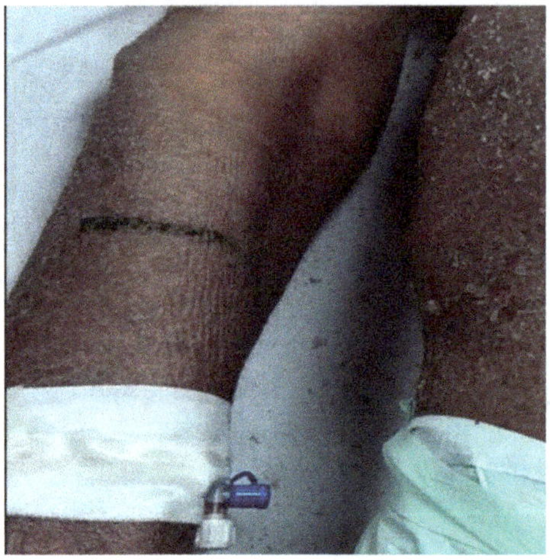

FIGURE 1: The right upper extremity image of the patient—before RT.

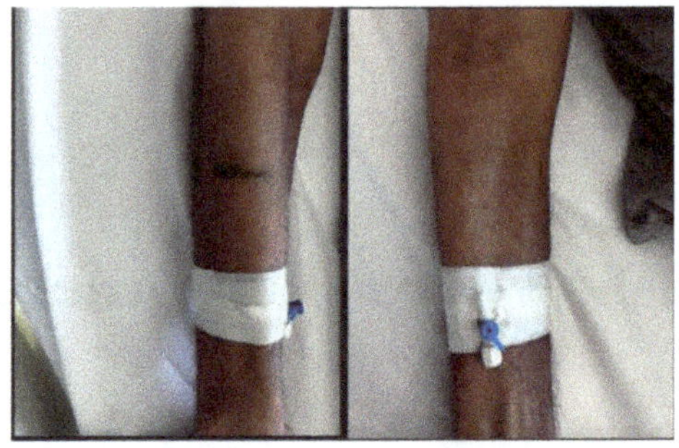

FIGURE 2: The right upper extremity image of the patient—after RT.

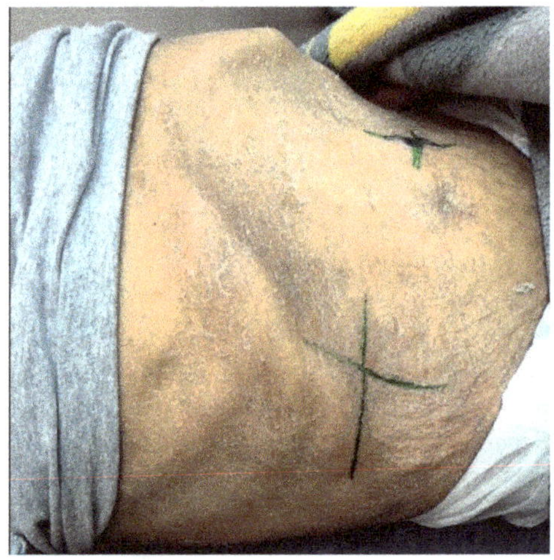

FIGURE 3: The abdominal image of the patient—before RT.

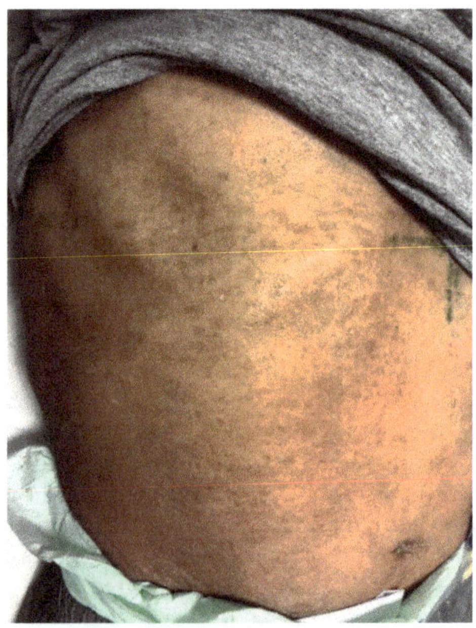

FIGURE 4: The abdominal image of the patient— after RT.

treatment, which was administered before RT, improved the patient's complaints of pruritus and hypothermia. The most complained areas of the patient were bilateral flexor and the upper anterior hemibody. RT was started on the flexor part of the bilateral arms with the most complaints. RT was applied with Elekta Versa HD device, SSD 100 cm, 6 MeV electron energy, 0 gantry angle, using a 20 × 20 applicator. The fraction (frc) dose was 2 Gy, and a total dose of 6 Gy was given. Clinical relief was observed after the first treatment (Figure 2). Following the response, RT was planned for the upper anterior hemibody (Figure 3). Because of the large RT area, right and left dual center radiotherapy was applied. For the right upper anterior hemibody radiotherapy, a 3200 gantry angle of 6 MeV electron energy with an SSD of 100 cm was used. Also, for the left upper hemibody radiotherapy, a 25 × 25 applicator at a 400 gantry angle with the same energy at SSD 100 cm was used. The 2 Gy was given per fraction, and the upper anterior hemibody received a total dose of 6 Gy. Significant clinical relief was observed with 6 Gy radiotherapy and medical treatment recommended by a dermatologist (Figure 4). The patient died due to multiorgan failure 2 months later, and no recurrence was observed in the RT areas.

3. Discussion

TSEI and TSI are technically difficult for patients with cutaneous lymphomas. Numerous approaches have been developed to solve "field problems" associated with such a large treatment volume. There is no "ideal" or even standard treatment for extensive skin irradiation. The current recommendations and treatment guidelines suggest several possible options for treatment [4].

Radiotherapy has been used for many years for patients with MF. Radiotherapy is not only effective treatment for the early-stage disease but also contributes to palliative treatment when the disease is advanced. For advanced MF, TSEI is involved in palliation of symptoms such as itching, pain, or dandruff. To date, experiences have shown that the effective dose of RT in the curative treatment of MF is 30 Gy or higher [5, 6]. In the literature, 20–30 Gy/10 frc or 8 Gy/1 frc treatments have been applied for palliative purposes. In advanced MF, the remission of symptoms has been reported in 36–96% of these treatments [6, 7]. Despite the promising results, an important reason why TSEI is not frequently applied in clinical practice is the concern of acute and late side effects [8]. Acute side effects are erythema, edema, hyperpigmentation, and fatigue. Additionally, an increase in the risk of superinfection can be observed [9, 10]. The acute reaction occurs intensely in the second week of treatment. These symptoms are temporary and usually resolve within 2–3 weeks of treatment. Hospitalization may be required according to the prevalence of symptoms [11, 12]. Hyperkeratosis, hyper- and de-pigmentation, and hypohidrosis caused by sweat gland atrophy are late side effects that can be observed due to RT [10]. In our case, no acute side effects were observed.

Historically, total doses of 30 Gy and above were administered. Although the treatment results were successful, severe skin side effects were especially observed. Therefore, low-dose RT started to be tried after 2010 [13–15]. Kroeger et al. achieved adequate treatment results with fewer grade 2 skin toxicities with low-dose (12 Gy) TSEI compared to conventional doses [16]. Additionally, the low total dose is important in terms of the need for a second treatment and improved quality of life [17, 18]. Today, for TSEI, a total dose of 12–36 Gy is often preferred as 4–6 Gy per week, and complete response rates are 90% and above some series [19–21]. After the effectiveness of low dose, phase 2 studies for ultra-low- dose have been tried and ongoing [22].

There is no standard dose and administration schedule of low-dose and ultra-low-dose TSEI for palliative purposes. Since studies on low-dose TSEI are not common in the literature, treatment standards are limited. Besides, there is currently no randomized trial comparing low- and high-dose TSEI. In a study conducted in Copenhagen Dermatology Department, it was reported that 4 Gy low-dose TSEI given in 4 fractions caused partial remission in IB-II MF, but the remission was short-term [9, 23]. In the study of Funk et al., TSEI was applied with doses of 29 Gy and above, and complete remission was observed in 50% of the patients and the remission was permanent for 1–18 months [10]. In our patient, the response was obtained at ultra-low dose (6 Gy), so treatment was terminated, and the patient was followed up closely. In case of recurrence, a second treatment was planned. However, the patient developed cystitis 2 months after the end of treatment and did not improve despite medical treatment. Then, he died of a sudden deterioration of multiple organ failure. No complaints were observed in the RT area during this period. Our case is one of the lowest dose-fractionated palliative wide-field irradiations in the literature.

4. Conclusion

In this case evaluation, full palliation was achieved in the advanced MF patient with fractionated 6 Gy hemibody RT for the remaining 2 months of life.

References

[1] K. Olek-Hrab and W. Silny, "Diagnostics in mycosis fungoides and Sezary syndrome," *Reports of Practical Oncology & Radiotherapy*, vol. 19, no. 2, pp. 72–76, 2014.

[2] D. K. Parida and G. K. Rath, "Advantages and implications of high dose rate (HDR) total skin electron irradiation (TSEI) for the management of Mycsis Fungoides. Indian experience," *Reports of Practical Oncology & Radiotherapy*, vol. 19, no. 2, pp. 104–108, 2014.

[3] B. J. King, S. C. Lester, S. N. Tolkachjov, M. D. P. Davis, L. E. Gibson, and J. A. Martenson, "Skin-directed radiation therapy for cutaneous lymphoma: the mayo clinic experience," *Journal of the American Academy of Dermatology*, vol. 82, no. 3, pp. 634–641, 2020.

[4] M. D. Evans, C. Hudon, E. B. Podgorsak, and C. R. Freeman, "Institutional experience with a rotational total skin electron irradiation (RTSEI) technique-a three decade review (1981–2012)," *Reports of Practical Oncology & Radiotherapy*, vol. 19, no. 2, pp. 120–134, 2014.

[5] F. W. Hensley, G. Major, C. Edel, H. Hauswald, and M. Bischof, "Technical and dosimetric aspects of the total skin electron beam technique implemented at Heidelberg University Hospital," *Reports of Practical Oncology & Radiotherapy*, vol. 19, no. 2, pp. 135–143, 2014.

[6] F. Y. Moraes, A. Carvalho Hde, S. A. Hanna, J. L. F. Da Silva, and G. N. Marta, "Literature review of clinical results of total skin electron irradiation (TSEBT) of mycosis fungoides in adults," *Reports of Practical Oncology & Radiotherapy*, vol. 19, no. 2, pp. 92–98, 2014.

[7] https://www.nccn.org/professionals/physician_gls/default.aspx.

[8] J. Kaźmierska, "Clinical results of the total skin electron irradiation of the mycosis fungoides in adults. Conventional fractionation and low dose schemes," *Reports of Practical Oncology & Radiotherapy*, vol. 19, no. 2, pp. 99–103, 2013.

[9] M. R. Kamstrup, L. Specht, G. L. Skovgaard, and R. Gniadecki, "A prospective, open-label study of low-dose total skin electron beam therapy in mycosis fungoides," *International Journal of Radiation Oncology Biology Physics*, vol. 71, no. 4, pp. 1204-1207, 2008.

[10] A. Funk, F. Hensley, and R. Krempien, "Palliative total skinelectron beam therapy (TSEBT) for advanced cutaneous T-celllymphoma," *European Journal of Dermatology*, vol. 18, no. 3, pp. 308–312, 2008.

[11] P. Maignon, P. Truc, G. Dalac et al., "Radiotherapy of advancedmycosis fungoides: indications and results of total skin electron beam and photon beam irradiation," *Radiotherapy and Oncology*, vol. 54, no. 1, pp. 73–78, 2000.

[12] N. Eros, M. Marschalkó, A. Bajcsay, C Polgár, J Fodor, and S Kárpáti, "Transient leukonychia after total skin electron beam irradiation," *Journal of the European Academy of Dermatology and Venereology*, vol. 25, no. 1, pp. 115–117, 2011.

[13] M. Chowdhary, A. Song, N. G. Zaorsky, and W. Shi, "Total skin electron beam therapy in mycosis fungoides-a shift towards lower dose?" *Chinese Clinical Oncology*, vol. 8, no. 1, p. 9, 2019.

[14] I. Georgakopoulos, E. Papadavid, K. Platoni et al., "Clinical application of total skin electron beam (TSEB) therapy for the

management of T cell cutaneous lymphomas. The evolving role of low dose (12 Gy) treatment schedule," *Clinical and Translational Radiation Oncology*, vol. 15, pp. 26–30, 2018.
[15] A. Taverniers, A. Du-Thanh, M. Charissoux, C. Kerr, and O. Dereure, "Low-vs. middle-dose total skin electron beam therapy for mycosis fungoides: an efficiency-based retrospective survey of skin response," *Acta Dermato Venereologica*, vol. 99, no. 6, pp. 544–550, 2019.
[16] K. Kroeger, K. Elsayad, C. Moustakis, U. Haverkamp, and H. T. Eich, "Low-dose total skin electron beam therapy for cutaneous lymphoma," *Strahlentherapie und Onkologie*, vol. 193, no. 12, pp. 1024–1030, 2017.
[17] K. Elsayad, K. Kroeger, B. Greve et al., "Low-dose total skin electron beam therapy: quality of life improvement and clinical impact of maintenance and adjuvant treatment in patients with mycosis fungoides or Sezary syndrome," *Strahlentherapie und Onkologie*, vol. 196, no. 1, pp. 77–84, 2020.
[18] A. Song, A. Gochoco, T Zhan et al., "A prospective cohort study of Ccondensed low dose total skin electron beam therapy for mycosis fungoides: reduction of disease burden and improvement in quality of life," *Journal of the American Academy of Dermatology*, pp. 30130–30134, 2020.
[19] J. A. Miccio, L. D. Wilson, B. H. Kann et al., "Cutaneous T-cell lymphoma: trends in radiation doses and patterns of care 2004–2015," *Anticancer Research*, vol. 39, no. 1, pp. 253–259, 2019.
[20] T. O. Thomas, P. Agrawal, J. Guitart et al., "Outcome of patients treated with a single-fraction dose of palliative radiation for cutaneous T-cell lymphoma," *International Journal of Radiation Oncology Biology Physics*, vol. 85, no. 3, pp. 747–753, 2013.
[21] K. J. Neelis, E. C. Schimmel, M. H. Vermeer, N. J. Senff, R. Willemze, and E. M. Noordijk, "Low-dose palliative radiotherapy for cutaneous B-and T-cell lymphomas," *International Journal of Radiation Oncology Biology Physics*, vol. 74, no. 1, pp. 154–158, 2009.
[22] https://clinicaltrials.gov/ct2/show/NCT03398161.
[23] L. M. Lindahl, M. R. Kamstrup, P. M. Petersen et al., "Total skin electron beam therapy for cutaneous T-cell lymphoma: a nationwide cohort study from Denmark," *Acta Oncologica*, vol. 50, no. 8, pp. 1199–1205, 2011.

15

Desmoplastic Melanoma Arising after 1,064 nm q-Switched Nd:YAG Laser of a Suspected Solar Lentigo

Leah Cohen,[1] **Sonali Nanda**,[2] **and Martin Zaiac**[1,2,3]

[1]*Department of Dermatology, Florida International University Herbert Wertheim College of Medicine, Miami, FL, USA*
[2]*Department of Dermatology and Cutaneous Surgery, University of Miami Miller School of Medicine, Miami, FL, USA*
[3]*Chairman of the Department of Dermatology, Florida International University Herbert Wertheim College of Medicine, Miami, FL, USA*

Correspondence should be addressed to Martin Zaiac; drmartyz@aol.com

Academic Editor: Kowichi Jimbow

Objectives. To present a case of desmoplastic melanoma (DM) arising after laser therapy of a suspected solar lentigo with the 1,064 nm Q-switched (QS) Neodymium:Yttrium-Aluminum-Garnet (Nd:YAG) laser and discuss the safety of treating suspected solar lentigines with laser therapy. *Methods.* Case presentation with discussion. *Results.* We describe a patient who developed DM after 1,064 nm QS Nd:YAG laser therapy to a suspected solar lentigo. *Conclusions.* Limited generalizable studies regarding the safety of laser therapy for solar lentigines exist, specifically for the 1,064 nm QS Nd:YAG laser. Therefore, we recommend caution is taken when considering laser therapy for these lesions, as well as strong consideration for histologic confirmation prior to therapy.

1. Introduction

Solar lentigines, or "age spots," are a common benign cosmetic complaint, present in 90% of the Caucasian population over 60 years old [1]. Removal of these lesions is one of the most frequently performed cosmetic procedures in laser centers around the United States [2]. The use of many Q-switched (QS) lasers including 532 nm Neodymium:Yttrium-Aluminum-Garnet (Nd:YAG) lasers, ruby lasers, and alexandrite lasers are an option for treatment of solar lentigines [3]. While the 1,064 nm QS Nd:YAG laser has demonstrated efficacy in treating melasma and nevus of Ota, to our knowledge no studies have addressed its efficacy for solar lentigines [3]. We report a case of a desmoplastic melanoma (DM) arising after 1,064-nm QS Nd:YAG laser therapy for a suspected solar lentigo of the inferior eyelid. This case introduces an important discussion regarding the safety of treating suspected solar lentigines with laser therapy.

2. Case Report

A 72-year-old woman presented with a two-year history of a light brown pigmented lesion located on the lateral segment of her right inferior eyelid. She had no history of nevi, rashes, or scaling of the area. The patient had a past medical history significant for a basal cell carcinoma, melasma, and numerous solar lentigines of the face and neck. She admitted to significant sun exposure and tanning in the past but denied any family history of skin cancer. Three months earlier, she had received laser therapy to the face and neck for skin rejuvenation, using the fractional resurfacing laser at a wavelength of 1,550 nm. Her only reaction to laser therapy was slight erythema and mild swelling. Otherwise, she healed well.

On examination, the lesion was a flat, well-circumscribed macule, measuring 3 mm x 2 mm, colored tan to dark brown involving the lateral segment of the right inferior eyelid (Figure 1). It appeared similar to many other lentigines on the patient's sun-exposed areas and was clinically correlated to be a solar lentigo. Due to the low clinical suspicion for malignant lesions and sensitive area, biopsy was not obtained. The patient sought cosmetic treatment of the right inferior eyelid lesion and the 1,064 nm QS Nd:YAG laser was used, pulse durations were not recorded.

Three months after targeted laser treatment of the right inferior eyelid patch, the patient returned complaining of

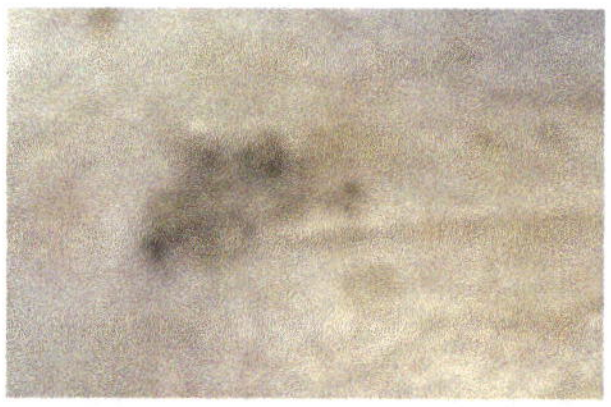

Figure 1: Initially the lesion resembled many other lesions in the patient's sun-exposed skin areas. The lesion was a 3 mm x 2 mm macule colored tan to dark brown involving the lateral segment of the right inferior eyelid.

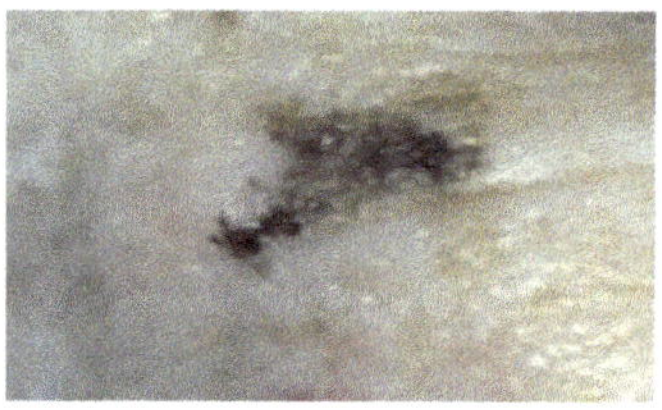

Figure 2: Presentation of lesion after 1,064 nm QS Nd:YAG laser therapy: 4 mm x 2 mm asymmetric macule colored tan to dark brown to black involving the lateral segment of the right inferior eyelid.

recurrence of the lesion, which appeared to have grown to be a 4 mm x 2 mm asymmetric macule colored tan to dark brown to black (Figure 2). A shave biopsy was taken and returned positive for atypical lentiginous and nested melanocytic proliferation with severe atypia, extending to the lateral margin. The lesion was subsequently excised and final pathology was reported as a desmoplastic melanoma, Clark's level IV, Breslow's thickness 2.5 mm with negative margins. Subsequent follow-up appointments at 2 months, 3 months, 6 months, and 8 months were all negative for clinical recurrence.

3. Discussion

We have described a patient who, after receiving 1,064 nm QS Nd:YAG laser treatment of a suspected solar lentigo, developed DM. This case produces several important clinical questions. Was the pigmented lesion at initial presentation a true solar lentigo? If it was a solar lentigo, could it have undergone transformation after laser treatment? Is the 1,064 nm QS Nd:YAG laser an appropriate choice for suspected solar lentigines?

Our current understanding is that there is significant improvement of the appearance of solar lentigines with low-fluence QS 1,064 nm Nd:YAG laser therapy, with many patients experiencing clearance without significant unwanted pigmentary changes or other side effects [3, 4]. A retrospective review of twelve patients with multiple solar lentigines treated with the 1,064 nm QS Nd:YAG laser found that 58% of patients reached near total improvement while 25% reached moderate improvement, with no side effects reported [3]. Despite promising results, this review is one of the only published assessments of the 1,064 nm QS Nd:YAG laser for solar lentigines and is limited by small sample size, retrospective analysis, and lack of histologic confirmation at diagnosis. As our applications of laser therapies expand, it is important to document their side effects to characterize their safety profiles.

When considering the possibility of misdiagnosis, we must consider the broad differential diagnosis of solar lentigines, which includes early seborrheic keratoses, pigmented actinic keratoses, and benign melanocytic nevi, as well as lentigo maligna (LM), a type of melanoma in situ [2]. As solar lentigines are a clinical diagnosis with a wide differential, whose definition may vary between physicians, it is logical that a variety of cosmetic treatments may be performed on these lesions [5]. Several reports have documented LM arising after laser therapies to a pigmented lesion [2, 5, 6]. In a retrospective review of biopsy-proven LM, Hibler et al. concluded that 7.4% of patients with LM had prior cosmetic therapy, 29.7% of which had received laser therapy of some type [5]. The authors also describe eight patients who had a history of benign biopsy prior to their eventual diagnosis of LM, suggesting a possible sampling error during biopsy [5].

Just as LM after laser therapy has been documented, several case series describe invasive melanoma after laser therapy. Zisper et al. describes twelve patients who were treated with ablative lasers, four of which developed nodular malignant melanoma, four developed LM, and four developed other subtypes [7]. Only four of the twelve cases were biopsied prior to laser therapy. When histology was reevaluated after the diagnosis of melanoma, two of the four cases had evidence for pathological misdiagnosis [7]. Most recently, Delker et al. identified eleven patients who developed melanoma after laser therapy; however, specific lasers used were not mentioned [8]. Of the eleven cases, three were LM, one was melanoma in situ, two were superficial spreading, two were nodular, and one was an unknown subtype; 82% had no histologic assessment performed on lesions prior to laser therapy. To our knowledge, there is only one case report documenting a case of DM after laser treatment [9]. Lee et al. describe the development of DM one to two years after treatment with a Nd:YAG laser of an unknown type.

4. Conclusion

The diagnosis of melanoma after laser treatment of a pigmented lesion in the same area is not conclusive evidence that a misdiagnosis occurred [2], nor is it conclusive of malignant transformation or, if performed, a misrepresentative biopsy. These three possibilities must be understood so that we can better characterize similar occurrences in the future. By establishing the outcomes associated with laser therapies, physicians and patients can better understand the risk of laser treatment of pigmented lesions. Two issues arise at the heart of this case, the first being that the solar lentigo is a clinical diagnosis, for which the differential diagnosis includes both benign and malignant pigmented entities, and the second is that few evaluations of the 1,064 nm QS Nd:YAG laser for solar lentigines exist. Therefore, we recommend using laser therapies for the treatment of clinically diagnosed solar lentigines with caution. Physicians should consider performing a biopsy of pigmented lesions prior to laser therapy, and if lesions recur after laser therapy, the possibility of malignancy should be considered and followed by immediate biopsy.

Abbreviations

QS Nd:YAG: Q-switched Neodymium:Yttrium-Aluminum-Garnet
DM: Desmoplastic melanoma
LM: Lentigo maligna.

References

[1] A. R. Rhodes, T. J. Harrist, and K. Momtaz-T, "The PUVA-induced pigmented macule: a lentiginous proliferation of large, sometimes cytologically atypical, melanocytes," *Journal of the American Academy of Dermatology*, vol. 9, no. 1, pp. 47–58, 1983.

[2] K. Stankiewicz, G. Chuang, and M. Avram, "Lentigines, laser, and melanoma: a case series and discussion," *Lasers in Surgery and Medicine*, vol. 44, no. 2, pp. 112–116, 2012.

[3] J.-H. Nam, H.-S. Kim, G.-Y. Lee, and W.-S. Kim, "Beneficial effect of low fluence 1,064 nm Q-Switched neodymium:Yttrium-Aluminum-Garnet laser in the treatment of senile lentigo," *Annals of Dermatology*, vol. 29, no. 4, pp. 427–432, 2017.

[4] C. Kaminaka, F. Furukawa, and Y. Yamamoto, "The clinical and histological effect of a low-fluence Q-Switched 1,064-nm Neodymium:Yttrium-Aluminum-Garnet laser for the treatment of melasma and solar lentigenes in asians prospective, randomized, and split-face comparative study," *Dermatologic Surgery*, vol. 43, no. 9, pp. 1120–1133, 2017.

[5] B. P. Hibler, K. L. Connolly, E. H. Lee, A. M. Rossi, and K. S. Nehal, "Lentigo maligna melanoma with a history of cosmetic treatment: prevalence, surgical outcomes and considerations," *Lasers in Surgery and Medicine*, vol. 49, no. 9, pp. 819–826, 2017.

[6] N. Ikoma, Y. Umezawa, T. Mabuchi, S. Tamiya, T. Matsuyama, and A. Ozawa, "Lentigo maligna occurring in a patient with the past history of laser therapy," *The Tokai Journal of Experimental and Clinical Medicine*, vol. 33, no. 2, pp. 75–77, 2008.

[7] M. C. Zipser, J. Mangana, P. A. Oberholzer, L. E. French, and R. Dummer, "Melanoma after laser therapy of pigmented lesions - circumstances and outcome," *European Journal of Dermatology*, vol. 20, no. 3, pp. 334–338, 2010.

[8] S. Delker, E. Livingstone, T. Schimming, D. Schadendorf, and K. G. Griewank, "Melanoma diagnosed in lesions previously treated by laser therapy," *The Journal of Dermatology*, vol. 44, no. 1, pp. 23–28, 2017.

[9] E. H. Lee and K. J. Busam, "Desmoplastic melanoma presenting after laser treatment: a case report and tale of cautiona," *Dermatologic Surgery*, vol. 37, no. 11, pp. 1689–1692, 2011.

16

Clinical and Histopathological Findings in a Patient of Darier–White Disease with Acrokertasosis Verruciformis of Hopf

Vikash Paudel,[1] **Manish Bhakta Pradhan**,[1] **Brijesh Shrestha**,[2] **and Sumit Paudel**[1]

[1]*Department of Dermatology and Venereology, National Medical College, Birgunj, Nepal*
[2]*Department of Pathology, National Medical College, Birgunj, Nepal*

Correspondence should be addressed to Vikash Paudel; vikashpoudel@iom.edu.np

Academic Editor: Sergio A. Cuevas Covarrubias

Darier disease (DD) is a rare genodermatoses characterized by greasy hyperkeratotic papules in seborrheic regions and nail and oral changes. Histologically, it presents as suprabasal clefts with acantholytic and dyskeratotic cells. Acrokertasosis verruciformis of Hopf (AKVH) is considered an allelic variant with clinical overlap where Church spires are seen histologically without dyskeratoses. Patients are susceptible to various viral and bacterial skin infections requiring prevention and treatment of infection. Nonspecific treatment includes patient counseling on exacerbating factors. Although there are no curative treatments for DD, topical corticosteroids and systemic retinoids may be used to control inflammation and hyperkeratosis. We are reporting a rare case with clinical and histological findings of DD with AKVH in a 17-year-old boy with keratotic papules, presented on the hands and feet, nose, and ears without mucosal involvement.

1. Introduction

Darier disease (DD) or Darier–White disease is an autosomal dominant genodermatosis, characterized by greasy hyperkeratotic papules in the seborrheic area and nail and mucous membrane changes [1]. First described by Prince Marrow (1886) and reported independently by Darier and White (1889), there is a mutation in the ATPA2 gene [2, 3]. Acrokeratosis verruciformis of Hopf (AKVH) is an autosomal dominant disorder of keratinization, described by Hopf (1931) [4] and is characterized by multiple flat-topped, papules on the hands and feet, punctate keratosis, and varying degrees of nail involvement [5]. DD and AKV are regarded as genetic evidence of unitary origin with allelic similarities, and it is suggested that patients with DD frequently show lesions that are indistinguishable from AKVH, both clinically and histopathologically [6–8]. We are reporting a rare case of DD with AKVH in a 17-year-old male who was treated with oral isotretinoin with a favorable outcome.

2. Case Report

A 17-year-old adolescent male, presented with generalized pruritic eruptions for 3 months. Initially, the lesions started from the neck later to progress over the face and trunk. No family history of atopy or such illness was found. On examination, there were firm, greyish, warty and greasy papules, and plaques scattered over the forehead, scalp, postauricular and preauricular regions, external ear, neck, nasolabial folds, anterior chest, and scapular area (Figures 1(a) and 1(b)).

Small-sized warty papules were also noted over the dorsum of the bilateral hands and feet (Figures 2 and 3). Oral mucosa appeared to be normal.

Routine investigations were within normal limits. Skin punch biopsies were taken from the neck and dorsum of the left hand for histopathological examination. Clinical and laboratory findings were compatible with DD and AKVH, respectively. However, genetic analyses and functional analyses of the mutation could not be done because of

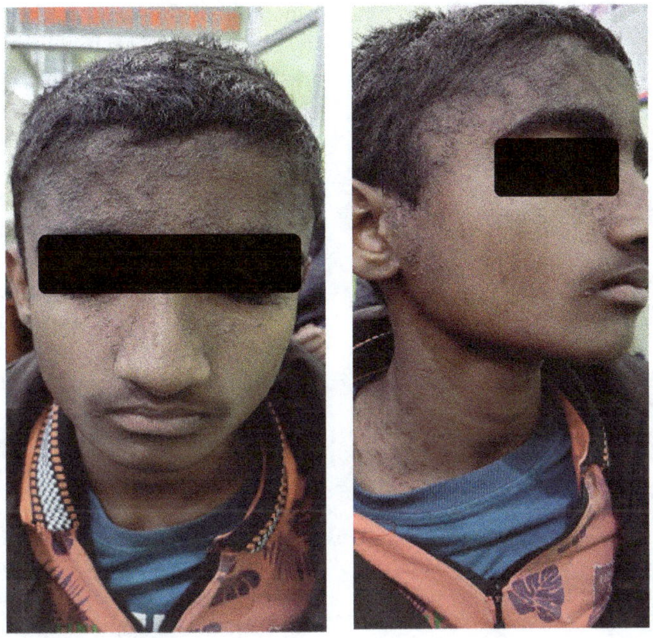

(a) (b)

Figure 1: (a, b) Multiple flat-topped brownish verrucous plaques over the forehead, neck, and the periauricular area.

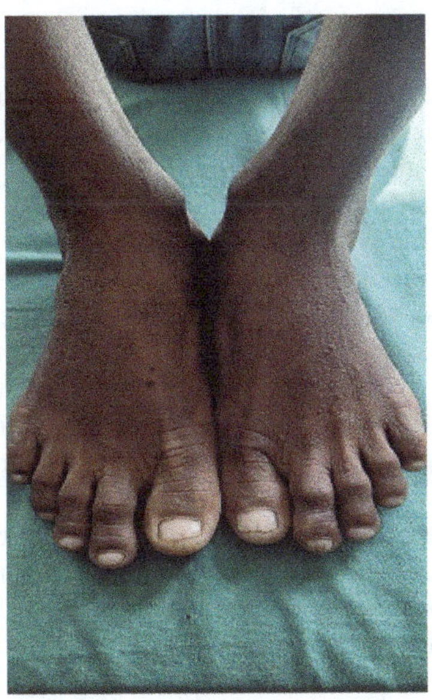

Figure 2: Multiple keratotic papules over the dorsum of bilateral feet.

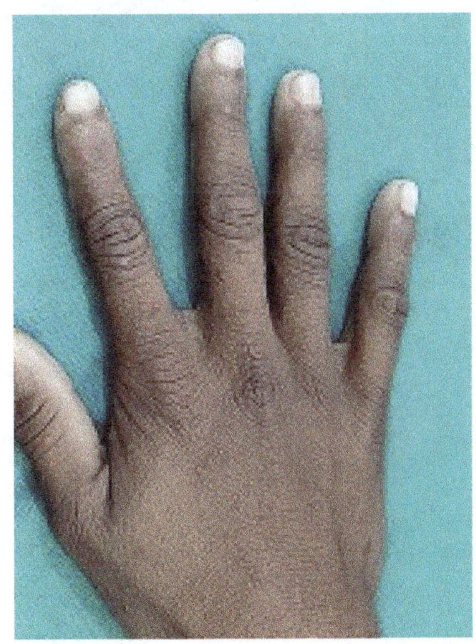

Figure 3: Multiple keratotic papules over the dorsum of the hand.

economic constraints, thus allelic similarities between the two could not be established.

Histopathological examination of the lesion from the neck shows acantholysis and dyskeratosis represented by corps rods and corps grains (Figure 4). Microscopic examination of the lesion from the dorsum of the left hand shows a focal area of hyperkeratosis, papillomatosis, and acanthosis with church spire appearance which was compatible with AKVH (Figure 5).

The patient was treated with isotretinoin 20 mg once daily, 5% salicylic acid and tretinoin 0.025% sunscreen, and urea-based moisturizers. Within two weeks of therapy, the lesions were flattened and crusted lesions were reduced. The patient was under follow-up for 3 months with improvement in the lesion, later the patient was lost.

3. Discussion

Darier's disease is a rare autosomal dominant genodermatosis caused by a mutation in the ATPA2 gene, at chromosome 12q23–12q24, which encodes the sarcoplasmic endoplasmic reticulum Ca^{2+} ATPase type 2 protein (SERCA2). The main function of SERCA2 is transporting Ca^{2+} from cytosol to the lumen of the endoplasmic

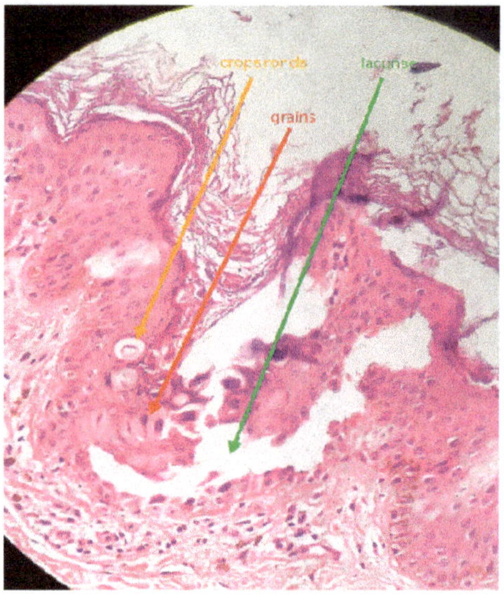

Figure 4: H&E stain with 20×: acantholysis and dyskeratosis represented by corps ronds and corps grains in DD.

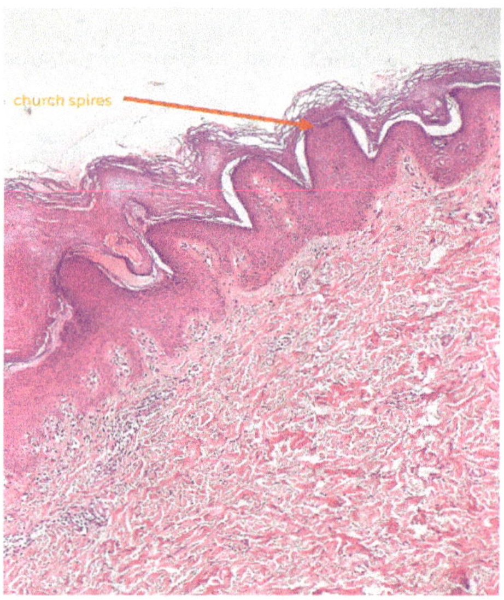

Figure 5: H&E stain with 10×: focal areas of hyperkeratosis, papillomatosis, and acanthosis with church spire appearance in AKVH.

reticulum [5]. A defect of SERCA2 leads to a deficiency of Ca^{2+} at the cell membrane, resulting in impaired cell-to-cell adhesion and apoptosis [5, 9]. The prevalence of this disorder in the population is 1 : 100,000. The sex incidence is equal, although the males appear to be more severely affected than females [10].

The clinical features of DD include the presence of multiple, hyperkeratotic papules distributed in seborrheic areas, as in our patient. The other clinical characteristics include flexural vegetative lesions, wart-like papules on the dorsal side of the hands and feet, palmer plantar pits, with red and white longitudinal bands, the distal wedge shape of the nail plate, and cobblestone papules on the oral mucosa. The patient might present with a foul offensive odor as well due to bacterial contamination. The oral mucosa is affected in 50% of the cases and lesions are usually asymptomatic [11]. Oral mucosal involvement and typical nail involvement were not present in our patient.

AKVH patients include mutations in ATP2A2, suggesting that this condition may be a variant of DD. However, it has been disputed for years that AKV and DD are separate entities or part of the same disease process. The main argument in favor of AKV and DD being separate entities is the existence, as in this family, of pure pedigrees where members only have features of AKV. In favor of AKVH being part of the DD spectrum is the presence of mixed pedigrees, and it is notable that 50% of Darier's patients have acral warty papules representing AKVH [7].

It is characterized by multiple flat-topped, flesh-colored papules on the hands and feet, punctate keratosis on the palms and soles, with varying degrees of nail involvement [7]. Our patient has similar lesions over the dorsum of the hand suggestive of AKVH.

Histopathological features of Darier's disease include acantholysis and dyskeratosis represented by "corps ronds" and "grains" (Figure 4). Corps ronds are located in the granular cell layer of the epidermis as central round dyskeratotic basophilic masses surrounded by a clear halo-like zone. Electron microscopy demonstrates loss of desmosomes, breakdown of keratin intermediate filament attachment, and perinuclear aggregation of keratin intermediate filaments [8]. Histopathological features of AKVH include papillomatosis with circumscribed epidermal elevations known as "church spire," acanthosis, hyperkeratosis, and hypergranulosis without parakeratosis (Figure 5) [8]. The histopathological findings in our patient were compatible with AKVH as well.

The differential diagnosis includes seborrheic dermatitis, acne vulgaris, acanthosis nigricans, confluent reticulate papillomatosis, and prurigo pigmentosa. Histologically, the disease needs differentiation from Hailey Hailey disease, Grover's disease, and pemphigus vulgaris. Immunofluorescence of skin biopsy differentiates different acantholytic disorders [5].

Treatment of DD remains a challenge due to a lack of validated curative treatment guidelines. Several treatment modalities have been reported in the literature including systemic/topical retinoids, corticosteroid, cyclosporine, fluorouracil, derma-abrasion, electro surgery, ablative lasers, photodynamic therapy, and surgical excision; however, they provide limited effectiveness [12]. Systemic retinoids have proven better in achieving some reduction of symptoms in 90% of patients. They reduce hyperkeratosis, smoothen papules, and reduce odor. Thus, isotretinoin was used in our patient with a good outcome. Sunscreen and emollients are also crucial [12]. Therefore, it is important to ensure a multidisciplinary approach in the management of patients with Darier's disease.

Though our case is supported by its clinical picture and histologic finding, its main limitation is the lack of genetic, molecular and functional analyses to confirm and correlate the allelic similarities between DD and AKVH.

Regardless of the clinical severity and treatment option, the patient should receive genetic counseling with information on the inherited condition and risk of transmission to the offspring. A biopsy is fundamental to allow a final diagnosis based on this result. Patients should be informed of the complications of this disorder and the care required. These patients should be treated by a multidisciplinary team.

Acknowledgments

The authors would like to acknowledge all the staff of the Department of Dermatology and the Department of Pathology, National Medical College and Teaching Hospital.

References

[1] S. M. Burge, "Darier's disease, keratins and proteases: a review," *Journal of the Royal Society of Medicine*, vol. 82, no. 11, pp. 673–676, 1989.

[2] J. Darier, "Vegetative follicular psorospermosise," *Annals of Dermatology and Syphiligraphy*, vol. 10, pp. 597–612, 1889.

[3] J. White, "A case of keratosis (ichthyosis) follicularis," *Journal of Cutan Genitourin Disease*, vol. 7, pp. 210–219, 1889.

[4] G. Hopf, "II. Über eine bisher nicht beschriebene disseminierte Keratose (Akrokeratosis verruciformis)," *Dermatology*, vol. 60, no. 4, pp. 227–250, 1931.

[5] C. Kositkuljorn and P. Suchonwanit, "Darier's disease: report of a case with facial involvement," *Case Report Dermatology*, vol. 11, no. 3, pp. 327–333, 2019.

[6] M. Harman, M. Durdu, and I. İbiloğlu, "Acrokeratosis verruciformis of Hopf exhibiting Darier disease-like cytological features," *Clinical and Experimental Dermatology*, vol. 41, no. 7, pp. 761–763, 2016.

[7] J. Dhitavat, S. Macfarlane, L. Dode et al., "Acrokeratosis verruciformis of Hopf is caused by mutation in ATP2A2: evidence that it is allelic to Darier's disease," *Journal of Investigative Dermatology*, vol. 120, no. 2, pp. 229–232, 2003.

[8] J. H. Herndon and J. D. Wilson, "Acrokeratosis verruciformis (Hopf) and Darier's disease: genetic evidence for a unitary origin," *Archives of Dermatology*, vol. 93, no. 3, 1966.

[9] H. Alain, "Acantholytic disorders of the skin: Darier-White disease, acrokeratosis verruciformis, Grover disease, and Hailey-hailey disease," *Fitzpatrick's Dermatology in General Medicine*, McGraw-Hill, New York, NY, USA, 2006.

[10] M. R. Judge, W. H. McLean, and C. S. Munro, "Disorders of keratinization," *Rook's Textbook of Dermatology*, Wiley-Blackwell Ltd, Hoboken, NY, USA, 2010.

[11] S. M. Cooper and S. M. Burge, "Darier's disease: epidemiology, pathophysiology, and management," *American Journal of Clinical Dermatology*, vol. 4, no. 2, pp. 97–105, 2003.

[12] R. N. Haber and N. G. Dib, "Management of Darier disease: a review of the literature and update," *Indian Journal of Dermatology, Venereology and Leprology*, vol. 87, no. 1, pp. 14–21, 2021.

17

Cutaneous Lymphadenoma: A Case of Recurrence after Shave Excision

Fateme Rajabi,[1,2] Kambiz Kamyab,[3] and Alireza Firooz[1]

[1]*Center for Research & Training in Skin Diseases and Leprosy, Tehran University of Medical Sciences, Tehran, Iran*
[2]*Network of Dermatology Research (NDR), Universal Scientific Education and Research Network (USERN), Tehran, Iran*
[3]*Department of Dermatopathology, Razi Hospital, Tehran University of Medical Sciences, Tehran, Iran*

Correspondence should be addressed to Alireza Firooz; firozali@tums.ac.ir

Academic Editor: Jacek Cezary Szepietowski

Cutaneous lymphadenoma (CL) is a rare skin tumor supposedly derived from the pilosebaceous unit. Since its description in 1987, fewer than 60 cases have been documented. Herein we report a case of CL presenting as a small nodule on the forehead of a young female. The lesion recurred two years after shave excision of a similar lesion. The histopathological examination revealed interconnected islands, sheets, and trabeculae consisting of two distinct types of cells within a sclerotic stroma, a peripheral rim of palisading basophilic cells, and central epithelial cells with eosinophilic to clear cytoplasm. A dense infiltration with prominent lymphocytes and few plasma cells dominated the stroma and permeated the epithelial nests. This case represents the recurrence of this type of skin tumor after shave excision and thus highlights the importance of complete margin-free excision of such lesions.

1. Introduction

Cutaneous lymphadenoma (CL) is a rare adnexal tumor that usually presents as an asymptomatic skin-colored nodule on the head and neck region [1]. Though the clinical features of this tumor are fairly nonspecific with numerous clinical differential diagnoses, the histopathological findings are characteristic. It consists of well-circumscribed epithelial nests embedded in a desmoplastic stroma with heavy infiltration of lymphocytes [2]. The nests are composed of two cell lines, a peripheral rim of small basaloid cells and an aggregate of clear cells. CL is an overlooked diagnosis that is often mistaken for basal cell carcinoma, trichoblastoma, and lymphoepithelioma-like carcinoma of the skin (LELC) [3]. Herein, we describe a case of CL presenting as a skin-colored nodule on the forehead of a young female that recurred after shave excision.

2. Case Presentation

An otherwise healthy 21-year-old woman presented for evaluation of a skin lesion on her forehead which had first appeared about seven years earlier. It had gradually grown to a 3–4 mm papule over four years when it was removed via shave excision. Approximately six months before visiting our department the lesion reemerged with a considerably faster growth rate that resulted in a 5–6 mm papule. Physical examination revealed a smooth skin-colored superficial papule with a central crust between the eyebrows (Figure 1). An excisional biopsy with a 3 mm margin was performed for histopathologic evaluation.

The histopathological examination revealed a dermal nodule of interconnected islands, sheets, and trabeculae of epithelial cells within a sclerotic stroma (Figure 2). The epithelial cells had eosinophilic to clear cytoplasm and mild

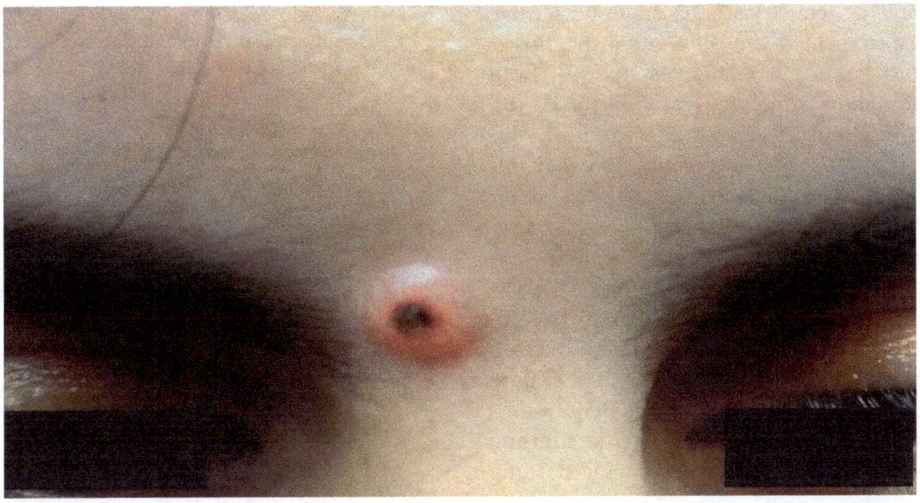

FIGURE 1: Clinical photograph of an indolent, asymptomatic nodule on the forehead.

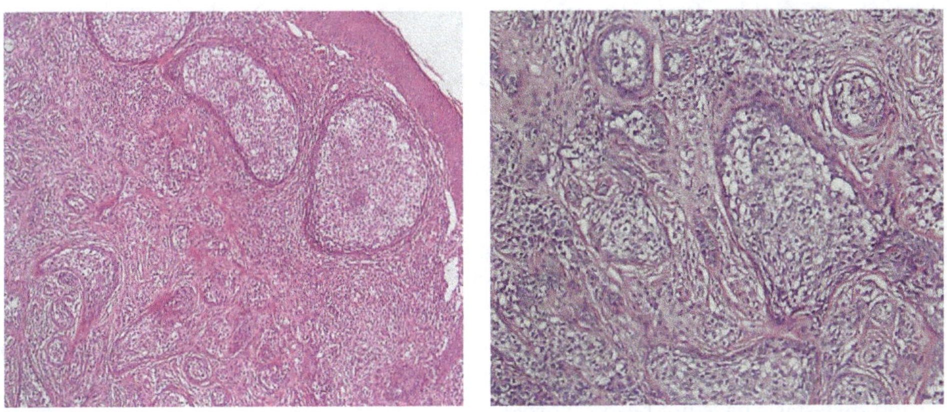

(a) (b)

FIGURE 2: (a) Histopathological findings demonstrate ill-defined interconnected islands of epithelial cells within a sclerotic stroma (4x). (b) The epithelial cells have eosinophilic to clear cytoplasm and mild pleomorphic vesicular nuclei (10x). A peripheral rim of palisading basophilic cells surrounds the epithelial islands. A prominent lymphocytic infiltration and few plasma cells that spill over to the epithelial nests is also present (hematoxylin-eosin).

pleomorphic vesicular nuclei. A peripheral rim of palisading basophilic cells surrounded the epithelial islands. A sclerotic stroma with dense infiltration of inflammatory cells contained the islands. The infiltration prominently consisted of lymphocytes and few plasma cells that permeated the epithelial nests. These histopathological findings were in favor of CL.

3. Discussion

CL is a rare skin tumor supposedly derived from the pilosebaceous unit. The tumor was first described by Santa Cruz and Barr in 1987 [4]. Since then fewer than 60 cases have been documented under different names such as cutaneous lymphoepithelial tumor, epithelial-lympho-histiocytic tumor, and adenomatoid trichoblastoma. The tumor usually affects middle-aged individuals, males more often than females, but it could affect all walks of life as even congenital lesions have been described [3, 5]. The tumor usually presents as an indolent, erythematous, or skin-colored, small nodule within the head and neck region.

The characteristic histopathology of lymphadenoma consists of a well-circumscribed but un-encapsulated nodule of epithelial nests embedded in a desmoplastic stroma both of which are heavily infiltrated by lymphocytes. The epithelial lobules can connect to the epidermis and extend down to the subcutaneous fat. The lobules are composed of two cell lines, a peripheral rim of small basaloid cells and an aggregate of large cells with faint eosinophilic cytoplasm, vesicular nuclei, and prominent nucleoli (clear cells). Ductal differentiation rimmed with central glassy cuticles, rudimentary follicular structures (papillary mesenchymal bodies), and compact keratinization are found on occasion [2]. The lymphocytic infiltration consists of mature B- and T-cells, few histiocytes (CD68+), and Langerhans cells (S100+, CD1a+) that can also form germinal center-like structures within the stroma [5, 6].

Though immunohistochemistry studies are not essential, they may help in distinguishing the differential diagnoses. The stroma of lymphadenoma is CD34 reactive [7]. Both basaloid and clear cells stain with cytokeratin AE1/AE3 [8]. The peripheral rim of basaloid cells also stains with BerEP4, a well-known BCC marker that is also positive in other follicular germinative cell-derived lesions such as trichoepithelioma and trichoblastoma [5, 9]. Nevertheless, lymphadenoma is distinguished from BCC based on its lack of peripheral palisading, mucin tinted retraction space, mitotic, and apoptosis figures [3]. Cytokeratin 20 (CK20) and CK17 have also been utilized to distinguish CL from BCC. The CK20+ Merkel cells often infiltrate the basaloid islands of CL but are usually absent in BCC. The BCC lesions demonstrate diffuse CK17 staining, whereas the tumoral islands in CL show a peripheral rim or patchy staining pattern [10].

Other histopathological differential diagnoses include clear cell syringoma, lymphoepithelioma-like carcinoma of the skin (LELC), and dermal thymus. Clear cell syringoma lacks the prominent lymphocytic infiltration and consists of a sclerotic stroma in which clear cells form tadpole-shaped ducts and islands. Syringoma is S-100, CEA, EMA, lysozyme, GCDFP-15, and GCDFP-24 positive [1]. The LELC is also composed of epithelial nests and lymphocytic infiltration, but it has a single linage of polygonal epithelioid cells with prominent cytological atypia that are derived from sweat glands. LELC is positive for EMA, and p63, and negative for S-100 [11]. The dermal thymus represents an ectopically located thymic tissue that is almost always associated with the branchio-oculofacial syndrome. Histologically, it consists of lymphoid tissue and Hassall's corpuscles [2].

Simple excision is currently the treatment of choice in CL. Since recurrence and metastasis have not been reported to date, the reemergence of the lesion, in this case, might be attributed to the insufficient margin of shave excision [3]. Additionally, if the tumor margins are not clinically well defined, Mohs surgery is particularly useful in such cases to ensure complete removal of the lesion. Mohs surgery might also be beneficial in cases that are located in anatomically sensitive areas where tissue preservation is critical [12].

Consent

A written consent form was obtained from the patient.

References

[1] A. Ghanadan and M. Khosravi, "Cutaneous syringoma: a clinicopathologic study of 34 new cases and review of the literature," *Indian Journal of Dermatology*, vol. 58, no. 4, p. 326, 2013.

[2] H. Hiraumi, K. Tabuchi, and S.-i. Kitajiri, "Dermal thymus: case report and review of the literature," *American Journal of Otolaryngology*, vol. 22, no. 4, pp. 294–296, 2001.

[3] R. Yu, S. Salama, and S. Alowami, "Cutaneous lymphadenoma: a rare case and brief review of a diagnostic pitfall," *Rare Tumors*, vol. 6, no. 2, pp. 53-54, 2014.

[4] D. Santa-Cruz, "Lymphoepithelial tumor of the skin," *Journal of Cutaneous Pathology*, vol. 14, p. 369, 1987.

[5] A. Fernandez-Flores, I. Nicklaus-Wollenteit, D. Sathishkumar et al., "Congenital cutaneous lymphadenoma," *Journal of Cutaneous Pathology*, vol. 44, no. 11, pp. 954–957, 2017.

[6] F. Aloi, C. Tomasini, and M. Pippione, "Cutaneous lymphadenoma," *The American Journal of Dermatopathology*, vol. 15, no. 4, pp. 353–357, 1993.

[7] A. Alsadhan, M. Taher, and M. Shokravi, "Cutaneous lymphadenoma," *Journal of the American Academy of Dermatology*, vol. 49, no. 6, pp. 1115-1116, 2003.

[8] M. Murphy, T. Brierley, J. Pennoyer, D. Rozenski, and J. M. Grant-Kels, "Lymphotropic adamantinoid trichoblastoma," *Pediatric Dermatology*, vol. 24, no. 2, pp. 157–161, 2007.

[9] A. P. Sunjaya, A. F. Sunjaya, and S. T. Tan, "The use of BEREP4 immunohistochemistry staining for detection of basal cell carcinoma," *Journal of Skin Cancer*, vol. 2017, Article ID 2692604, 10 pages, 2017.

[10] A. Goyal, J. F. Solus, M. P. Chan et al., "Cytokeratin 17 is highly sensitive in discriminating cutaneous lymphadenoma (a distinct trichoblastoma variant) from basal cell carcinoma," *Journal of Cutaneous Pathology*, vol. 43, no. 5, pp. 422–429, 2016.

[11] C. M. Clark, C. Muro-Cacho, and M. B. Ridley, "An uncommon cutaneous lesion," *JAMA Otolaryngology-Head and Neck Surgery*, vol. 144, no. 4, pp. 377-378, 2018.

[12] A. Hanlon, A. Clayton, and T. Stasko, "Mohs micrographic surgery for cutaneous lymphadenoma," *Dermatologic Surgery*, vol. 38, no. 9, pp. 1552–1554, 2012.

18

Grade IV Sacral Sore Treated with an Ointment Rich in PUFAs, Ceramides and Antimicrobial Peptides

Marta Cassini and Irina Saretzky

University of Buenos Aires, Buenos Aires, Argentina

Correspondence should be addressed to Irina Saretzky; irinasares@yahoo.com.ar

Academic Editor: Ravi Krishnan

This report presents the case of a 57-year-old male patient with a history of hypertension, obesity, dyslipidemia, and coronary disease that after a prolonged postcoronary surgery hospitalization developed a sacral butterfly-shaped sore, with asymmetric involvement of the base of both buttocks, grade III on the left and grade IV on the right sides. The lesion was very painful and had a negative impact on the patient's sleep and mood. Following the initial surgical debridement and treatment with collagenase ointment, the wound showed delayed healing, an increase in necrotic tissue, and purulent discharge, requiring a second surgical debridement that revealed a deeper involvement of the wound. After a month with poor therapeutic response, it was decided to change the treatment to the application of gauzes embedded in an ointment rich in polyunsaturated fatty acids (PUFAs), ceramides, and antimicrobial peptides, Curefini® ointment. After 30 days of treatment, a 50% reduction of the initial wound diameter was obtained with a positive impact on the patient's quality of life, together with a reduction of incidental and spontaneous local pain resulting in better night rest and a return of appetite and strength. During the treatment course, the patient did not suffer any local or systemic infection in connection with the wound. After one month, the patient could discontinue the use of opioid analgesics. A 95% closure of the lesion was achieved in 45 days. This case highlights the therapeutic efficacy of the treatment of cavitated wounds with a product based on natural ingredients that helps reduce pain and promotes granulation and reepithelialization.

1. Introduction

Chronic wounds are defined as wounds nonresponsive to initial therapy or persistent in the face of appropriate care, with no significant progress towards healing in 30 days [1]. Chronic wounds have several distinctive features that affect their ability to heal in a timely manner. Alterations in cellular function and biochemical balances can keep a chronic wound "stuck" in the inflammatory, proliferative phase of healing. Cells in a chronic wound become senescent and do not respond to chemical messengers. Cytokines and growth factors, essential to the healing of the wound, become ineffective in senescent cells. Chronic wound fluid contains chronic inflammatory cells as a result of the prolonged inflammatory proliferative phase. The effect is dramatic. Apoptosis, the genetic code to normal cell death, is inhibited and delayed. There is defective extracellular matrix remodeling, failure in reepithelialization and wound-edge migration and an increase in senescent fibroblasts [2].

Pressure ulcers are considered chronic cutaneous wounds as the healing process is prolonged and slow, with a second-intention healing strategy. These lesions are usually located in the skin and underlying tissues on bony prominences and are caused by sustained pressure over time, deformation, friction, and rubbing [3].

Pressure ulcers represent a major problem in the health care system, with great epidemiologic, economic, and socio-family impact [4]. Approximately 65% of pressure ulcers originate in hospital stays, affecting mostly patients above 65 years of age and producing a negative impact on their nutritional and metabolic status and alteration in bowel movement, in mobility, cognitive, and perceptual capacity, and on the skin barrier [5].

Hospital-acquired pressure ulcers are considered as one of the healthcare quality indicators, and it is estimated that 55 to 77% of cases could be avoided [6]. Early detection of patients at risk of developing a pressure injury needs to be implemented from the time of admission. Age, incontinence, and body mass index (BMI) are well-established risk factors. Having a BMI <19 kg/square meter and age above 65 are the most significant risk factors [7, 8]. Incidence is lower in overweight (BMI 25–30 kg/square meter) and obese (BMI >30 kg/square meter) patients [9].

The Braden Scale assesses the risk of developing a pressure injury based on criteria related to activity, mobility, skin moisture, nutritional status, friction, and rubbing, as well as the ability to feel pain and discomfort in different parts of the body as a result of pressure [10, 11]. Charlson's Comorbidity Index permits the assessment of comorbidity factors related to the mortality risk of hospitalized patients [12]. Use of this index to predict the mortality of patients with pressure ulcers has shown moderate to high risk when comorbidities include vascular disease (myocardial infarction, congestive heart failure, peripheral vascular disease, and cerebrovascular disease), diabetes, renal disease, chronic pulmonary disease, and metastatic cancer [13].

Another important aspect in risk evaluation can be the categorization by related risk groups; this means clustering groups of surgical patients and nonsurgical patients during hospitalization, with the surgical group being the one that bears the highest risk [14]. Surgical patients are at higher risk of developing pressure ulcers due to factors such as longer immobilization, anesthesia and/or surgery, and preexisting medical conditions [15, 16]. In the United States, patients with hospital-acquired pressure ulcers imply longer hospital stays and higher indirect costs [17]. The prevalence of hospital-acquired pressure ulcers in surgical patients amounts to approximately 8.5% or higher, depending on the type and duration of the surgery [18]. Many hospitals use the Braden Scale to assess surgical patients' risk of developing pressure ulcers; this evaluation can be done one day before or after the surgery [19]. A low total value on the Braden Scale means a higher risk of developing pressure ulcers [20]. The Braden Scale has proven at least 70% sensitivity and specificity to identify the risk of developing pressure ulcers in hospitalized patients [21]. However, this scale does not include the abovementioned risk variables and comorbidities. Thus, it is suggested not to use it alone to predict pressure ulcer risk in surgical patients [22].

Once the pressure ulcer has formed, the selection of an appropriate therapeutic strategy will determine the time of evolution, the type of response of the injured tissue, related infectious complications, and the total cost of medication and related procedures.

In the treatment of cavitated wounds, different therapeutic options focus on stimulating granulation at the dermis level to achieve coverage of underlying structures such as muscles, bones, or tendons. Crevices and tunneling present in this type of lesion pose a therapeutic challenge as does the management of wound discharges and the prevention of site contamination by feces or urine, which require advanced care by staff skilled in the management of smart dressings and wound devices. The presence of odor, peri-ulcer inflammation, and local pain need to be considered when selecting a therapeutic strategy. Currently, calcium alginate is frequently used, as well as negative pressure systems or grafts for cavitated wounds. The choice will depend on the availability of financial and human resources and hospital infrastructure.

Advanced wound care, proper diagnostic understanding in each individual case, and management of the patient and of his/her family context are all necessary conditions to achieve good clinical results.

Insufficient availability of skilled human resources as well as the high cost of materials required for advanced care of wounds in developing countries calls for the development of easy-to-implement, reproducible, and economical strategies that can be supervised by telemedicine.

In this article, we present the clinical case of a cavitated, grade IV wound treated with gauzes embedded in an ointment based on natural components derived from cod liver oil, sunflower oil, sweet almond oil, and bee wax, showing the high capacity of the ointment to favor granulation with appropriate control of the inflammatory process, thus avoiding the build-up of bacterial colonies and providing quick relief of local pain. The article stresses that the ease of application of the product for advanced care of grade IV cavitated wounds permitted continuity of treatment in remote locations by nonspecialized personnel.

2. Case Presentation

We present a case of a 57-year-old male patient with a history of hypertension, dyslipidemia, obesity, and coronary disease that underwent double bypass surgery, with a 27-day-postop interment period during which he developed a sacral pressure ulcer with asymmetrical compromise on both sides of the intergluteal cleft, grade III and grade IV pressure ulcers on the left and right sides, respectively, according to the NUAP/EUAP classification [23].

At home, the patient felt weak, could barely move, and complained of intense local pain in the sacral area that disabled him to sit down or sleep well. The patient's wife incidentally discovered that a skin brownish lesion was present at both sides of the intergluteal fold, motivating a new medical consult with a plastic surgeon three days after. According to the patient's report, no advanced wound care treatment was established during his hospitalization and he lost 10 kg of weight.

The patient's photographs showed a sacral ulcer involving the intergluteal cleft in a butterfly shape, with necrotic tissue 10 cm diameter on each side. Involvement of the deep tissues was not evident at first sight, but the left side seemed to have more superficial involvement (Figure 1(a)). The treating physician decided to initiate autolytic debridement with chloramphenicol/collagenase ointment plus secondary gauze dressing with petrolatum, cleaning with polyhexanide solution twice daily.

After 10 days of evolution, the first surgical toilette was performed with debridement of necrotized tissue; no swabs or culture specimens were collected. An ulcerative

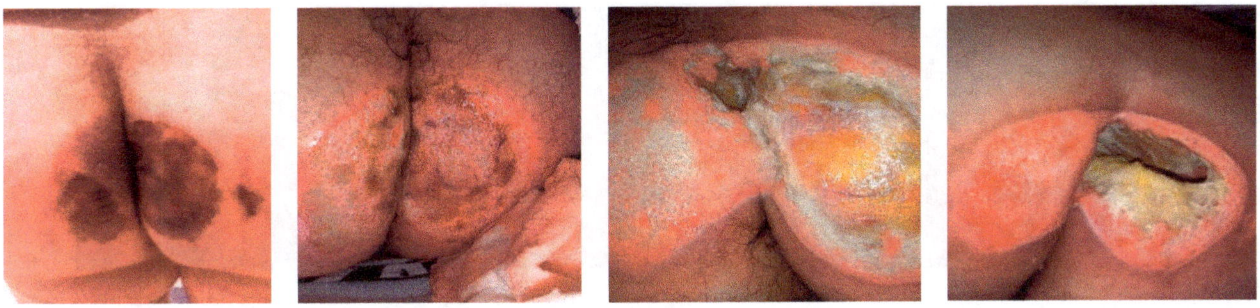

(a) (b) (c) (d)

FIGURE 1: Wound progression before Curefini® treatment. (a) Day 1: the patient is discharged from hospital after 27 days. Chloramphenicol/collagen is initiated as local treatment. (b) Day 10: the first surgical debridement is performed. Chloramphenicol/collagenase local treatment continues. (c) Day 18: topical treatment with chloramphenicol/collagenase continues. (d) Day 20: the second surgical debridement is performed, initiated with iodoform gauze, antibiotics PO, and oral opioids.

granulation bed was observed in the deep dermis with active borders and some brownish red areas on both sides. No local erythema, temperature, or purulent discharge was observed (Figure 1(b)). The patient received prophylactic antibiotic therapy with ciprofloxacin 500 mg PO bid for five days and continued with chloramphenicol/collagenase treatment at home.

After 18 days of chloramphenicol/collagenase local treatment, an ulcerative bed was involving sectors up to the hypodermis with fatty tissue exposure and cavitation at the right median and paramedian sacral level, reaching the muscular plane with no evident bone exposure (Figure 1(c)). Neither the probe to bone nor the lumbosacral IRM was performed. A fetid, purulent discharge was found on the gauze. No fever or shivering was reported. It was decided to schedule a new surgical toilette which was performed on day 20.

On day 20, a second surgical debridement was performed. Physical examination showed a left-side grade III pressure sore with granulation tissue at the wound bed and active reepithelialization borders; on the right side, a cavitated grade IV sore was observed, with hypodermis fat exposure, increased depth of the cavity with no bone exposure, and negative probe to bone (Figure 1(d)).

Following the debridement, according to the patient's medical report, no soft tissue culture specimens were collected and empiric systemic antibiotic treatment was indicated: amoxicillin/clavulanate 875/125 mg PO bid for ten days and local treatment with iodoform gauze dressings inside the cavity, with the indication to change every 48 hours. The patient complained of an increase in local pain and received tramadol 50 mg PO every 8 hours.

On day 30, the treating physician proposed a skin graft; however, the patient decided to get a second opinion from a wound care specialist. At this time point, the authors contacted the patient for the first time. During the interview, the patient was said to be concerned about the evolution of the wound, was said to be unwilling to have a surgical procedure and later hospitalization since his home is located 500 km away from the hospital, and had reported continuous pain and impossibility to sit or find a good position to sleep and regarding his mood, he seemed to be more depressed.

As independent wound care specialists, we suggested the patient and his family a new local treatment consisting of gauzes embedded in an ointment made of cod liver oil, sunflower seed oil, sweet almonds, virgin beeswax, and vitamins A and D, Curefini® [24,25]. One month after being discharged from the Coronary Unit, the patient started topical treatment with a sterile gauze lubricated with Curefini®, filling the cavity. The surface of both buttocks was covered with the sterile gauze embedded with Curefini®, with the indication to change it every 12 hours.

On day 42, after 12 days of topical treatment with natural ointment, pain improved significantly, oral opioids were tapered until total discontinuation, and the patient tolerated the sitting position for brief periods. After Curefini® local treatment was established, the granulation and reepithelialization processes were reactivated and hypodermis fat tissue was covered with new skin (Figure 2(a)).

On day 60, after 30 days of treatment with Curefini®, a 50% reduction in transverse wound diameter was observed, along with granulation tissue in the cavity bed and advanced epithelialization border (Figure 2(b)).

On day 75 after discharge from the hospital, with a 45-day-continuous period of Curefini® treatment, 95% closure of the lesion was achieved and a large crater ulcer was replaced by a transverse fissure in the right intergluteal fold of only 4 cm in depth, which continued to be treated locally with a gauze impregnated with the ointment (Figure 2(c)).

At this point, the patient starts to walk without difficulty or pain, maintains a correct diet with normal bowel movements, has a restorative sleep, and shows a tranquil mood.

Control after 3 months of Curefini® treatment showed the cavitation was completely filled, although a certain degree of scar retraction is observed in the surrounding tissue with some hypertrophy. No remnant fistula trajectory or tunnel is observed.

3. Discussion

During the last decade, the therapeutic approach to cavitated pressure ulcers has made great progress with the advancement of new technologies such as negative pressure, which

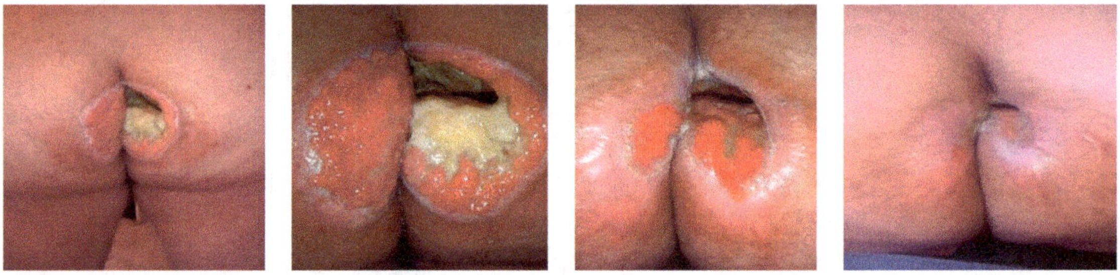

(a) (b) (c) (d)

FIGURE 2: Wound progression with Curefini® treatment. (a) Day 42: after 12 days of Curefini® local treatment. (b) Day 60: after 30 days of Curefini®. (c) Day 75: after 45 days of Curefini® local treatment. (d) Follow-up after three months.

promotes the filling of deep wounds [26]. Negative pressure cannot be applied in the presence of cancer tissue in the wound, to untreated osteomyelitis, in wounds with organ or vessel exposure, or to areas with poor blood flow. In some trials, its use in infected grade IV sacral ulcers has proved advantageous in terms of the recovery time as compared to conventional treatments, achieving recovery time duration of approximately 6 weeks [27]. However, in developing countries, this type of device continues to have a high cost, not only because of the elements required but also because of the skilled staff required for correct application and removal.

Other options are flaps and grafts close to the anal region, but these may lead to complications such as infection and necrosis. Usually, the sacral and perianal regions create difficulties for the adjustment and fixation of any device. Combined techniques and strategies, such as flaps plus a negative pressure system, tend to work well, although they also imply greater therapeutic demands [28].

A low-cost option for the treatment of cavitated wounds is calcium alginate, alone or in combination with micronized silver, with high absorptive and hemostatic capacity and some bactericidal properties. Calcium alginate may be applied in rope dressings that are easily introduced in tunneled wounds and can easily integrate naturally into the tissue. The dressings can be changed every 72 hours. When this product dissolves, it releases a gel-type discharge from the wound bed with a special smell that may be mistaken with infection. It requires a secondary dressing [29].

In the case of our patient, the treatment strategy was conditioned by previous established therapeutic actions, distance from the medical center, and economic limitations. On the one hand, during a 20-day period of time since patient discharge, no soft tissue culture specimens were collected and empiric broad-spectrum antibiotic treatment was indicated. We assume that this choice was aimed at preventing and/or treating a possible but not proven soft tissue local infection. In such cases, wound irrigation and debridement of necrotic tissue are the most important factors in the prevention of infection and can substantially decrease the incidence of invasive wound infection. Antibiotic prophylaxis is not generally recommended (recommendation 1C). However, in patients with systemic signs of infection, compromised immune status, severe comorbidities, associated severe cellulitis, and severe and deep wounds, a broad-spectrum antibiotic effective against aerobic and anaerobic organisms is always required (recommendation 1C) [30]. According to the medical history, the patient did not show any signs of systemic compromise like fever or shivering, but bad odor and purulent discharge were observed locally. No visible bone was found in the physical exam, the probe to bone was negative, and the C-reactive protein alteration or leukocytosis ruled out osteomyelitis. Nevertheless, we think that a magnetic resonance imaging (MRI) scan would have helped to better understand the complete structures compromised beneath and that a deep tissue biopsy and culture should have been collected. Due to the lack of resources and the large distance from a high-complexity health center, those were not performed [31]. On the other hand, intense local pain led the patient to refuse any kind of aggressive treatment at the wound site. Oral opioids were indicated by the plastic surgeon.

Pain associated with chronic wounds has been postulated to be related to the stimulation of nociceptors by complex inflammatory environments [32]. Molecular studies investigating keratinocyte biology and wound healing have shown that functionally active μ-opiate receptors are present on human keratinocytes [33]. The activation of these receptors by μ-opiate receptor agonist β-endorphin in cultured keratinocytes results in upregulation of type II transforming growth factor-β (TGF-β) receptor and cytokeratin 16 (CK16) [34]. The type II TGF-β receptor plays an important role in wound healing, and it is expressed in regenerating epithelial cells in acute wounds and at the margin of chronic wounds. CK16 is a filament protein that is not expressed in normal skin but appears in the suprabasal compartment of the epidermis during wound healing. Additional experiments using cultured keratinocytes show that CK16 response can be blocked by incubation together with the μ-opiate receptor antagonist naltrexone [34, 35]. These findings suggest that, hypothetically, the clinical use of opioids in patients with chronic wounds might be beneficial in upregulating molecular pathways contributing to wound healing and may be associated with improved clinical outcomes. Other studies have suggested that opioid use may negatively impact wound healing by reducing immune activation and impacting tissue oxygenation and angiogenesis [36, 37]. In contrast, untreated pain may affect tissue perfusion and oxygenation [38, 39]. The Wound

Etiology and Healing Study (WE-HEAL) (IRB 041408, NCT 03152078) investigates the relationship between patient-reported pain, opioid exposure, and wound outcome in the clinical care of a longitudinal cohort of patients with chronic wounds. This study corroborates at a cellular and molecular level that opioid exposure may impact keratinocyte biology and wound healing, resulting in delayed wound healing in patients with chronic wounds. It also concludes that opioid exposure was a strong predictor of wound size and that patients who received opioids above 10 mg per day had slower rates of healing than those with no exposure or dosing less than 10 mg per day [40].

Since the patient completed a 20-day empiric antibiotic therapy, the ulcer appeared to be clean after the last surgical debridement, and the patient showed no systemic compromise, it was decided to use a gentile wound care strategy, with a less-aggressive debridement technique aimed at reducing incidental pain. It was decided to use a natural ingredient ointment embedded in sterile gauzes. Its main components are polyunsaturated fatty acids (PUFAs) from cod liver oil, sunflower oil, sweet almond oil, antimicrobial peptides from virgin beeswax, and vitamins A and D. A clear knowledge of the action of its main components in the healing process and the ease of application, added to the low cost, led to the selection of this product, also taking into consideration the patient's home distance from the hospital for regular controls that were conducted by videos and photos sent by his wife and weekly telephone calls. Curefini® ointment is a formula enriched with polyunsaturated fatty acids (PUFAs), omega 3, and omega 6, contained in its pure source oils. PUFAs reduce the local inflammatory process in the wound by inhibiting the production of inflammatory eicosanoids and competitive inhibition of the formation of arachidonic acid. PUFAs also have antibacterial action [41]. Sunflower seed oil contains large amounts of linoleic acid, which has anti-inflammatory and antibacterial properties and promotes restoration of the skin barrier [42]. Sweet almond oil is restorative to the skin barrier and has antipruritic properties [43]. Beeswax is known for its healing, antibacterial, and anti-inflammatory properties [44, 45]. The combination of cod liver oil and medicinal beeswax has been successfully used in wound treatment in veterinary medicine [46, 47]. Curefini® has been previously tested on a porcine model for second-degree burns and showed the ability to control the inflammatory process and promote the development of a more-resistant skin layer in the affected area [25].

Vitamins A and D participate in normal skin function and collaborate as antioxidant cofactors.

Vitamin D is a pleiotropic molecule that has widespread effects not only on calcium homeostasis but also on cellular differentiation, proliferation, and immune responsiveness [48, 49]. 1,25-dihydroxyvitamin D (1, 25D3), the active form of vitamin D, has been widely studied for its immunomodulatory properties and is known to suppress inflammation in a variety of tissues, largely through its influence on antigen-presenting cell differentiation, lymphocyte proliferation, innate immune receptor signaling, and cytokine and chemokine expression [50–52]. In addition to its beneficial effects during inflammatory events, vitamin D also induces the expression of antimicrobial peptides [53–55], potentially providing enhanced protection during infection and wound healing.

Vitamin A is a family of retinoids that are available as preformed vitamin A (retinol, retinaldehyde, and retinoic acid) or as pro-vitamin A (carotenoids). Vitamin A is an essential fat-soluble micronutrient that cannot be synthesized by the human body and must be obtained from the diet. It is available in eggs, fish oils, liver, dairy products, yellow and orange fruits, and dark-green leafy vegetables. Vitamin A promotes cell mitosis and increases epithelial thickness, the number of Langerhans cells, and glycosaminoglycan synthesis in the skin. Studies have shown that vitamin A functions as a hormone, altering the activity of epithelial cells, melanocytes, fibroblasts, and endothelial cells through its action on the family of retinoic acid receptors (RARs) [56, 57]. It maintains the health of epithelial cells on the surface of the skin and the mucous membranes. It stimulates the immune system, maintains mucosal and epithelial integrity, and increases collagen and extracellular matrix formation, fibroplasia, and synthesis of collagen, glycoprotein, and proteoglycan [58–60]. It enhances the epithelialization of cell membranes, the rate of collagen synthesis, and cross-linking of newly formed collagen and antagonizes the inhibitory effects of glucocorticoids on cell membranes [61]. Vitamin A requirements are exceedingly in demand during serious injury or stress. Burns, fractures, and even elective surgery can lead to decreased serum levels of vitamin A, retinol-binding protein (RBP), retinyl esters, and β carotene. Also, liver storage of vitamin A can be depleted by large doses of corticosteroids [62]. Vitamin A is known for its ability to stimulate epithelial growth, fibroblasts, and granulation tissue. Many dermatologic conditions have been treated using topical formulas. Moreover, early in the inflammatory phase, vitamin A facilitates epithelial cell differentiation in open wounds by increasing the number of monocytes and macrophages and thus acts as an anti-inflammatory agent [63]. It seems that vitamin A has the potential to be provided topically or orally. Wounds can be acute (such as the trauma of lacerations, crush wounds, or burns) or they can be chronic (such as diabetic foot ulcerations). Vitamin A can promote and enhance various aspects of wound healing via the stimulation of angiogenesis, collagen synthesis, epithelialization, and fibroplasia. Local (topical) and systemic supplementation with vitamin A has been proven to increase dermal collagen deposition [64]. Topical administration of vitamin A has numerous dermatology indications, but its application directly on wounds has not been established as a treatment modality, despite some data suggesting it helps with diabetic foot ulcers and venous leg ulcers [65, 66].

Curefini® is an OTC product approved by the FDA and is currently in use in pediatric patients with recessive dystrophic epidermolysis bullosa [46, 67]. Its use in adults with second-degree burns has recently been reported with promising results regarding cosmetic and functional achievements [47, 68]. Curefini's main components are petrolatum, sunflower oil, cod liver oil, and sweet almond oil. Medical beeswax is present in the formula in a lower proportion than the previously mentioned oils. Curefini PUFA's component gives anti-inflammatory properties that facilitate a controlled wound inflammatory environment, enhance reepithelialization and granulation processes, and allow for autolytic debridement and gentile mechanical detritus removal t on each gauze change. Antibacterial peptides present in the beeswax component bring additional antibacterial properties [69–72]. Regarding the anti-inflammatory activity of Curefini®, a remarkable clinical aspect is that patients with second-degree burns report immediate pain reduction [68] with its use. Although our patient had a chronic wound, the Curefini® anti-inflammatory action allowed us to taper opioid therapy with no need for further pain relief replacement.

There are commercial products that share some of the components present in Curefini® ointment. For example, L-Mesitran contains medical-grade honey (MGH) as the main active ingredient and shows promising results in treating severe wounds in pediatric patients [72]. This honey-based wound care product contains 48% medical-grade honey, hypoallergenic lanolin, vitamin C, vitamin E, zinc oxide, and essential oils. Several studies have demonstrated that the supplements in L-Mesitran enhance the antimicrobial properties of its raw honey. In the pediatric case series presented by Smaropoulos [72], we note similar rates of response in wound healing reactivation and no infectious complications as with Curefini®. Both in adult and pediatric patients, the Curefini® restorative action relies on its preponderant PUFA composition provided by fish oil, sweet almond oil, and sunflower oil. Additionally, it has antimicrobial activity thanks to the bee wax component, but not as the main active compound. Vitamins A and D, as explained before, contribute with an excellent restorative and antioxidant action.

No comparison trials of Curefini® vs. other related formulas have been done. However, this case report highlights that Curefini® can be a reliable treatment for grade IV sacral pressure ulcers in adult patients.

4. Conclusion

This case highlights the therapeutic efficacy of treatment with a natural ingredient-based product on cavitated wounds that helps to reduce pain and promote granulation and reepithelialization of the skin. We remark that despite the location of a cavitated sacral wound near the anus and patient depositions, no local or systemic infectious events were detected. Its use should be considered a treatment of choice in developing countries where the distance from the hospital, economic limitations, and lack of wound care specialists are key conditions for a successful outcome.

References

[1] The Wound Healing Society, "Chronic Wound Care Guidelines," 2017, https://woundheal.org/files/2017/final_pocket_guide_treatment.pdf.

[2] C. Gokoo, "A primer on wound bed preparation," *The Journal of the American College of Certified Wound Specialists*, vol. 1, no. 1, pp. 35–39, 2009.

[3] National Pressure Ulcer Advisory Panel (NPUAP) announces a change in terminology from pressure ulcer to pressure injury and updates the stages of pressure injury|the National Pressure Ulcer Advisory Panel—NPUAP, https://www.npuap.org/national-pressure-ulcer-advisory-panel-npuap-announces-a-change-in-terminology-from-pressure-ulcer-to-pressure-injury-and-updates-the-stages-of-pressure-injury/.

[4] J. Meddings, H. Reichert, M. A. M. Rogers, T. P. Hofer, L. F. McMahon Jr., and K. L. Grazier, "Under pressure: financial effect of the hospital-acquired conditions initiative-a statewide analysis of pressure ulcer development and payment," *Journal of American Geriatrics Society*, vol. 63, no. 7, pp. 1407–1412, 2015.

[5] C. Zuñiga-Castro, N. A. Espinoza-Cáceres, and M. Á Fernandez-Pacheco, "Level of risk and incidents of pressure ulcers in hospitalized patients in the medical services of a national hospital," *Revista Enfermeria Herediana*, vol. 7, no. 2, Article ID 155, 2015.

[6] J. M. R. Prieto, L. A. Areosa, M. Romero, M. Romero, F. G. Collado, and A. R. Pizano, "Adverse events related to pressure ulcers: an avoidable problem?" *Enfermería Dermatológica*, vol. 4, no. 11, pp. 21–26, 2010.

[7] M. Baumgarten, D. J. Margolis, A. R. Localio et al., "Pressure ulcers among elderly patients early in the hospital stay," *The Journals of Gerontology Series A: Biological Sciences and Medical Sciences*, vol. 61, no. 7, pp. 749–754, 2006.

[8] C. VanGilder, G. MacFarlane, S. Meyer, and C. Lachenbruch, "Body mass index, weight, and pressure ulcer prevalence: an analysis of the 2006-2007 international pressure ulcer prevalence surveys," *Journal of Nursing Care Quality*, vol. 24, no. 2, pp. 127–135, 2009.

[9] D. J. Drake, M. Swanson, G. Baker et al., "The association of BMI and Braden total score on the occurrence of pressure ulcers," *The Journal of Wound, Ostomy and Continence Nursing*, vol. 37, no. 4, pp. 367–371, 2010.

[10] N. Bergstrom, B. Braden, M. Kemp, M. Champagne, and E. Ruby, "Multi-site study of incidence of pressure ulcers and the relationship between risk level, demographic characteristics, diagnoses, and prescription of preventive interventions," *Journal of the American Geriatrics Society*, vol. 44, no. 1, pp. 22–30, 1996.

[11] N. Bergstrom, B. Braden, M. Kemp, M. Champagne, and E. Ruby, "Predicting pressure ulcer risk: a multisite study of the predictive validity of the Braden scale," *Nursing Research*, vol. 47, no. 5, pp. 261–269, 1998.

[12] M. E. Charlson, P. Pompei, K. L. Ales, and C. R. Mackenzie, "A new method of classifying prognostic comorbidity in longitudinal studies: development and validation," *Journal of Chronic Diseases*, vol. 40, no. 5, pp. 373–383, 1987.

[13] A. Flattau and A. E. Blank, "Risk factors for 90-day and 180-day mortality in hospitalised patients with pressure ulcers," *International Wound Journal*, vol. 11, no. 1, pp. 14–20, 2014.

[14] R. F. Averill, N. Goldfield, J. S. Hughes et al., *Development of the All Patient Refined DRGs (APR-DRGs) Research Report*, 3M Health Information Systems, Wallingford, CT, USA, 2003.

[15] D. Tschannen, O. Bates, A. Talsma, and Y. Guo, "Patient-specific and surgical characteristics in the development of pressure ulcers," *American Journal of Critical Care*, vol. 21, no. 2, pp. 116–125, 2012.

[16] J. L. Lumbley, S. A. Ali, and L. S. Tchokouani, "Retrospective review of predisposing factors for intraoperative pressure ulcer development," *Journal of Clinical Anesthesia*, vol. 26, no. 5, pp. 368–374, 2014.

[17] J. Dreyfus, J. Gayle, P. Trueman, G. Delhougne, and A. Siddiqui, "Assessment of risk factors associated with hospital-acquired pressure injuries and impact on health care utilization and cost outcomes in US hospitals," *American Journal of Medical Quality*, vol. 33, no. 4, pp. 348–358, 2018.

[18] M. Primiano, M. Friend, C. McClure et al., "Pressure ulcer prevalence and risk factors during prolonged surgical procedures," *AORN Journal*, vol. 94, no. 6, pp. 555–566, 2011.

[19] F. Aloweni, S. Y. Ang, S. Fook-Chong et al., "A prediction tool for hospital-acquired pressure ulcers among surgical patients: surgical pressure ulcer risk score," *International Wound Journal*, vol. 16, no. 1, pp. 164–175, 2018.

[20] B. J. Braden and J. Maklebust, "Preventing pressure ulcers with the Braden scale: an update on this easy-to-use tool that assesses a patient's risk," *American Journal of Nursing*, vol. 105, no. 5, pp. 70–72, 2005.

[21] J. Stausberg, "The Braden Scale and Care Dependency Scale each demonstrate at least 70% sensitivity and specificity for identifying inpatients at risk of pressure ulcer," *Evidence-Based Nursing*, vol. 14, no. 1, pp. 20-21, 2011.

[22] W. He, P. Liu, and H. L. Chen, "The Braden scale cannot be used alone for assessing pressure ulcer risk in surgical patients: a meta-analysis," *Ostomy/Wound Management*, vol. 58, no. 2, pp. 34–40, 2012.

[23] National Pressure Ulcer Advisory Panel, "European pressure ulcer advisory panel and pan pacific pressure injury alliance," in *Prevention and Treatment of Pressure Ulcers: Clinical Practice Guideline*, H. Emily, Ed., Cambridge Media, Perth, Australia, 2014.

[24] G. Manzur, M. Cassini, M. Natale, L. Valinotto, I. Massimo, and H. Massimo, "Evaluation of topical therapy with the use of ointment made with natural ingredients in patients with recessive dystrophic epidermolysis bullosa," in *Proceedings of the Debra Congress International*, Zermatt Switzerland, August 2018.

[25] S. C. Davis, J. Lie, J. Gil, J. Vades, and M. Solis, *Study Report Second Degree Burn Porcine Model with Curefini vs. Petrolatum Vehicle and Non Adherent Gauze*, University of Miami, Miller School of Medicine. Departament of Dermatology and Cutaneous Surgery, Coral Gables, Fl, USA, 2014.

[26] V. K. Agarwal, D. Kumar, S. Kansal, and C. Khanna, "Negative pressure wound therapy versus conventional wound therapy in pressure sores," *International Journal of Science and Research (IJSR)*, vol. 6, no. 3, pp. 794–798, 2017.

[27] R. K. Batra and V. Aseeja, "VAC therapy in large infected sacral pressure ulcer grade IV-can be an alternative to flap Reconstruction?" *Indian Journal of Surgery*, vol. 76, no. 2, pp. 162–164, 2014.

[28] F. X. Hu, X. X. Hu, X. L. Yang et al., "Treatment of large avulsion injury in perianal, sacral, and perineal regions by island flaps or skin graft combined with vacuum assisted closure," *BMC Surgery*, vol. 19, no. 1, Article ID 65, 2019.

[29] K. Y. Lee and D. J. Mooney, "Alginate: properties and biomedical applications," *Progress in Polymer Science*, vol. 37, no. 1, pp. 106–126, 2012.

[30] M. Sartelli, X. Guirao, T. C. Hardcastle et al., "2018 WSES/SIS-E consensus conference: recommendations for the management of skin and soft-tissue infections,," *World Journal of Emergency Surgery*, vol. 13, no. 1, Article ID 58, 2018.

[31] D. Wong, P. Holtom, and B. Spellberg, "Osteomyelitis complicating sacral pressure ulcers: whether or not to treat with antibiotic therapy," *Clinical Infectious Diseases: An Official Publication of the Infectious Diseases Society of America*, vol. 68, no. 2, pp. 338–342, 2019.

[32] C. Stein and S. Küchler, "Targeting inflammation and wound healing by opioids," *Trends in Pharmacological Sciences*, vol. 34, no. 6, pp. 303–312, 2013.

[33] M. Bigliardi-Qi, P. L. Bigliardi, S. Büchner, and T. Rufli, "Characterization of mu-opiate receptor in human epidermis and keratinocytes," *Annals of the New York Academy of Sciences*, vol. 885, pp. 368–371, 1999.

[34] M. Bigliardi-Qi, P. L. Bigliardi, A. N. Eberle, S. Büchner, and T. Rufli, "Beta-endorphin stimulates cytokeratin 16 expression and downregulates mu-opiate receptor expression in human epidermis," *Journal of Investigative Dermatology*, vol. 114, no. 3, pp. 527–532, 2000.

[35] M. Bigliardi-Qi, L. T. Sumanovski, S. Büchner, T. Rufli, and P. L. Bigliardi, "Mu-opiate receptor and Beta-endorphin expression in nerve endings and keratinocytes in human skin," *Dermatology*, vol. 209, no. 3, pp. 183–189, 2004.

[36] J. L. Martin, R. Charboneau, R. A. Barke, and S. Roy, "Chronic morphine treatment inhibits LPS-induced angiogenesis: implications in wound healing," *Cellular Immunology*, vol. 265, no. 2, pp. 139–145, 2010.

[37] J. L. Martin, L. Koodie, A. G. Krishnan, R. Charboneau, R. A. Barke, and S. Roy, "Chronic morphine administration delays wound healing by inhibiting immune cell recruitment to the wound site," *American Journal of Pathology*, vol. 176, no. 2, pp. 786–799, 2010.

[38] O. Akca, "Pain and tissue oxygenation," *Critical Care Medicine*, vol. 43, no. 10, pp. e462–e463, 2015.

[39] L. O. Hoiseth, J. Hisdal, I. E. Hoff, O. A. Hagen, S. A. Landsverk, and K. A. Kirkeboen, "Tissue oxygen saturation and finger perfusion index in central hypovolemia: influence of pain," *Critical Care Medicine*, vol. 43, no. 4, pp. 747–756, 2015.

[40] V. K. Shanmugam, K. S. Couch, S. McNish, and R. L. Amdur, "Relationship between opioid treatment and rate of healing in chronic wounds," *Wound Repair and Regeneration*, vol. 25, no. 1, pp. 120–130, 2017.

[41] L. H. Terkelsen, A. Eskild-Jensen, H. Kjeldsen, J. H. Barker, and V. E. Hjortdal, "Topical application of cod liver oil ointment accelerates wound healing: an experimental study in wounds in the ears of hairless mice," *Scandinavian Journal of Plastic and Reconstructive Surgery and Hand Surgery*, vol. 34, no. 1, pp. 15–20, 2000.

[42] S. R. Marques, C. A. Peixoto, J. B. Messias, A. R. d. Albuquerque, and V. A. d. Silva Jr, "The effects of topical application of sunflower-seed oil on open wound healing in lambs," *Acta Cirurgica Brasileira*, vol. 19, no. 3, pp. 196–209, 2004.

[43] M. Hajhashemi, M. Rafieian, H. A. Rouhi Boroujeni et al., "The effect of aloe vera gel and sweet almond oil on striae gravidarum in nulliparous women," *Journal of Maternal-Fetal and Neonatal Medicine*, vol. 31, no. 13, pp. 1703–1708, 2018.

[44] F. Fratini, G. Cilia, B. Turchi, and A. Felicioli, "Beeswax: a minireview of its antimicrobial activity and its application in medicine," *Asian Pacific Journal of Tropical Medicine*, vol. 9, no. 9, pp. 839–843, 2016.
[45] L. Cornara, M. Biagi, J. Xiao, and B. Burlando, "Therapeutic properties of bioactive compounds from different honeybee products," *Frontiers in Pharmacology*, vol. 8, Article ID 412, 2017.
[46] M. S. Addisu, "Effect of topical application of mixture of cod liver oil and honey on old (chronic) wounds and granulation tissue in donkeys," *Journal of Veterinary Medicine and Animal Health*, vol. 10, no. 3, pp. 78–88, 2018.
[47] J. Ahmed, J. A. Bannai, and R. K. Abdulsamad, "Topical application of mixture of honey with cod liver oil as a novel therapy to treat contaminated skin wounds in rabbits model," *Kufa Journal for Veterinary Medical Sciences*, vol. 8, no. 1, pp. 19–30, 2017.
[48] H. F. DeLuca, "The metabolism and functions of vitamin D," *Advances in Experimental Medicine and Biology*, vol. 196, pp. 361–375, 1986.
[49] M. Hewison, "Vitamin D and the immune system: new perspectives on an old theme," *Endocrinology and Metabolism Clinics of North America*, vol. 39, no. 2, pp. 365–379, 2010.
[50] J. H. White, "Vitamin D signaling, infectious diseases, and regulation of innate immunity," *Infection and Immunity*, vol. 76, no. 9, pp. 3837–3843, 2008.
[51] C. D. Tsoukas, D. M. Provvedini, and S. C. Manolagas, "1,25-Dihydroxyvitamin D3: a novel immunoregulatory hormone," *Science*, vol. 224, no. 4656, pp. 1438–1440, 1984.
[52] M. T. Cantorna, L. Snyder, Y.-D. Lin, and L. Yang, "Vitamin D and 1,25(OH)2D regulation of T cells," *Nutrients*, vol. 7, no. 4, pp. 3011–3021, 2015.
[53] T.-T. Wang, F. P. Nestel, V. Bourdeau et al., "Cutting edge: 1,25-dihydroxyvitamin D3 is a direct inducer of antimicrobial peptide gene expression," *Journal of Immunology*, vol. 173, pp. 2909–2912, 2004.
[54] P. T. Liu, S. Stenger, H. Li et al., "Toll-like receptor triggering of a vitamin D-mediated human antimicrobial response," *Science*, vol. 311, no. 5768, pp. 1770–1773, 2006.
[55] J. Schauber, R. A. Dorschner, A. B. Coda et al., "Injury enhances TLR2 function and antimicrobial peptide expression through a vitamin D-dependent mechanism," *Journal of Clinical Investigation*, vol. 117, no. 3, pp. 803–811, 2007.
[56] D. A. Bender, "Chapter 44, Micronutrients: Vitamins & Minerals," in *Harper's Illustrated Biochemistry*, V. W. Rodwell, Ed., McGraw-Hill, New York, NY, USA, 31st edition, 2018.
[57] J. Reichrath, B. Lehmann, C. Carlberg, J. Varani, and C. C. Zouboulis, "Vitamins as hormones," *Hormone and Metabolic Research*, vol. 39, no. 2, pp. 71–84, 2007.
[58] M. E. Posthauer, "What is the role of vitamins in wound healing?" *Advances in Skin & Wound Care*, vol. 20, no. 5, pp. 260–264, 2007.
[59] A. I. Rojas and T. J. Phillips, "Patients with chronic leg ulcers show diminished levels of vitamins A and E, carotenes, and zinc," *Dermatologic Surgery*, vol. 25, no. 8, pp. 601–604, 1999.
[60] M. Abdelmalek and J. Spencer, "Retinoids and wound healing," *Dermatologic Surgery*, vol. 32, no. 10, pp. 1219–1230, 2006.
[61] D. Schumann, "Preoperative measures to promote wound healing," *Nursing Clinics of North America*, vol. 14, pp. 683–699, 1979.
[62] T. Baumgartner, "Trace elements and wound healing," in *Nutrition and Wound Healing*, J. A. Molnar, Ed., p. 182, CRC Press, St. Louis, MO, USA, 2007.
[63] J. A. Molnar, M. J. Underdown, and W. A. Clark, "Nutrition and chronic wounds," *Advances in Wound Care*, vol. 3, no. 11, pp. 663–681, 2014.
[64] T. K. Hunt, "Vitamin A and wound healing," *Journal of the American Academy of Dermatology*, vol. 15, no. 4 Pt 2, pp. 817–821, 1986.
[65] D. Paquette, E. Badiavas, and V. Falanga, "Short-contact topical tretinoin therapy to stimulate granulation tissue in chronic wounds," *Journal of the American Academy of Dermatology*, vol. 45, no. 3, pp. 382–386, 2001.
[66] W. L. Tom, D. H. Peng, A. Allaei, D. Hsu, and T. R. Hata, "The effect of short-contact topical tretinoin therapy for foot ulcers in patients with diabetes," *Archives of Dermatology*, vol. 141, no. 11, pp. 1373–1377, 2005.
[67] C. Prialé-Zevallos, S. Santillana Lozano, L. Scerpalla-Crespo, R. Prialé-Miranda, and O. De la Peña-Brush, "Treatment of mucocutaneous lesions associated with patients with epidermolysis bullosa with a cream based on petrolatum and cod liver oil: report of three cases from the cities of lima and iquitos," *Dermatología Peruana*, vol. 25, no. 3, 2015.
[68] I. Saretzky, "Second degree burn treated with Curefini ointment and PVC film: an accessible wound care strategy in developing countries," *Wounds International*, vol. 12, no. 1, pp. 40–43, 2021.
[69] R. M. C. Hermanns, A. Thrasyvoulou, C. Tananaki, F. A. D. T. G. Wagener, and N. A. J. Cremers, "Defining the standards for medical grade honey," *Journal of Apicultural Research*, vol. 59, 2019.
[70] A. M. P. Oliveira, J. S. P. Devesa, and P. B. Hill, "In vitro efficacy of a honey-based gel against canine clinical isolates of Staphylococcus pseudintermedius and Malassezia pachydermatis," *Veterinary Dermatology*, vol. 29, no. 3, pp. 180–e65, 2018.
[71] N. Cremers, A. Belas, S. Santos Costa, I. Couto, H. de Rooster, and C. Pomba, "In vitro antimicrobial efficacy of two medical grade honey formulations against common high-risk meticillin-resistant staphylococci and Pseudomonas spp. pathogens," *Veterinary Dermatology*, vol. 31, 2019.
[72] E. Smaropoulos and N. A. J. Cremers, "Treating severe wounds in pediatrics with medical grade honey: a case series," *Clinical Case Reports*, vol. 8, no. 3, pp. 469–476, 2020.

19

Pityriasis Versicolor Resistant to Antifungal Drugs in a Patient in Lomé (Togo)

Julienne Teclessou[1], **Koussake Kombate**,[1] **Bayaki Saka**,[2] **Séfako Abla Akakpo**,[2] **and Palokinam Pitche**[2]

[1]*Department of, Dermatology and STDs, University Teaching Hospital of Campus, Togo*
[2]*Department of Dermatology and STDs, University Teaching Hospital of Sylvanus Olympio, Togo*

Correspondence should be addressed to Julienne Teclessou; tjulie06@yahoo.fr

Academic Editor: Alireza Firooz

Background. Pityriasis versicolor (PV) is a ubiquitous superficial skin mycosis that often affects young adults. It is often effectively treated with local or oral antifungal agents. Cases of PV resistance to antifungal agents have been reported rarely. We report a case of antifungal resistant PV. *Observation.* A 22-year-old patient was followed since the age of 17 years in a dermatology outpatient clinic for hyperpigmented scaly macular lesions of the trunk and upper limbs. The clinical diagnosis of PV was retained. The patient was treated by fluconazole 300 mg/week before being lost to follow-up. He was seen again in 2019 (about 2 years later) for the same symptomatology and treated again by fluconazole and ciclopirox olamine cream without improvement. He was again lost to follow-up and seen again six months later. A mycological sample was taken and *Aspergillus niger* was isolated. The patient was treated by itraconazole for 6 weeks. The evolution was marked by a clinical status quo. The patient was again put on salicylated petroleum jelly 10% associated with terbinafine cream and then lost to follow-up. *Conclusion.* The emergence of fungal resistance to antifungal drugs does not spare PV. It can therefore be resistant to several antifungal drugs, leaving clinicians and patients in despair.

1. Introduction

Pityriasis versicolor (PV) is a superficial skin infection caused by fungi. It is a common ubiquitous dermatosis affecting young adults mainly in tropical regions with prevalence up to 40% [1]. PV manifests as well-limited scaly macules that may be separated by spaces of healthy skin or coalesce into irregular patches [2]. The lesions may be hypopigmented or hyperpigmented and are located preferentially in seborrheic areas. Lesions usually predominate on the back [2]. The diagnosis of PV is easy, essentially clinical. Wood's light examination is a diagnostic tool but is positive in only one-third of cases [3]. Fungal elements (filament spores) can be demonstrated by microscopic examination.

Therapeutically, the treatment of PV is based on topical or oral azole (imidazole) antifungals. They can be combined with azole-based antifungal foaming gels (ketoconazole foaming gel) [4]. However, recurrences are frequently described after a well-managed treatment. The recurrence rate is estimated at 60% after one year and can reach 80% in the second year [5]. In general, the resistance of mycoses to antifungal agents has become a major concern in clinical practice over the last 30 years. This resistance in fungal species is unevenly distributed worldwide and involves several fungal species [6]. In Africa, cases of resistance of candida species have been reported [7].

PV, apart from recurrences, can be resistant to antifungal treatments that have already been proven to manage the condition. Helou et al. in 2014 had reported a case of PV resistant to antifungal drugs [8]. We report a clinical case.

2. Observation

This is a 22-year-old patient, followed since the age of 17 years in the dermatology department of the Campus Hospital of Lomé for PV. The onset dates back to 2017 when the

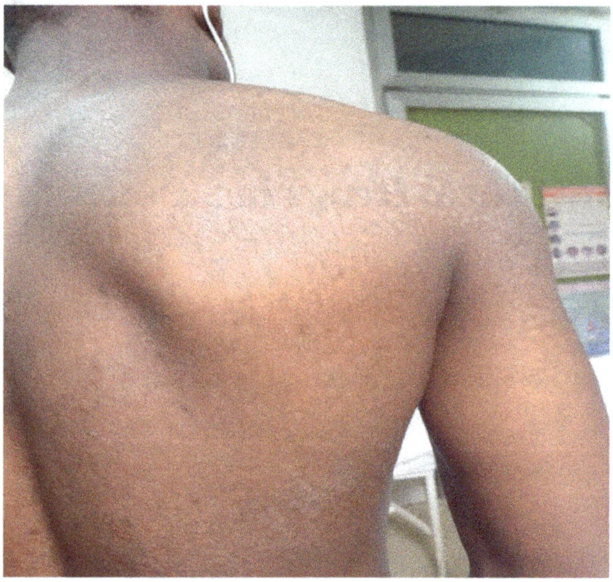

FIGURE 1: Scaly hypopigmented macular lesions of the trunk (months after the start of the second treatment).

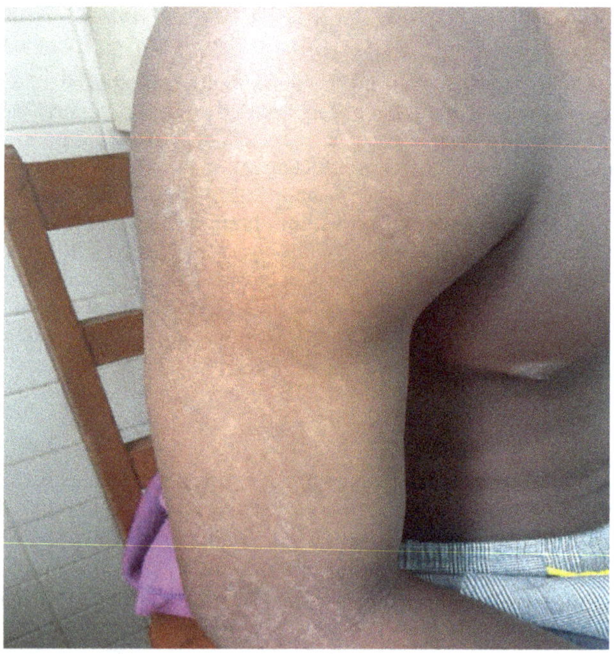

FIGURE 2: Pityriasis versicolor (six weeks after itraconazole treatment).

patient was seen on an outpatient basis for scaly hyperpigmented macular lesions with a positive chip sign. The lesions were located on the trunk and upper extremities and had been evolving for one year. There was no pruritus or pain. The clinical diagnosis of PV was retained and patient was treated by fluconazole 300 mg/week associated with ketoconazole foaming gel. The patient was then lost to follow-up. He was seen again two years later in October 2019 for the same symptoms. The interrogation allowed concluding that there was a discreet improvement of the lesions after the beginning of the treatment prescribed 2 years earlier followed by an aggravation. The treatment with fluconazole 300 mg/day was continued for 4 weeks and then replaced by ciclopirox olamine cream. The patient was seen once a month for 3 months without any improvement. He was again lost to follow-up. Six months later, the patient returned with the same symptoms (Figure 1). A mycological sample examination by microscopic in KOH identified a hyphae of *Aspergillus niger*. For technical reasons, the antifungigram (antifungal data) was not performed. Blood count, glycemia, and liver enzymes were normal. HIV serology was negative. The patient was treated by itraconazole 200 mg daily for 6 weeks. The evolution was marked by a clinical status quo of the lesions with persistence of scaly macules, the chip sign being always positive (Figure 2). The patient was then put on terbinafine cream and salicylated ointment 10%, in the course of treatment. The patient is lost again for more than 1 year.

3. Discussion

Two particularities are noted in this case: first, the persistence of lesions after a clinical diagnosis and a treatment by azoles; and secondly, the persistence of lesions after a mycological sampling and a treatment of isolated fungal species.

PV is a common dermatosis with an easy diagnosis based mainly on clinical findings. This clinical diagnosis can be supplemented by sampling of the scales (by Scotch or curette scraping) for mycological examination to identify the responsible fungal species. In our case, the diagnosis was based on clinical signs. However, given the persistence of the lesions after several well-conducted antifungal treatments, a direct microscopy examination in KOH was performed to identify the causal agent. Wood's light is also a diagnostic feature of the condition. However, it is not positive in all cases [8]. In our case, Wood's light examination was not performed for technical reasons.

PV can be managed by both general practitioners and dermatologists. Treatment is based on topical or oral antifungal agents. Most systemic or topical antifungal agents used in the treatment of PV are effective according to the study by Hu and Bigby [9]. Thus, topical fungistatic or fungicidal azoles are often used successfully in the treatment of PV [3]. In our case, these antifungals were also used unsuccessfully. Although our patient's follow-up was interrupted several times by periods of loss to sight, each time we started treatment we always had a sufficient follow-up period to assess the efficacy of the treatment.

Oral ketoconazole, the first available oral treatment for PV with multiple regimens [3], was the first-line treatment in our patient. It was offered at a regimen of 300 mg per week, close to the 400 mg per week regimen [10]. Also, itraconazole is an effective treatment with low toxicity used in the treatment of PV [11–13]. It is a triazole that has a broad spectrum of activity compared to fluconazole [6]. In contrast to fluconazole, itraconazole has been shown to be effective in fungal infections caused by *Aspergillus niger* [6]. In the absence of a scotch test performed at the start of treatment in our patient, we treated with fluconazole. But, the isolation of the *Aspergillus* strain prompted the initiation of itraconazole. We did not notice any improvement in the patient after the start of itraconazole. This leads us to conclude that there is resistance to the treatment. Few cases of PV resistance to antifungal drugs have been reported in the literature. Helou et al. in 2014 reported a similar case of PV resistant to antifungal drugs [8]. Several similarities can be noted with our case, notably the use of fluconazole from the first consultation, the persistence of the lesions, and then the use of itraconazole.

In our case, as in Helou et al.'s case, we were unable to assess the effect of salicylated petroleum jelly on the lesions as our patient was again lost to follow-up.

This observation again shows an increasing increase in antifungal resistance to the increasingly described fungal species [14]. Other antifungal agents such as Rilopirox (a synthetic pyridine derivative) and lanoconazole (an azole) known to be effective in the management of PV [5] were not prescribed in our patient due to their availability.

Resistant PV also poses a psychological problem for patients. Indeed, the unsightly appearance of the lesions could be a source of social rejection for the patient, especially when he is an adolescent or young adult. Our patient, aged 22, was seen several times in the department despite repeated therapeutic failure and periods of loss of sight. This could be explained by the unsightly aspect of the lesions and the permanent quest for healing.

4. Conclusion

Pityriasis versicolor is a ubiquitous superficial cutaneous mycosis with an easy diagnosis based essentially on clinical findings. Most cases of PV respond to conventional antifungal treatments. However, the emergence of fungal resistance to antifungal agents does not spare PV. Thus, cases of PV resistant to several antifungals may be noted and cause despair to clinicians and patients.

References

[1] J. C. Szepietowski, E. Baran, and E. Wild, "Tinea versicolor: a prospective study," *Korean journal of medical mycology*, vol. 5, pp. 108–112, 2000.

[2] R. A. Schwartz, "Superficial fungal infections," *The Lancet*, vol. 364, no. 9440, pp. 1173–1182, 2004.

[3] A. K. Gupta, R. Batra, R. Bluhm, and J. Faergemann, "Pityriasis versicolor," *Dermatologic Clinics*, vol. 21, no. 3, pp. 413–429, 2003.

[4] D. El Euch, I. Riahi, M. Mokni, A. Ben Osman, S. Mezlini, and H. Abidi, "[Ketoconazole foaming gel in tinea versicolor (report of 60 cases)]," *Tunisie Medicale*, vol. 77, no. 1, pp. 38–40, 1999.

[5] J. Faergemann, "The role of Malassezia yeasts in skin diseases," *Mikologia Lekarska*, vol. 11, pp. 129–133, 2004.

[6] P. Vandeputte, S. Ferrari, and A. T. Coste, "Antifungal resistance and new strategies toControl fungal infections," *International Journal of Microbiology*, vol. 2012, pp. 1–26, 2012.

[7] C. G. Yapo-kouadio, A. V. Bonouman-Ira, N. A. D. Aka, G. S. P. Dou, K. D. Zika et al., "Resistance ofVaginal Candida albicans to antifungal drugs in abidjan (Cote d'Ivoire)," *Revue Bio-Africa*, vol. 16, pp. 7–12, 2017.

[8] J. Helou, G. Obeid, R. Moutran, and I. Maatouk, "Pityriasis versicolor: a case of resistance to treatment," *International Journal of Dermatology*, vol. 53, no. 2, pp. e114–e116, 2013.

[9] S. W. Hu and M. Bigby, "Pityriasis versicolor: a systematic review of interventions," *Archives of Dermatology*, vol. 146, no. 10, pp. 1132–1140, 2010.

[10] H. E. Jones, "Pityriasis versicolor with ketoconazole [reply to letter]," *Journal of the American Academy of Dermatology*, vol. 20, 1989.

[11] O. Köse, H. B. Taştan, A. R. Gür, and Z. Kurumlu, "Comparison of a single 400 mg dose versus a 7-day 200 mg daily dose of itraconazole in the treatment of tinea versicolor," *Journal of Dermatological Treatment*, vol. 13, no. 2, pp. 77–79, 2002.

[12] A. Shemer, N. Nathansohn, B. Kaplan, H. Trau, N. Newman, and H. Trau, "Itraconazole versus ketoconazole in the treatment of tinea versicolor," *Journal of Dermatological Treatment*, vol. 10, no. 1, pp. 19–23, 1999.

[13] F. Montero-Gei, M. E. Robles, and P. Suchil, "Fluconazole vs. itraconazole in the treatment of tinea versicolor," *International Journal of Dermatology*, vol. 38, no. 8, pp. 601–603, 1999.

[14] A. I. Rubin, B. Bagheri, and R. K. Scher, "Six novel antimycotics," *American Journal of Clinical Dermatology*, vol. 3, no. 2, pp. 71–81, 2002.

20

Giant Protruding High-Grade Undifferentiated Pleomorphic Sarcoma Arising in a Keloid Scar on the Abdominal Wall

Hideyuki Kinoshita,[1] Toshinori Tsukanishi,[1] Takeshi Ishii,[1] Hiroto Kamoda,[1] Yoko Hagiwara,[1] Sumihisa Orita,[2] Kazuhide Inage,[2] Naoya Hirosawa,[2] Seiji Ohtori,[2] and Tsukasa Yonemoto[1]

[1]*Department of Orthopedic Surgery, Chiba Cancer Center, 666-2 Nitonacho, Chuo-ku, Chiba 260-8717, Japan*
[2]*Department of Orthopaedic Surgery, Graduate School of Medicine, Chiba University, 1-8-1 Inohana, Chuo-ku, Chiba 260-8670, Japan*

Correspondence should be addressed to Hideyuki Kinoshita; kinoshi1783@yahoo.co.jp

Academic Editor: Sergio A. Cuevas Covarrubias

Undifferentiated pleomorphic sarcoma (UPS) is a high-grade, aggressive, soft tissue sarcoma that is often fatal. Although there are reports describing associations of sarcoma and skin lesions such as burns, radiation, and trauma, to our knowledge, UPS development in a keloid scar has not been reported. Herein, we present the case of a 76-year-old woman who had undergone surgery for endometrial cancer, 5 years before. She presented with a protruding lesion that was continuous to a keloid scar on the abdominal wall. The tumor appeared clinically malignant as it was protruding and doubled in size within three weeks, reaching approximately 6 × 6 × 2 cm. Since the tumor was diagnosed as UPS after pathological evaluation by needle biopsy, wide resection was performed. Intraoperatively, the tumor was apparently continuous to the keloid, protruding and pedunculated outside the body, and had not invaded the abdominal cavity. Histopathological examination of the resected tumor showed evidence of UPS and no suspicion of metastasis of endometrial cancer. No recurrence, metastases, or other complications were noted 6 months after surgery. The current case study reminds us that keloids may cause high-grade sarcoma such as UPS, and careful follow-up is required.

1. Introduction

Undifferentiated pleomorphic sarcoma (UPS) is a high-grade, aggressive, soft tissue sarcoma, and the preferred name for the sarcoma is, previously called, malignant fibrous histiocytoma (MFH) [1]. Since UPS has a high rate of lung metastasis and is sometimes fatal, early diagnosis is imperative. There are many reports describing associations between sarcomas, such as osteosarcoma and UPS and skin lesions, such as burns, radiation, and trauma [2]. Keloid is a benign fibroproliferative disorder of the skin that presents in scar tissue when a wound heals. Although keloid scars can be difficult to be differentiated from dermatofibrosarcoma protuberans (DFSP) [3], there are no reports of UPS development in a keloid scar.

Here, we present an unusual case of high-grade undifferentiated pleomorphic sarcoma arising in a keloid scar.

2. Case Presentation

A 76-year-old woman with a 4-month history of a tumor protruding from the abdominal wall presented to our orthopedic outpatient department. She had a medical history of partial resection for endometrial cancer 5 years before. Although the skin developed keloid scars after the resection, the clinical course was good with no recurrence or wound infection. However, 4 months prior to presentation, a tumor emerged from the keloid scar on the abdominal wall and protruded outside the skin, growing rapidly. On physical examination, a protruding lesion continuous with the keloid scar was noted on the abdominal wall, measuring

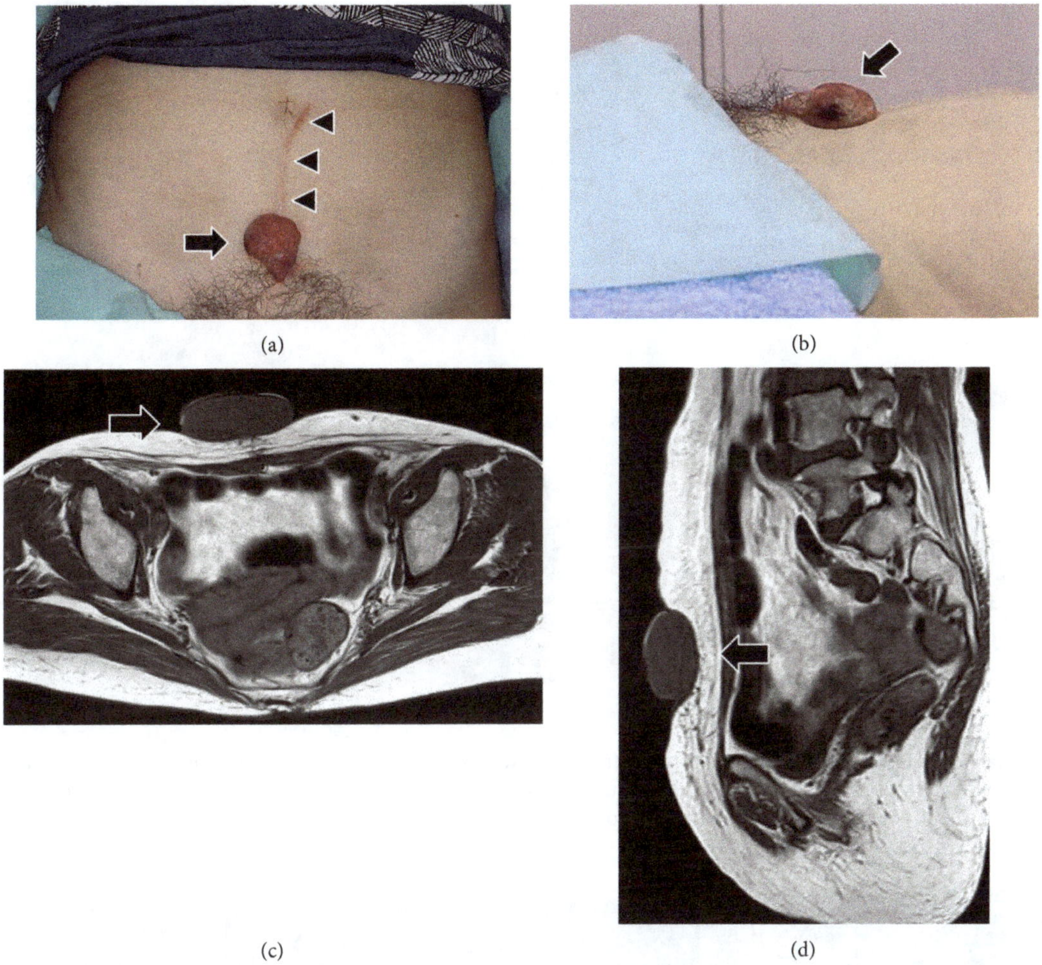

Figure 1: Frontal (a) and lateral (b) view of the large protruding tumor (arrow) located on the abdominal wall. The lesion measured $3 \times 3 \times 2$ cm at the first visit. A keloid scar (arrowhead) is visible on the abdominal wall due to partial resection of endometrial cancer. Axial (c) and sagittal (d) view of magnetic resonance imaging revealing a tumor protruding subcutaneously with no continuity to the abdominal cavity (arrow).

approximately $3 \times 3 \times 2$ cm (Figures 1(a)-1(b)). The needle biopsy specimen was characterized by high cellularity and marked nuclear pleomorphism and accompanied by abundant mitotic activity and a spindle cell morphology, suggesting pleomorphic and spindle cell sarcoma. Furthermore, magnetic resonance imaging (MRI) 1 week later revealed a tumor measuring $5 \times 4 \times 3$ cm protruding subcutaneously with no continuity to the abdominal cavity (Figures 1(c)-1(d)). The tumor rapidly increased in size to $6 \times 6 \times 2$ cm and protruded further in the following two weeks (Figures 2(a)-2(b)). Wide resection of the tumor including the keloid scar and fat layer immediately above the rectus sheath was performed. Intraoperatively, the tumor was apparently continuous to the keloid, protruding outside the body, and pedunculated (Figure 2(c)). Furthermore, we observed that the tumor had not invaded the abdominal cavity (Figure 2(d)). The resected tumor was continuous to the keloid, measuring approximately $6.2 \times 6 \times 3.2$ cm (Figure 3(a)). Histopathological examination following hematoxylin and eosin staining revealed short pleomorphic spindle cells and polygonal cells with a storiform pattern, accompanied by abundant mitotic activity, similar to the histology obtained on needle biopsy (Figure 3(b)). Moreover, the tumor was negative for smooth muscle actin, h-caldesmon, cytokeratin AE1/AE3, CAM5.2, and CD34 (Figures 3(c)-3(d)), and there was no suspicion of metastasis of the endometrial cancer, suggesting a diagnosis of high-grade UPS. The postoperative period was uneventful. In the 6 months of follow-up, the patient did not experience any recurrence, metastasis, novel keloid scars, or other complications.

3. Discussion

The UPS tumor category, previously known as pleomorphic MFH, is a heterogeneous group of disorders. It is the fourth most common soft tissue sarcoma and has a slight male preponderance. It is mainly composed of mesenchymal lineages that belong to established sarcoma subgroups such as liposarcoma, leiomyosarcoma, and fibrosarcoma [1]. UPS is common in the deep soft tissue of the extremities and rarely occurs on the body surface of the skin with a stalk. The

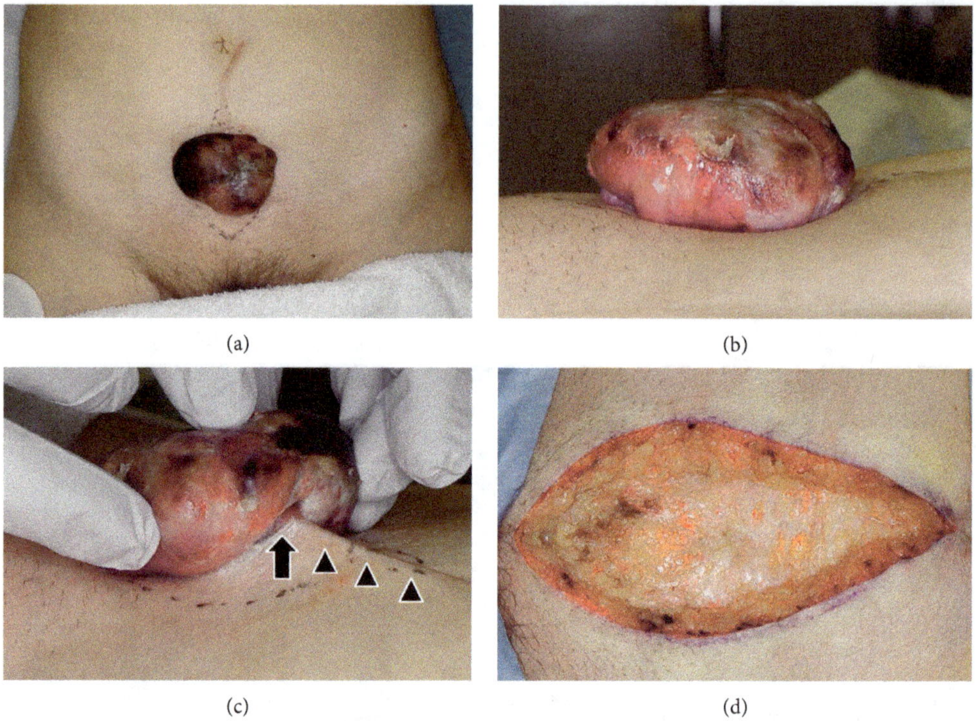

Figure 2: Frontal (a) and lateral (b) view of the tumor after three weeks. The tumor has rapidly increased in size to 6 × 6 × 2 cm and protruded further. (c) The tumor is observed to be continuous with the keloid scar (arrowhead), protruding outside the body, and pedunculated (arrow). (d) Intraoperatively, the tumor had not invaded the abdominal cavity.

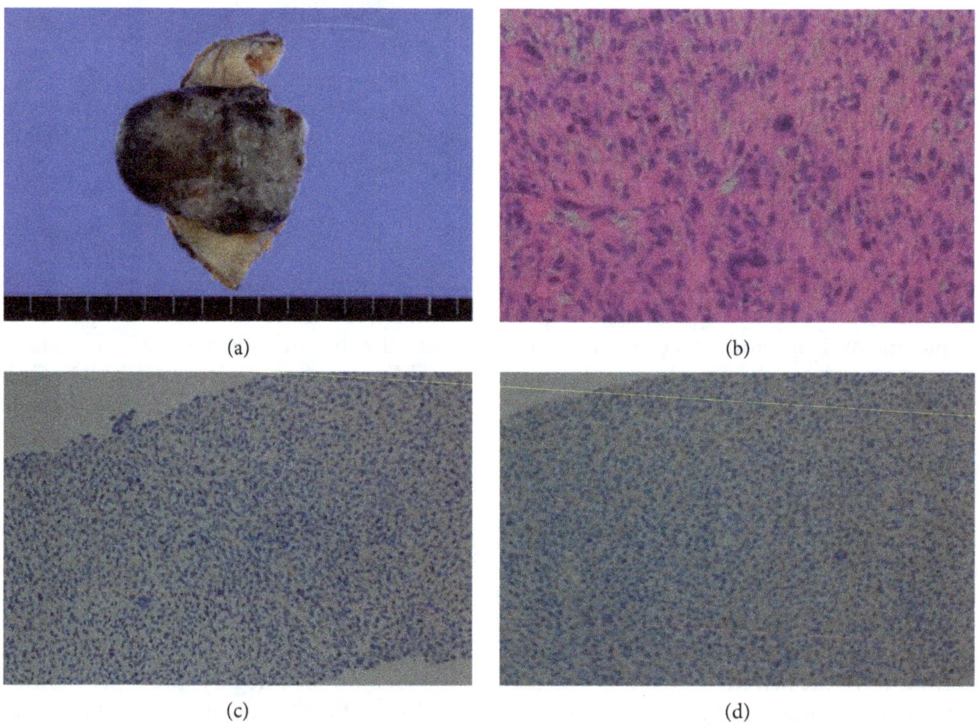

Figure 3: (a) Gross view of the resected tumor. The tumor is observed to be continuous to the keloid and measures approximately 6.2 × 6 × 3.2 cm. (b) Histopathological examination following hematoxylin and eosin (HE) staining revealing short pleomorphic spindle cells and polygonal cells with a storiform pattern, accompanied by abundant mitotic activity, suggesting undifferentiated pleomorphic sarcoma. The tumor is negative for cytokeratin AE1/AE3 (c) and CAM5.2 (d) on immunohistochemical staining.

etiology of UPS remains unknown. Histologically, UPS has pleomorphic spindle cells with abundant mitotic figures, associated regions of necrosis, and hemorrhage, while UPS is negative for S-100, CD34, and cytokeratin on immunostaining. Although wide surgical excision is the best procedure for UPS, postoperative multidisciplinary treatment with chemotherapy and radiation therapy is often required, depending on the tumor size, grade, and stage.

There are many reports on sarcoma and skin lesions such as burns, radiation, and trauma. An 80-year review of the literature on burn cases showed 412 case reports of neoplasm arising in burn scars [2]. Furthermore, Kowal-Vern and Criswell reported that, among neoplasms arising in burn scars, although squamous cell carcinoma (SCC) was the most common at 71% cases, 5% of them were sarcomas [4]. Radiation can also induce sarcomas although this is rare. In most cases, radiotherapy for cancer treatment leads to radiation-induced sarcoma (RIS). Although radiation-induced malignancies may cause any subtypes of sarcoma, osteosarcoma and UPS are the most common among them. Radiation may also develop other malignancies, including leukemia, lymphoma, and solid tumors from other germ layers [5]. Significant trauma has been also reported to be a rare risk factor for the development of neoplasia. Witwicki et al. reported that sarcoma arose at a fracture site after internal fixation and open reduction [6].

The pathogenesis of malignancies accompanied with skin lesions such as burns and trauma is not precisely understood. Initially, it was hypothesized that the tissue damaged by burn and trauma released toxins, inducing cellular mutations [7]. Another theory regarding the occurrence of skin malignancy after trauma is the displacement of live epithelial cells into the deep tissue with a concurrent inability of the tissue damaged by trauma to regulate for the invading cells [8]. Furthermore, Nakanishi et al. reported that SCCs, which commonly harbor p53 mutations, are the commonest malignancy arising in burn scars [9]. In contrast, the etiology of RIS has been elucidated. The increase in ionizing radiation induces an increase in DNA breaking, eventually leading to the replication of aberrant cells. Sarcomas arisen from the mesenchymal origin indicates one of the highest proportions of radiation-induced cancers, probably because of a massive amount of active dividing tissue over a large surface area. [10].

Keloids are fibroproliferative disorders of the skin that result from abnormal healing of injured or irritated skin [11]. Although keloids are thought to be derived from epigenetic alterations in fibroblast DNA and acetylation of histone proteins, keloid scar formation and progression is complex and poorly understood. Differential diagnoses of keloids include complications of acne, hyperplastic scars, and keloidal dermatofibroma. DFSP can be misdiagnosed as a keloid scar [3].

To our knowledge, this is the first case to report UPS development in a keloid scar. Although our patient had a history of endometrial cancer, suggesting the possibility of recurrent disease, the present case had no continuity from the abdominal cavity on MRI. Furthermore, there was no pathological evidence of any recurrence or metastasis of endometrial cancer. In addition, as a clinical finding, a tumor continuous to the keloid was observed; therefore, the tumor was thought to have originated from the area of the keloid.

In conclusion, we reported a rare case of high-grade UPS arising in a keloid scar. Keloids may cause high-grade sarcomas such as UPS, and careful follow-up is required.

Consent

Written informed consent was obtained from the patient for publication of this case report and the accompanying images.

References

[1] F. C. Kelleher and A. Viterbo, "Histologic and genetic advances in refining the diagnosis of "undifferentiated pleomorphic sarcoma"," *Cancers (Basel)*, vol. 5, no. 1, pp. 218–233, 2013.

[2] T. J. Pan, L. Pantanowitz, and K. R. Weiss, "High-grade leiomyosarcoma arising in a previously replanted limb," *Case Reports in Oncological Medicine*, vol. 2015, Article ID 172603, 4 pages, 2015.

[3] M. Ucak, "A rare case of misdiagnosis: recurrence of dermatofibrosarcoma protuberans that was treated surgicallyas a keloid," *Medical Archives*, vol. 72, no. 1, pp. 74-75, 2018.

[4] A. Kowal-Vern and B. K. Criswell, "Burn scar neoplasms: a literature review and statistical analysis," *Burns*, vol. 31, no. 4, pp. 403–413, 2005.

[5] S. C. Kamran, A. Berrington de Gonzalez, A. Ng, D. Haas-Kogan, and A. N. Viswanathan, "Therapeutic radiation and the potential risk of second malignancies," *Cancer*, vol. 122, no. 12, pp. 1809–1821, 2016.

[6] T. Witwicki, A. Daniluk, and W. Dulowski, "2 cases of sarcoma developing at the site of fracture and metallic osteosynthesis," *Wiadomości Lekarskie*, vol. 29, no. 4, pp. 339–343, 1976.

[7] A. R. Kadir, "Burn scar neoplasm," *Annals of Burns and Fire Disasters*, vol. 20, no. 4, pp. 185–188, 2007.

[8] Z. Neuman, N. Ben-Hur, and J. Shulman, "Trauma and skin cancer," *Plastic and Reconstructive Surgery*, vol. 32, no. 6, pp. 649–656, 1963.

[9] H. Nakanishi, Y. Tomita, H. Yoshikawa, N. Sato, T. Ochi, and K. Aozasa, "Frequentp53Gene mutations in soft tissue sarcomas arising in burn scar," *Japanese Journal of Cancer Research*, vol. 90, no. 3, pp. 276–279, 1999.

[10] E. J. Vick, C. T. Clark, and J. M. Lewis, "Radiation-induced sarcoma following prolonged coronary stent placement," *Case Reports in Surgery*, vol. 2018, Article ID 2903801, 5 pages, 2018.

[11] C. H. Tsai and R. Ogawa, "Keloid research: current status and future directions," *Scars, Burns & Healing*, vol. 5, Article ID 2059513119868659, 2019.

21

Granuloma Multiforme: A Rare Granulomatous Disease

Yogesh Poudyal[1] **and Anita Shah**[2]

[1]*Sarnath Skin Centre, Shanti Path, Bhairahawa 32900, Nepal*
[2]*Department of Pathology, Universal College of Medical Sciences-Teaching Hospital, Ranigaon, Bhairahawa 32900, Nepal*

Correspondence should be addressed to Yogesh Poudyal; neverland791@yahoo.com

Academic Editor: Ravi Krishnan

Granuloma Multiforme (GM) is a reactive skin disorder with annular lesion and focal necrobiosis. It was first described in Nigeria (Africa), since than it was mostly described from various regions of Africa where leprosy was endemic. Outside Africa, this disease is rarely reported. Till 2016 only five cases were reported from India. This is the second case report from Nepal. A fifty-nine-year-old female, farmer by occupation, presented with annular and polycyclic plaques with elevated beaded border for one year. It was distributed over upper trunk, lower back, and arms, and was mildly pruritic. Histopathologically, loss of elastic fibres at focal area of upper dermis, with elastic fibres engulfed histiocytes were noted. GM was mostly noted from leprosy endemic areas of Africa. Clinically, it is very difficult to distinguish from granuloma annulare. This report adds the number of GM occurrence in Asia especially from area where leprosy is still prevalent. This report also emphasizes in resource poor settings where most diagnosis is made clinically, the granuloma annulare should be looked for very carefully in order not to miss GM.

1. Introduction

Granuloma Multiforme is a reactive skin disorder of unknown aetiology, characterized clinically by confluent annular lesions and histologically by focal necrobiosis and histiocytic granuloma [1]. It was first described by D. L. Leiker, which was endemic in Mkar, Nigeria. It was identified when lesion resembling leprosy was not responding to sulphone treatment, as this disease was misdiagnosed and treated as leprosy. Later this disease was noticed to be of high prevalence in South Eastern Nigeria, West Kenya, and Isle of Sumba in Indonesia [2]. Very few reports were found from other parts of the world. Even from India, till 2016 only five cases were reported [3].

2. Case Presentation

A fifty-nine-year-old female, from Western Terai region of Nepal, presented with slightly itchy lesion on trunk and arm for one year. The first lesion was noted on chest, then gradually new lesions were seen on the arm and lower back. It started as skin color small palpable lesion that gradually increased in size giving ring shape. There was no history of other disease and drug intake. She was a farmer by occupation.

On examination, there were multiple skin color and slightly erythematous annular and polycyclic plaques with elevated, beaded border with central clearing. Lesions were distributed over chest, forearm, upper, and lower back with size ranging from 2 cm to 10 cm in diameter (Figures 1–3). The sensation was intact and peripheral nerves were not thickened.

The clinical possibilities considered were granuloma annulare, leprosy, annular sarcoid, and actinic granuloma.

Complete haemogram, renal and liver function test, blood glucose level, and routine urine examination were within normal range.

The elliptical incisional biopsy was taken from the margin of lesion and sent for histopathological examination. It showed keratinized stratified squamous epithelium with normal maturation. There was loss of elastic fibres at focal area of upper dermis (Figure 4). The periphery of the lesion showed many multinucleated giant cell and histiocyte along with few lymphocyte and plasma cell. Engulfed elastic fibres by multinucleated giant cells were also noted (Figure 5).

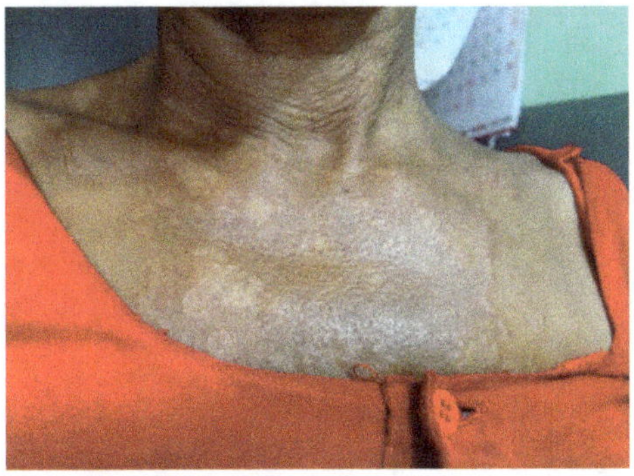

FIGURE 1: Annular and polycyclic plaques on chest.

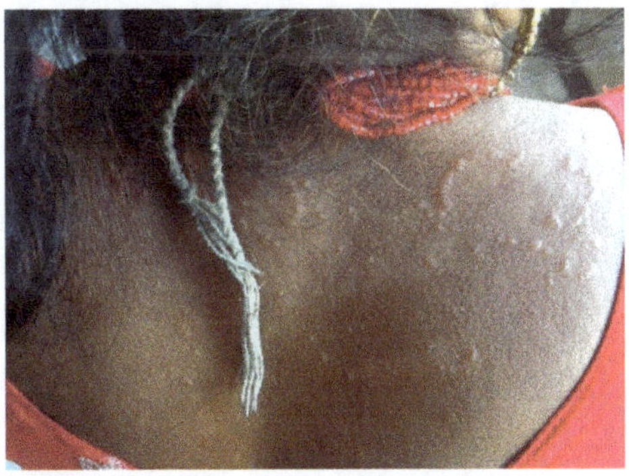

FIGURE 2: Annular and polycyclic plaques with beaded well defined border on upper back.

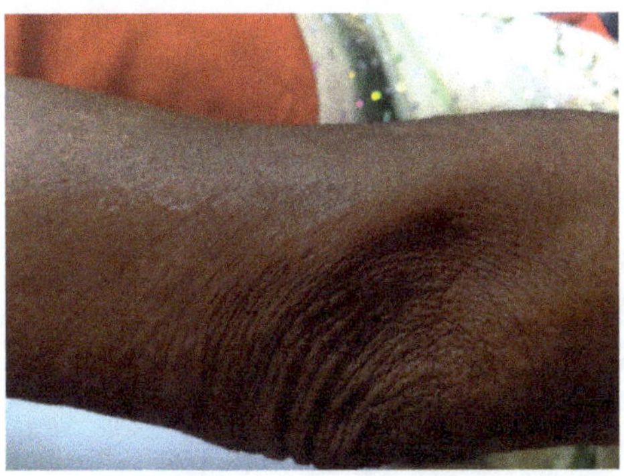

FIGURE 3: Annular plaques with well defined border on arm.

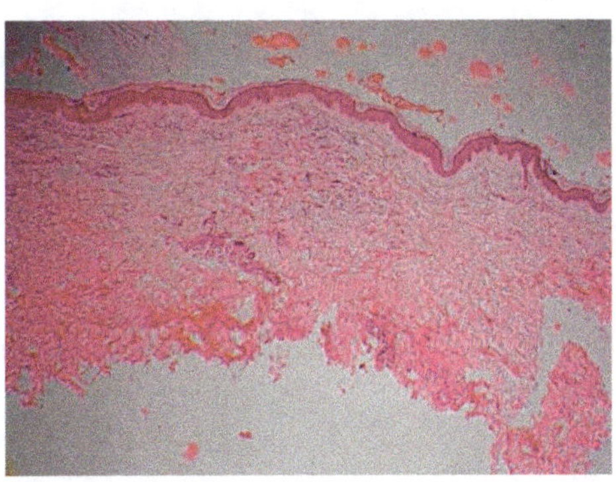

FIGURE 4: Multinucleated histiocytes abutting connective tissue with elastotic degeneration (H&E stain with 4x magnification).

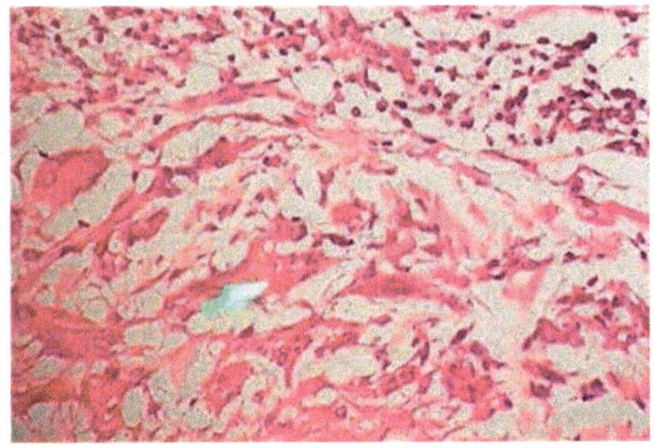

FIGURE 5: Multinucleated giant cell with ingested elastic fibres (arrowhead); (H&E stain 40x magnification).

The patient was prescribed topical steroid, but showed no improvement at follow up after six weeks.

3. Discussion

Granuloma Multiforme is found among adult over the age group of 40 years with the predilection for the female sex. The sun exposed sites of the upper trunk and arms are predominantly affected. The initial lesions are usually papules, which soon evolve to form annular and polycyclic lesions with papular or nodular edge. The lesion tends to last for months or years. It is pruritic and irritating, especially when new lesions are forming [1]. Scattered case reports of GM were seen in recent times from Congo [4], India [5], Tunisia [6].

Since the time first described, its important differential diagnosis has been leprosy. The absence of loss of sensation and normal peripheral nerves will easily rule out leprosy. Granuloma Annulare (GA) sometime without histopathological support can be very difficult to differentiate. GA has smaller lesion and is seen in children. The presence of palisading granuloma differentiates it from GM. Annular sarcoid will show naked granuloma histologically and infiltrated reddish brown plaque clinically. Actinic granuloma or Annular elastolytic giant cell granuloma can be differentiated by its asymptomatic nature and absence of necrobiosis in histology. Some authors believe Actinic granuloma and GM are the same entity.

The exact aetiology of this disease is not known. In past there were reports even suspecting droppings of bat, leaves as the aetiological factors but none were confirmed [2]. It is suggested that GM is due to cumulative damage to collagen by sunlight induced by chemical or biological agent in environment and potentiated by immunologic factor [7]. Like previous reports [3, 5, 7–9], our case too showed female gender with age above forty. The propensity in females is difficult to explain but we should remember that other photodermatosis like Lupus erythematosus also shows a strong predominance in women [7]. The occupation as farmer and residence at Western Terai region, where in summer temperature rises above 40°C, shows the possibility of photoexposure for a long time.

There is no effective therapy for this condition, but recent report has shown some response with dapsone [5].

This is the second reported case from Nepal [10]. Like most of the previous reports, we have a female above forty.

There are very few reported cases for this disease, this can be probably due to misdiagnosis as there is striking similarity of this case with Granuloma Annulare. Due to rarity of occurrence of GM, it might have been over looked in most instances. High degree of suspicion is required, while dealing with the granulomatous disorder of skin especially Granuloma Annulare. With this report and few others from India, it can be emphasized that this disease is not only confined to Africa, but also at Asian Subcontinent.

Disclosure

This case was earlier presented as an e-poster on DERMACON INTERNATIONAL 2019 (47th National Conference of Indian Association of Dermatologists, Venereologists & Leprologists), held at Bengaluru on 17th–20th January 2019.

References

[1] R. Kumari, D. M. Thappa, A. Chougule, and B. Adityan, "Granuloma multiforme: a report from India," *Indian Journal of Dermatology, Venereology and Leprology*, vol. 75, no. 3, pp. 296–299, 2009.

[2] D. L. Leiker, "Granuloma multiforme: a new disease," *Tropical Doctor*, vol. 2, no. 2, pp. 64–67, 1972.

[3] Y. K. Sharma, N. S. Ankadavar, G. Malik, and R. J. Patel, "A rare report of granuloma multiforme," *Indian Journal of Dermatology*, vol. 61, no. 1, p. 124, 2016.

[4] B. Chandenier, J. Guillemette, J. Labussiere et al., "First case of multiform granuloma from Congo," *Cahiers Sante*, vol. 5, no. 4, pp. 245–246, 1995.

[5] S. Bhatia, S. D. Shenoi, K. Pai, and P. S. Srilatha, "Granuloma multiforme: an uncommon differential for leprosy," *Tropical Doctors*, vol. 49, no. 1, pp. 55–58, 2018.

[6] S. Ziadi, M. Trimeche, B. Sriha et al., "Granuloma multiforme: first report in Tunisia," *Pathologica*, vol. 99, no. 6, pp. 443–445, 2007.

[7] S. Cherian, "Is granuloma multiforme a photodermatosis?," *International Journal of Dermatology*, vol. 33, no. 1, pp. 21–22, 1994.

[8] S. Cherian, "Granuloma multiforme in India," *International Journal of Leprology Other Mycobacterial Disease*, vol. 58, no. 4, pp. 719–721, 1990.

[9] S. G. Browne, "Granuloma multiforme in Eastern Nigeria," *International Journal of Leprology*, vol. 34, no. 1, pp. 27–29, 1996.

[10] S. Paudel and S. Marhatta, "Granuloma multiforme: first report from Nepal," *Nepal Journal of Dermatology, Venereology & Leprology*, vol. 17, no. 1, pp. 66–68, 2019.

22

Multiple Nonfamilial Unilateral Trichoepitheliomas: Report of a Case—Mini Review of the Literature

I. Mandekou-Lefaki,[1] G. Theodosiou,[2] F.-S. Delli,[3]
D. Oikonomou,[4] and M. Papageorgiou[3]

[1]*Dermatology, Geniki Kliniki–Euromedica Private Hospital, Thessaloniki, Greece*
[2]*Department of Dermatology, Skåne Univeristy of Skåne, Malmö, Sweden*
[3]*State Dermatology Clinic, Hospital for Skin and Venereal Diseases, Thessaloniki, Greece*
[4]*Plastic Surgery, Private Practice, Thessaloniki, Greece*

Correspondence should be addressed to G. Theodosiou; gregtheodosiou@yahoo.com

Academic Editor: Christos C. Zouboulis

Trichoepitheliomas are benign skin tumors with follicular differentiation that present most commonly as solitary lesions. They can also present as multiple centrofacial papules due to several mutations in the CYLD gene. Multiple unilateral trichoepitheliomas in a linear or dermatomal distribution may rarely be seen. Herein, we report a case of multiple unilateral trichoepitheliomas on the face of a healthy 34-year-old woman of Caucasian origin.

1. Case Report

A 34-year-old woman of Caucasian origin was referred to the outpatient clinic of our department with a rash on the right side of her face. At the age of five years, multiple asymptomatic skin-colored firm papules developed in a unilateral configuration on the right side of her face. The rash was asymptomatic but of cosmetic concern to the patient. The family history was unremarkable. The patient was otherwise healthy.

Physical examination showed skin-colored papules ranging from 2 to 8 mm in size localized on her mid-forehead, the right eyebrow, the eyelids, down the right cheek, and the right nasolabial fold (Figure 1). The lesions were nontender, smooth, and firm. No other skin lesions were noted. Contact polarized dermatoscopy revealed the presence of bright white linear streaks on an ivory-white background as well as yellow and light brown dots and clods (Figure 2)

Histological examination of a skin biopsy showed a well-demarcated dermal tumor composed of anastomosing lobules of basaloid cells of uniform size arrange in an organoid pattern. The cells were small, with regular nuclei, surrounded by prominent cellular stroma. Small keratinous cysts lined by stratified squamous epithelium were also noted. No connection with the overlying epidermis was noted (Figure 3).

A lesion in the nasolabial fold was excised in toto and the patient was started on topical treatment with imiquimod 5% cream. The patient applied a thin layer of imiquimod 5% cream prior to normal sleeping hours, left on the lesions for about 8 hours, and then removed by washing the area with mild soap and water, 3 times per week. At the follow-up visit, after three months of treatment with imiquimod 5% cream less than 25% of the lesions at the baseline examination were still present but we also observed a size reduction of the remaining lesions by 1 to 2 mm. The patient was satisfied from aesthetic point of view as she considered that the lesions were less prominent. No side effects were reported during treatment (Figure 4).

2. Discussion

Trichoepitheliomas (TE) are benign neoplasms differentiated toward the folliculosebaceous-apocrine germ, occurring mainly in early childhood or adolescence. Their prevalence

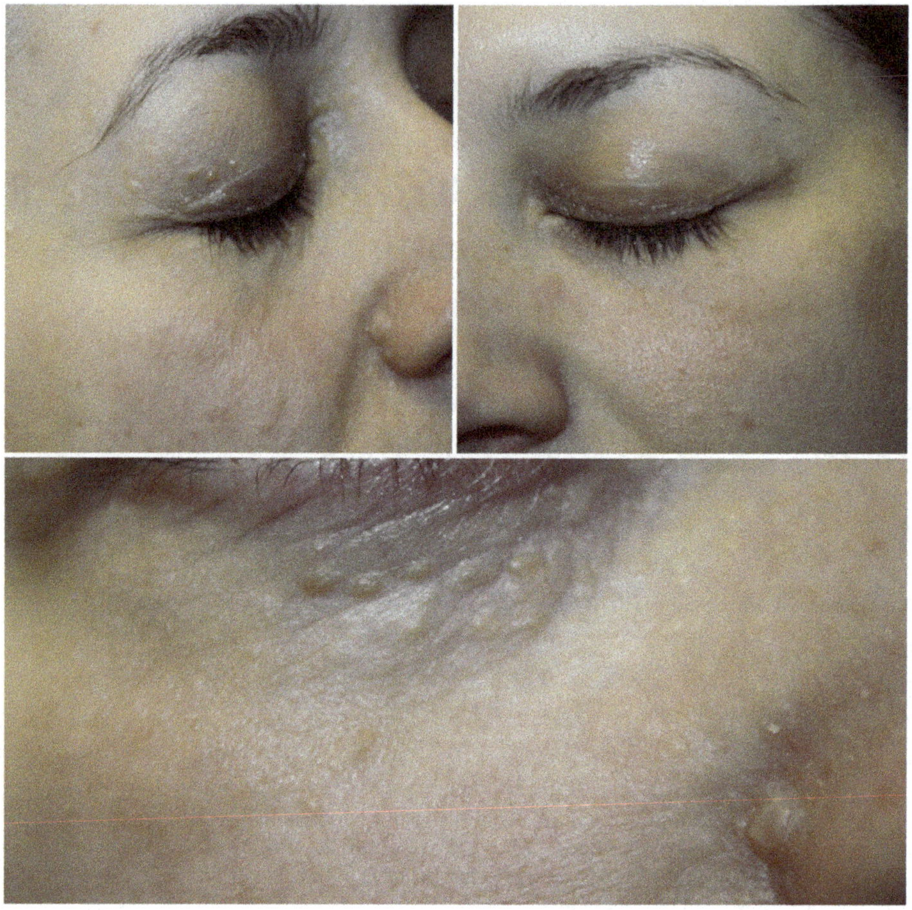

FIGURE 1: (a) Numerous skin-colored papules on the right side of the patient's face. (b) The left side of the face is free of lesions. (c) Closer view of the right side: multiple rounded whitish and skin-colored papules and nodules symmetrically distributed on the lower eyelid and the perinasal area.

remains unknown. Trichoepitheliomas increase slowly in size and number throughout life, often causing a significant cosmetic problem [1, 2].

TE are, as a rule, solitary. They present as a solitary skin-colored, round, smooth, firm papule or nodule frequently transversed by telangiectasias on any hair follicle-bearing location, with a predilection for the nose, upper lip, and cheeks. The size can vary from a few millimeters to several centimeters, but most trichoepitheliomas measure not over 1 cm in diameter. Rare presentations include a linear form and a large hemifacial plaque form. The solitary type occurs more frequently in adults [1].

Multiple familial trichoepitheliomas (MFT) usually begin in early childhood or adolescence as multiple round, firm, pink, or skin-colored, sometimes translucent, papules or nodules symmetrically distributed on the face particularly in the perinasal area but can also occur on the trunk and the extremities [2, 3]. MFT have an autosomal dominant mode of inheritance. Various mutations in the CYLD gene, a tumor suppression gene located on chromosome 16q12-q13, have been associated with inherited disorders characterized by multiple adnexal tumors such as trichoepitheliomas, cylindromas, and spiradenomas namely, Brooke-Spiegler syndrome (BSS), multiple familial trichoepithelioma, and familial cylindromatosis [4]. Multiple familial trichoepithelioma and familial cylindromatosis are considered phenotypic variants of BSS.

Multiple trichoepitheliomas have been reported as a rare feature of the Bazex-Dupré-Christol syndrome which is an X-linked dominant disorder characterized by congenital hypotrichosis, follicular atrophoderma, milia, basal cell carcinomas, and hypohidrosis [5, 6]. MFT are often cited feature of Rombo syndrome which is characterized by follicular atrophy, atrophoderma vermiculata, acral cyanosis, milia, hypotrichosis, and basal cell cancers. As a matter of fact, multiple trichoepitheliomas were reported only in one family member from the original case [7]. James Rasmussen described in 1975 a combination of multiple trichoepitheliomas, cylindromas, and milia. Although the term "Rasmussen's syndrome" is still in use, it is nowadays considered a variant of BSS [8].

Rare presentations include linear lesions on the face arranged along the Blaschko lines, and association with ungual fibromas [9–14]. Multiple nonfamilial trichoepitheliomas have also been reported. However, it is unclear whether genetic analyses were performed in these patients

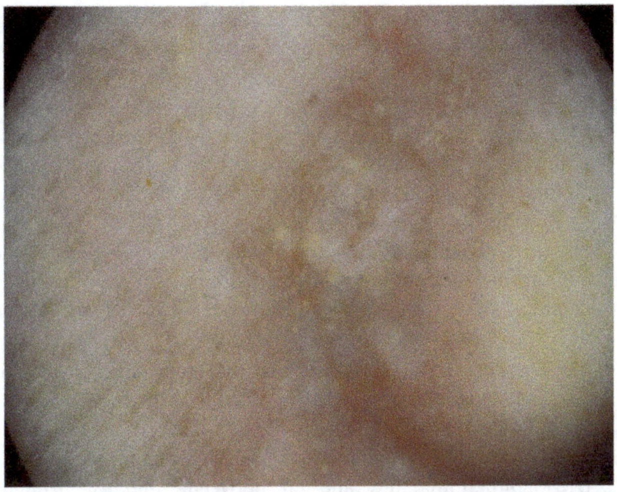

FIGURE 2: Polarized contact dermatoscopy: on a white-ivory background, bright white lines and yellow to light brown dots and clods.

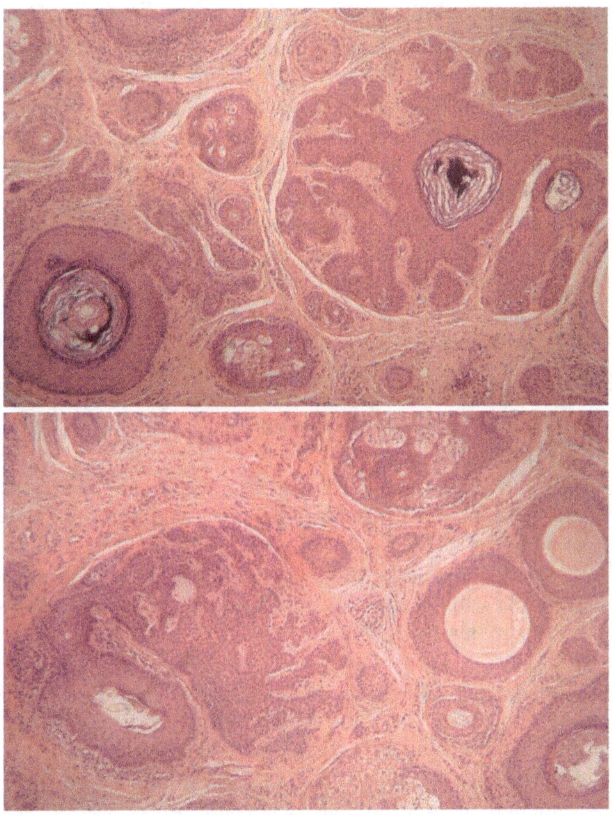

FIGURE 3: Histopathology: hematoxylin and eosin stain; original magnification x40: multiple horn cysts and aggregations of basaloid keratinocytes surrounded by a fibrous stroma.

[15, 16]. Only a few cases of unilateral multiple trichoepitheliomas have been reported in the literature most of which occurred in dark-skinned individuals [9–11].

Histologically, TE are symmetrical, well-circumscribed nonulcerated dermal neoplasms comprised mostly of follicular germitive cells that are usually arranged in a cribriform

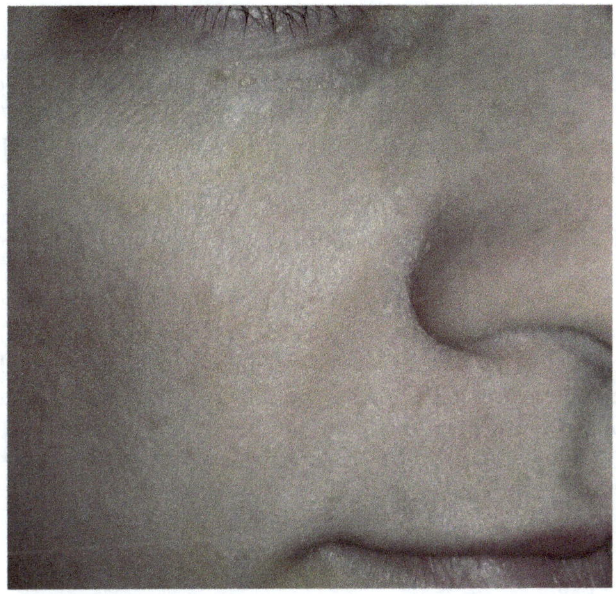

FIGURE 4: Marked improvement after a 3-month treatment with cream imiquimod 5%.

pattern. The epithelial cells are deeply basophilic and uniform and usually overlap each other. In addition to the predominant epithelial component, there is also a connective tissue component that resembles that of an embryonic perifollicular sheath. In short, it is abundant highly fibrocystic and constituted mostly of delicate fibrillary collagen. The histological features of the solitary and the multiple variants are identical [17].

Multiple trichoepitheliomas must be differentiated from other adnexal tumors such as eruptive syringomas and the angiofibromas of tuberous sclerosis. The main differential diagnosis for solitary trichoepithelioma is basal cell carcinoma (BCC). Absence of specific follicular stroma, asymmetry, or invasive growth and clefts between epithelial aggregations and the surrounding stroma are clues favoring a diagnosis of BCC. Malignant transformation of trichoepitheliomas is a very rare event, convincingly documented only in a handful of cases [18, 19].

Trichoepitheliomas, as a rule, cannot be differentiated from basal cell cancer solely on specific expression of cytokeratins. A panel of immunohistochemical markers composed of CD10, CK15, CK20, and D2-40 that could facilitate the differentiation trichoepithelioma and basal cell carcinoma has been proposed [20].

Multiple trichoepithelioma on the face present a major cosmetic concern and are typically difficult to treat. The management of trichoepitheliomas is challenging especially in patients with multiple facial lesions. Various treatment modalities have been efficacious in treating trichoepitheliomas, namely, surgery, electrodessication, CO_2 laser, Erbium–YAG laser, and imiquimod [21–23]. Successful use of topical sirolimus alone or in combination with CO_2 ablative laser has been also reported [24].

Imiquimod is an immunomodulating agent approved for the treatment of HPV infections, actinic keratoses, and basal cell carcinomas. Imiquimod induced a potent antiviral and antitumor effect by activating the Toll-like receptor 7 (TLR-7) subsequently leading to secretion of interferon-gamma (IFN-γ), tumor necrosis factor-a (TNF-a), IL-1a, IL-1b, IL-6, IL-8, IL-12, and GM-CSF. Many studies have tested the effect of imiquimod on several types of skin tumors with mixed results.

In our case, partial response and size reduction to topical therapy with imiquimod were achieved. This is in line with the finding of Alessi et al. who reported two patients with multiple trichoepitheliomas who showed partial response to topical treatment with imiquimod 5% for 32 weeks [25].

In our case, the combination of excision of the largest lesion with topical imiquimod treatment in the smaller lesions brought a satisfactory result for the patient.

References

[1] E. Calonje, "Tumors of the skin appendages," in *Rook's Textbook of Dermatology*, pp. 53.8-53.10, Wiley-Blackwell, 8th edition, 2010.

[2] J. C. Szepietowski, F. Wasik, G. Szybejko-Machaj, A. Bieniek, and R. A. Schwartz, "Brooke-Spiegler syndrome," *Journal of the European Academy of Dermatology and Venereology*, vol. 1, no. 5, pp. 346–349, 2001.

[3] S. Saggar, K. A. Chernoff, S. Lodha et al., "CYLD mutations in familial skin appendage tumours," *Journal of Medical Genetics*, vol. 45, no. 5, pp. 298–302, 2008.

[4] N. Nagy, K. Farkas, L. Kemény, and M. Széll, "Phenotype-genotype correlations for clinical variants caused by CYLD mutations," *European Journal of Medical Genetics*, vol. 58, no. 5, pp. 271–278, 2015.

[5] M. Goeteyn, M.-L. Geerts, A. Kint, and J. Weert, "The Bazex-Dupré-Christol syndrome," *JAMA Dermatology*, vol. 130, no. 3, pp. 337–342, 1994.

[6] A. Yung and J. A. Newton-Bishop, "A case of Bazex-Dupré-Christol syndrome associated with multiple genital trichoepitheliomas," *British Journal of Dermatology*, vol. 153, no. 3, pp. 682–684, 2005.

[7] G. Michaelsson, E. Olsson, and P. Westermark, "The Rombo syndrome: a familial disorder with vermiculate atrophoderma, milia, hypotrichosis, trichoepitheliomas, basal cell carcinomas and peripheral vasodilation with cyanosis," *Acta Dermato-Venereologica*, vol. 61, no. 6, pp. 497–503, 1981.

[8] J. E. Rasmussen, "A syndrome of trichoepitheliomas, milia, and cylindromas," *JAMA Dermatology*, vol. 111, no. 5, pp. 610–614, 1975.

[9] R. E. Geffner, J. B. Goslen, and D. J. Santa Cruz, "Linear and dermatomal trichoepitheliomas," *Journal of the American Academy of Dermatology*, vol. 14, no. 5, pp. 927–930, 1986.

[10] R. M. Strauss, W. J. Merchant, J. M. Stainforth, and S. M. Clark, "Unilateral naevoid trichoepitheliomas on the face of a child," *Clinical and Experimental Dermatology*, vol. 31, no. 6, pp. 778–780, 2006.

[11] A. Singh, D. M. Thappa, and C. Ratnakar, "Unilateral linear trichoepitheliomas," *International Journal of Dermatology*, vol. 38, no. 3, pp. 236-237, 1999.

[12] W. C. Lambert, D. L. Bilinski, M. Y. Khan, and R. H. Brodkin, "Trichoepithelioma in a systematized epidermal nevus with acantholytic dyskeratosis: its occurrence in a black man," *JAMA Dermatology*, vol. 120, no. 2, pp. 227–230, 1984.

[13] C. G. Schirren, B. Worle, P. Kind, and G. Plewig, "A nevoid plaque with histological changes of trichoepithelioma and cylindroma in Brooke-Spiegler syndrome. An immunohistochemical study with cytokeratins," *Journal of Cutaneous Pathology*, vol. 22, no. 6, pp. 563–569, 1995.

[14] M. Cramers, "Trichoepithelioma multiplex and dystrophia unguis congenita: a new syndrome?" *Acta Dermato-Venereologica*, vol. 61, no. 4, pp. 364-365, 1981.

[15] M. Sehrawat, V. Jairath, and V. Jain, "Nonfamilial multiple trichoepithelioma: few and far between," *Indian Journal of Dermatology*, vol. 61, no. 1, pp. 78–80, 2016.

[16] K. Sanaa and M. F. Zahra, "A rare case of sporadic multiple trichoepitheliomas," *Pan African Medical Journal*, vol. 21, p. 19, 2015.

[17] D. V. Kazakov, "Lesions with predominant follicular differentiation," in *Cutaneous Adnexal Tumors*, D. V. Kazakov, P. McKee, M. Michal, and D. Kacerovska, Eds., pp. 207–232, Lippincott Williams and Wilkins, Philadelphia, Penn, USA, 2012.

[18] N. Misago and Y. Narisawa, "Basal cell carcinoma in association with multiple trichoepitheliomas," *Dermatology*, vol. 202, no. 3, pp. 201–205, 2001.

[19] O. Bakry, I. Seleit, M. Abdelwahed, R. Hassan, and R. Samaka, "Multiple familial trichoepithelioma with malignant transformation," *Indian Journal of Dermatology*, vol. 58, no. 5, p. 409, 2013.

[20] A. J. Tebcherani, H. F. De Andrade, and M. N. Sotto, "Diagnostic utility of immunohistochemistry in distinguishing trichoepithelioma and basal cell carcinoma: evaluation using tissue microarray samples," *Modern Pathology*, vol. 25, no. 10, pp. 1345–1353, 2012.

[21] C. C. Ning, H. M. Sheu, Y. C. Chen, and S. C. Chao, "Successful treatment of linear trichoepithelioma with carbon dioxide laser," *Dermatol Sinica*, vol. 19, pp. 221–224, 2001.

[22] M. Shaffelburg and R. Miller, "Treatment of multiple trichoepithelioma with electrosurgery," *Dermatologic Surgery*, vol. 24, no. 10, pp. 1154–1156, 1998.

[23] J. S. McGee, M. F. Suchter, and S. S. Milgraum, "Multiple familial trichoepithelioma successfully treated with CO2 laser and imiquimod," *SKINmed Journal*, vol. 14, no. 6, pp. 467-468, 2016.

[24] J. H. Tu and J. M. Teng, "Use of topical sirolimus in the management of multiple familial trichoepitheliomas," *Dermatologic Therapy*, vol. 30, no. 2, p. e12458, 2017.

[25] S. S. Alessi, J. A. Sanches, W. R. Oliveira, M. C. Messina, E. R. Pimentel, and C. Festa Neto, "Treatment of cutaneous tumors with topical 5% imiquimod cream," *Clinics*, vol. 64, no. 10, pp. 961–966, 2009.

23

The use of Neodymium-Doped Yttrium Aluminum Garnet Laser for Treatment of Hypertrophic Port-Wine Stain

Brittany Miles,[1] **Andrew Armenta**,[1] **and James Mackey**[2]

[1]*University of Texas Medical Branch, Galveston, Texas, USA*
[2]*Deja You Medical Aesthetics, League City, Texas, USA*

Correspondence should be addressed to Brittany Miles; brlmiles@utmb.edu

Academic Editor: Thomas Berger

Port-wine stains (also called nevus flammeus) are congenital malformations of the capillaries and postcapillary venules. They occur in 0.1–2% of newborns without sex predilection. Although PWS lesions are flat early in life, with age, they become hypertrophic and darker. Pulsed dye laser therapy is the standard of care for treating these lesions, although other laser wavelengths have been utilized with varying degrees of success. We present the case of a gentleman with a hypertrophic PWS who had an excellent response to Nd:YAG laser treatment. The increased tissue penetration of longer laser wavelengths may be of benefit to patients with hypertrophic PWS, and further research into this concept is warranted.

1. Introduction

Port-wine stain (PWS), also called nevus flammeus, is the most common congenital malformation of the capillaries and postcapillary venules, previously called "fire marks" or misnamed "flat hemangioma." They occur in 0.1–2% of newborns without sex predilection but are less common in both Asians and African Americans [1]. At birth, the lesions are flat, but with age, they become hypertrophic and darker due to progressive vascular ectasia [2]. Histologic examination of these lesions reveals ectasia of the capillaries and postcapillary venules in the papillary and reticular dermis, with fibrosis and dilatation developing in later-stage lesions. They may occur anywhere on the body, but facial involvement is common and may be a significant source of psychological stress for the patient. It is often treated as a cosmetic condition, but depending on size and location, patients may show functional compromise of speaking, eating, or even vision. In approximately two-thirds of patients, vascular hyperplasia leads to the development of vascular nodules by the age of 50 [1]. Soft tissue hypertrophy usually occurs between 1 and 29 years of age, bony hypertrophy begins at an average age of 15 years, and nodules tend to develop in the age range of 15–53 years. Approximately 90% of PWS are located on the face in a trigeminal dermatome pattern. The majority of facial PWS (90%) are unilateral [3].

Interestingly, about 15–20% of children with PWS of the (V1) trigeminal dermatome are at risk for Sturge–Weber syndrome (SWS), a neurocutaneous disorder with vascular malformations in the cerebral cortex ipsilateral to PWS. Current literature suggests pathoanatomically redefining PWS as "a malformation resulting from differentiation-impaired endothelial cells with a progressive dilatation of immature venule-like vasculatures." Recent discoveries have identified somatic mutations in the guanine nucleotide-binding protein, *G* alpha subunit *q* (GNAQ) (R183Q), phosphatidylinositol 3-kinase (PI3K), and activation of mitogen-activated protein kinase (MAPK), and PI3K pathway in skin lesions of PWS/SWS improved our understanding of the pathogenesis of these malformations [4].

Since the early 80s, vascular-specific lasers have been considered the gold standard in treating PWS, and classically pulsed dye lasers are regarded as the treatment of choice. However, the concept of selective photothermolysis with

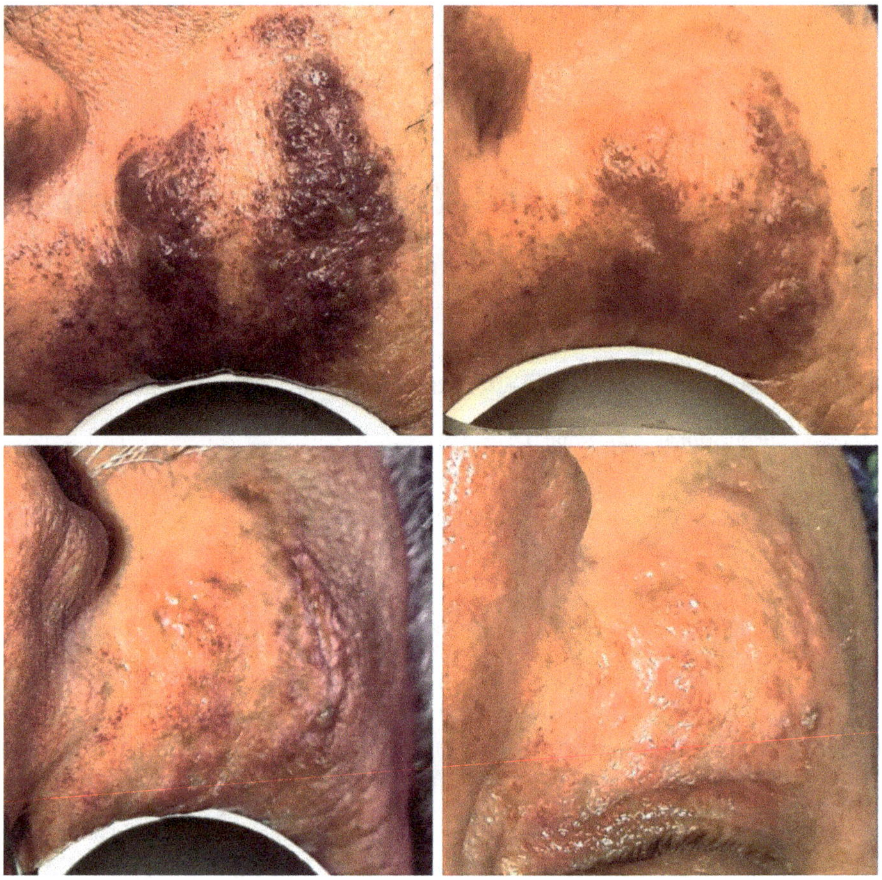

Figure 1: Port-wine stain after 3 Nd:YAG laser treatments.

these devices was most applicable to patients with specific vascular phenotypes in superficial dermal layers. Therefore, some patients with hypertrophic port-wine stains are recalcitrant to pulse dye lasers. Research has suggested that over the last decade, meaningful treatment outcomes have not significantly improved, despite numerous technical innovations and pharmacological interventions [5]. These interventions have included new PDL systems with longer wavelengths (585 and 595 nm), epidermal cooling modalities, longer pulse durations, different light sources, and novel approaches altogether such as photodynamic therapy, pharmacological interventions, and combinations of the aforementioned treatments [6]. The importance of advances in patient outcomes for PWS is clear: patients are often stigmatized due to disfigurement, and this can have a serious impact on self-esteem and contribute to significant psychological stress [7].

2. Case Report

A 60-year-old Caucasian male presented to our office for treatment of port-wine stain on his right cheek. The lesion had significant hypertrophy, and he had neither sought nor received prior treatment for condition. A pulsed dye laser was not available at our institution, so Nd:YAG laser was offered as an alternative treatment option with the patient's informed consent. Our previous experience with Nd:YAG therapy was for treatment of superficial vascular lesions, where it has an established track record in clinical practice [8]. After 3 treatments, the patient had dramatic improvement in appearance, with significant reduction in color and tissue hypertrophy (Figure 1).

3. Discussion

For treatment of port-wine stains, pulsed dye lasers have been regarded as the standard of care. This is primarily due to the excellent avidity of the 585 nm wavelength for oxyhemoglobin, and studies have shown the clinical benefit with low risk of side effects. However, the degree of lesion improvement and patient satisfaction vary significantly, and studies have shown that younger patients achieve better clearance with fewer treatments than older patients [9]. It has also been shown that patients with hypertrophic lesions experience higher complications and significantly less benefit from PDL therapy [10].

The 585 nm pulsed dye laser wavelength is excellent for treating superficial vascular lesions because of its high absorption coefficient for targeting oxyhemoglobin, but it has a significant shortcoming with regards to depth of tissue penetration. The 1064 nm wavelength may be less efficient against oxyhemoglobin as a target, but it has superior tissue penetration and a better ability to reach dermal vessels. This superior tissue penetration could potentially have a role in treating thicker, hypertrophied lesions such as the port-wine stains in older adult patients.

4. Conclusions

585 nm pulse dye lasers not only have an efficient wavelength for targeting oxyhemoglobin but also possess suboptimal tissue penetration for treatment of thicker lesions such as hypertrophic PWS. The 1064 nm Nd:YAG laser has better tissue penetration, but with decreased avidity for oxyhemoglobin. Instead of a one-size-fits-all approach to the treatment of PWS, it seems possible that patients may benefit from the use of different wavelengths depending on the degree of hypertrophy that is present in the vascular lesion. The optimal sequence of wavelengths is currently unclear, but we believe that a logical approach would be to use longer wavelengths initially, as this may decrease tissue hypertrophy and congestion, such that subsequent treatment with shorter wavelengths may be more successful.

References

[1] A. K. Greene, S. F. Taber, K. L. Ball, B. L. Padwa, and J. B. Mulliken, "Sturge-weber syndrome," *Journal of Craniofacial Surgery*, vol. 20, no. Suppl 1, pp. 617–621, 2009.

[2] K. Minkis, R. G. Geronemus, and E. K. Hale, "Port wine stain progression: a potential consequence of delayed and inadequate treatment?" *Lasers in Surgery and Medicine*, vol. 41, no. 6, pp. 423–426, 2009.

[3] J. W. Lee and H. Y. Chung, "Capillary malformations (portwine stains) of the head and neck," *Otolaryngologic Clinics of North America*, vol. 51, no. 1, pp. 197–211, 2018.

[4] W. Tan, M. Chernova, L. Gao et al., "Sustained activation of c-Jun N-terminal and extracellular signal-regulated kinases in port-wine stain blood vessels," *Journal of the American Academy of Dermatology*, vol. 71, no. 5, pp. 964–968, 2014.

[5] M. I. Raath, S. Chohan, A. Wolkerstorfer, C. M. A. M. Horst, G. Storm, and M. Heger, "Port wine stain treatment outcomes have not improved over the past three decades," *Journal of the European Academy of Dermatology and Venereology*, vol. 33, no. 7, pp. 1369–1377, 2019.

[6] J. K. Chen, P. Ghasri, G. Aguilar et al., "An overview of clinical and experimental treatment modalities for port wine stains," *Journal of the American Academy of Dermatology*, vol. 67, no. 2, pp. 289–304, 2012.

[7] S. Michael Kalick, "Toward an interdisciplinary psychology of appearances," *Psychiatry*, vol. 41, no. 3, pp. 243–253, 1978.

[8] N. S. Sadick, "Long-term results with a multiple synchronized-pulse 1064 nm Nd:YAG laser for the treatment of leg venulectasias and reticular veins," *Dermatologic Surgery*, vol. 27, no. 4, pp. 365–369, 2001.

[9] J. G. Morelli, W. L. Weston, J. C. Huff, and J. J. Yohn, "Initial lesion size as a predictive factor in determining the response of port-wine stains in children treated with the pulsed dye laser," *Archives of Pediatrics and Adolescent Medicine*, vol. 149, no. 10, pp. 1142–1144, 1995.

[10] T. Passeron, A. Salhi, J.-M. Mazer et al., "Prognosis and response to laser treatment of early-onset hypertrophic port-wine stains (PWS)," *Journal of the American Academy of Dermatology*, vol. 75, no. 1, pp. 64–68, 2016.

A Case Report of Improved Palmoplantar Pustulosis following Periodontal Treatment and Possible Association with Diminished Systemic Subclinical Inflammation

Akiko Yamashita[1] **Tomomi Sano,**[2] **Misaki Iwashita,**[1] **and Fusanori Nishimura**[1]

[1]*Department of Periodontology, Division of Oral Rehabilitation, Faculty of Dental Science, Kyushu University, Fukuoka, Japan*
[2]*Department of Cell Biology and Pharmacology, Faculty of Dental Science, Kyushu University, Fukuoka, Japan*

Correspondence should be addressed to Akiko Yamashita; yamashita.akiko.339@m.kyushu-u.ac.jp

Academic Editor: Ravi Krishnan

Palmoplantar pustulosis (PPP) is a recurrent pustular dermatosis located on the palms and soles. Focal infection may exacerbate the symptoms of PPP, but the etiology is not fully clear. A 56-year-old woman with PPP was diagnosed with severe chronic periodontitis. Initial treatment for periodontitis combined with topical application of antibiotics and surgical treatment was performed. In this case, attention was paid to the relevance of systemic inflammation caused by periodontitis with the clinical symptoms of PPP. With periodontal treatment, the symptoms of PPP and periodontitis, high-sensitivity C-reactive protein (hs-CRP) level, and periodontal inflamed surface area (PISA) improved. This case highlights the importance of comprehensive dental examinations, including those for oral infections, such as periodontitis and other unrecognized sources of infection, and dental treatment in the overall management of PPP.

1. Introduction

Palmoplantar pustulosis (PPP) is a type of intractable, chronic, and recurrent pustular dermatosis located on the palms and soles [1]. Approximately 95% of patients are smokers at the time of onset [1, 2]. The disease usually takes a relapsing course and is often refractory to treatment [1]. PPP patients tend to have comorbidities, with an increased risk of autoimmune thyroid disease, type 2 diabetes, and so on [1]. PPP is a chronic skin disease that has a large impact on a patient's quality of life. Although the etiology of psoriasis, including PPP, has not been fully clarified, epidemiologic studies have suggested that the disease is often exacerbated by focal infections, such as tonsillitis, periodontitis, and metal allergy [3–5]. Currently, PPP is considered a type of psoriasis in most countries [6]. In contrast, it is considered a distinct disease entity from psoriasis in some countries because of the differences in genetic polymorphisms between the two [7]. Although many case reports have suggested a relationship between periodontitis and psoriasis, less than ten reports have described the relationship between periodontitis and PPP alone [2, 5]. According to a review, patients with periodontitis have a significantly elevated risk of psoriasis [8]. However, the role of the resolution of periodontal inflammation in PPP has not been well documented. Here, we report a case of PPP in a patient with suspected intraoral disease deteriorating factors who showed dramatic improvement in symptoms after periodontal therapy. The novelty of this report is that we particularly focused on inflammation and discussed the relationship between periodontitis and PPP from the standpoint of systemic inflammation, as assessed by the high-sensitivity C-reactive protein (hs-CRP) and related periodontal inflamed surface area (PISA).

2. Case Presentation

A 56-year-old woman with PPP was referred to a dentist with suspected intraoral disease deteriorating factors

(Figure 1(a)). She had discovered the symptom 2 years before on her palms and soles, smoking 10 cigarettes per day for 30 years. She did not have any arthralgia, suggestive of concomitant pustulotic arthro-osteitis (PAO). Since her symptoms did not improve spontaneously, she visited the dermatologist and was diagnosed with PPP and treated with topical steroids. The dermatologist also recommended that she undergo a patch test to diagnose a metal allergy, but it is physically difficult. Because her symptoms did not improve, she visited another doctor. The next doctor prescribed biotin, vitamin C, *Clostridium butyricum*, and oriental medicine (Asian ginseng and jumihaidokuto). Her symptoms eventually became refractory to treatment. The doctor noted her oral condition, and her medical history revealed oral discomfort, including gingival bleeding and swelling. Subsequently, the dermatologist suspected intraoral disease deteriorating factors and referred her to the Kyushu University Hospital Periodontology Clinic to investigate the possible association of PPP with her oral condition.

Her medical records were unremarkable, except for severe chronic periodontitis. It was severe (stage IV and grade C) (Figures 2(a) and 2(b)). She had not received any prior comprehensive periodontal treatment. Upon her visit at our centre, we performed a regular examination and measured hs-CRP, white blood cell (WBC) count, and calculated PISA. Figure 3 shows the results of the initial dental examination and the changes in each parameter according to the treatment. At the initial examination, the hs-CRP level, WBC count, PISA, and proportion of the probing pocket depth of over 4 mm were 2650 ng/mL, 6660/μl, 1103.4 mm^2, and 45.3%, respectively.

Because her hs-CRP level was relatively high, we first aimed to determine whether this elevation was due to periodontitis. We started the normal initial preparation with the topical application of antibiotics (minocycline hydrochloride ointment) to carefully observe the effects of anti-infectious periodontal treatment on PPP. We removed dental plaque and calculus and administered antibiotics in every pocket with a depth of >4 mm once a week for 1 month. A few months after the initiation of periodontal treatment, her palms, soles, and intraoral symptoms improved slightly. After initial preparation and reevaluation, we performed surgical treatment, including tooth extraction and correction of the irregular shape of the alveolar bone. Periodontitis showed further improvement 3 months after periodontal surgery (Figure 3). The symptoms of PPP gradually improved, and complete remission was observed in the supportive periodontal therapy (SPT) phase. Figure 3 shows the changes in laboratory and clinical examination data. In the SPT phase, the hs-CRP level, WBC count, PISA, and proportion of the probing pocket depth of >4 mm were 565 ng/mL, 6020/μl, 77.2 mm^2, and 1.1%, respectively. The patient also showed improvement in PPP and periodontitis. After periodontal treatment, the patient continued SPT once every 3 months. In addition, although more than 2 years had passed after complete remission, no recurrence was observed (Figure 1(b)).

3. Discussion

PPP is considered a chronic inflammatory disease of the skin that severely impacts the patient's quality of life. Although the exact etiology of PPP is completely unknown, associations with thyroid disease, smoking, and focal infections, such as tonsillitis, periodontitis, and metal allergy, have been suggested [3–5]. A dermatologist recommended that the patient undergo a dental checkup because of suspected intraoral disease deteriorating factors. A dental examination revealed severe periodontitis.

Although the most contributory factor in the relationship between PPP and dentistry is a dental metal allergy, only 33% of the patients showed a positive response after metal removal from the oral cavity [9]. In addition, infection control has been reported to improve PPP[9] symptoms. Periodontitis is the focus of focal infection.

With periodontal treatment, her PPP symptoms improved dramatically. After she was referred to our dental clinic, she stopped using the corticosteroid ointment. Furthermore, the doses of the other medications were unchanged. Smokers account for 95% of PPP patients [1]. Smoking is regarded as a strong risk factor for PPP [1]. Based on previous observations, smoking cessation is strongly recommended and may result in fewer pustules and lesser scales and erythema [1]. Furthermore, smoking exacerbates periodontitis and can affect the onset, progression, and recurrence of periodontitis [10]. It has been reported that hs-CRP is significantly higher in current smokers than in never and past smokers [11]. Therefore, we strongly recommended smoking cessation, but she has not quit smoking so far. There is a possibility that the continuation of oriental medicine and biotin might have improved her physical condition, leading to the improvement of PPP. However, along with the remission of inflammation, the symptoms dramatically improved as assessed by hs-CRP and PISA. The hs-CRP level is a highly sensitive low-grade inflammatory marker, and periodontitis is associated with elevated hs-CRP, decreasing with successful therapy [12]. On the other hand, PISA quantifies the degree of inflamed periodontal area, thereby quantifying the inflammatory burden posed by periodontitis [13]. It is beginning to be introduced as a new parameter of inflammation. Hs-CRP also decreased with periodontal treatment and showed a tendency to correlate with PISA in this case. It is considered that PISA at the second examination increased temporarily because the patient's tooth brushing condition before the examination was poor, and there were many points of bleeding on probing (BOP) at the time of periodontal tissue examination. The PISA increased as the BOP area expanded. In contrast, antibiotics were administered as needed during the period of aggressive periodontal treatment. However, antibiotics were not administered 3 months prior to the fourth examination. Therefore, the hs-CRP level in the fourth examination might have been higher than in the second and third examinations. As a result of additional examination after the fourth examination, hs-CRP was almost the same. It is considered that hs-CRP can be maintained within the normal range compared with the initial value. These findings suggest that

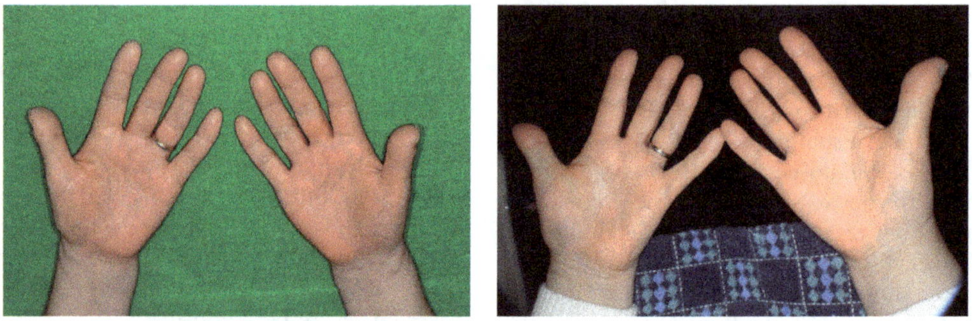

(a) (b)

Figure 1: Appearances of the palm at (a) first visit and (b) 1 year after periodontal treatment. (a) Scaly erythemas with tiny pustules were scattered on the palm. (b) Marked improvement was observed after periodontal treatment.

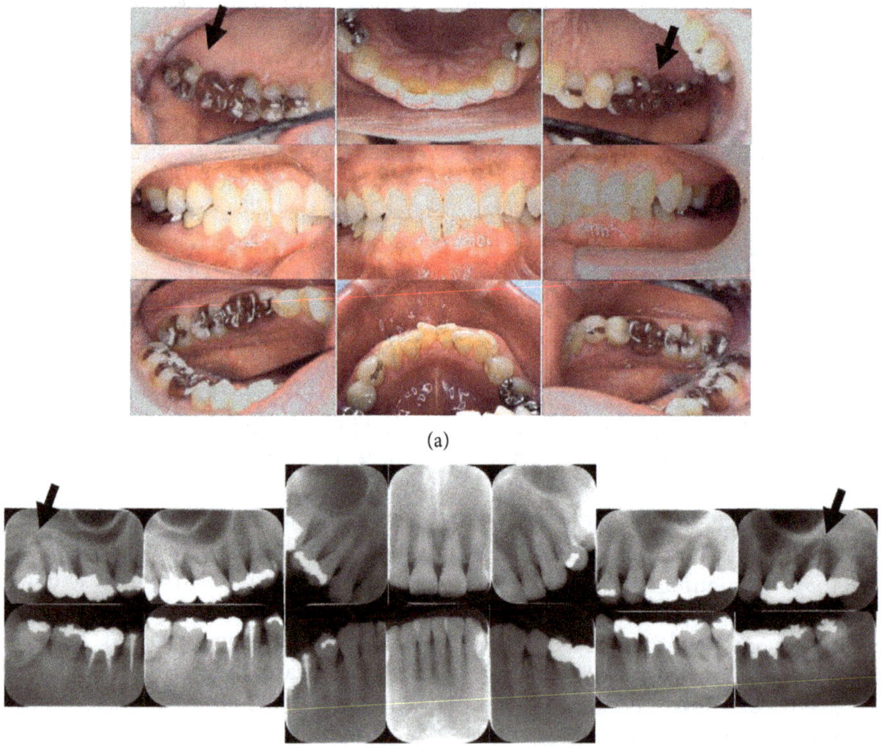

(a)

(b)

Figure 2: Appearance of the patient's periodontal tissues at the first visit (a) and radiograph of the periodontium (b). Note the severe alveolar bone resorption and so-called "floating teeth" due to severe periodontitis (b) and moderate gingival inflammation (a). "Floating teeth" were indicated by arrows. In addition, many metal restorations are observed.

severe periodontitis caused intraoral inflammation, increased PISA, and systemic inflammation, as indicated by increased hs-CRP. Furthermore, this inflammation participates in the deterioration of the PPP. Both conventional CRP and hs-CRP measure the same proteins. Conventional CRP measurements could not detect amounts below 0.1 mg/dL (1000 ng/ml). However, hs-CRP can measure trace amounts of CRP, which are normally undetectable. In this patient, the values at any examination were within the conventional CRP reference.

Previous studies have suggested that bacterial infection plays an important role in PPP. Some findings suggest that the immune responses to heat-shock proteins induced by chronically infected bacteria, such as periodontal bacteria, could also be etiological factors for PPP[3]. Some researchers have reported that the IL-23/IL-17 inflammatory pathway is important in the pathology of PPP [14]. Notably, several studies have reported that IL-17 is associated with periodontitis, psoriasis, and other immune-mediated inflammatory diseases [15, 16].

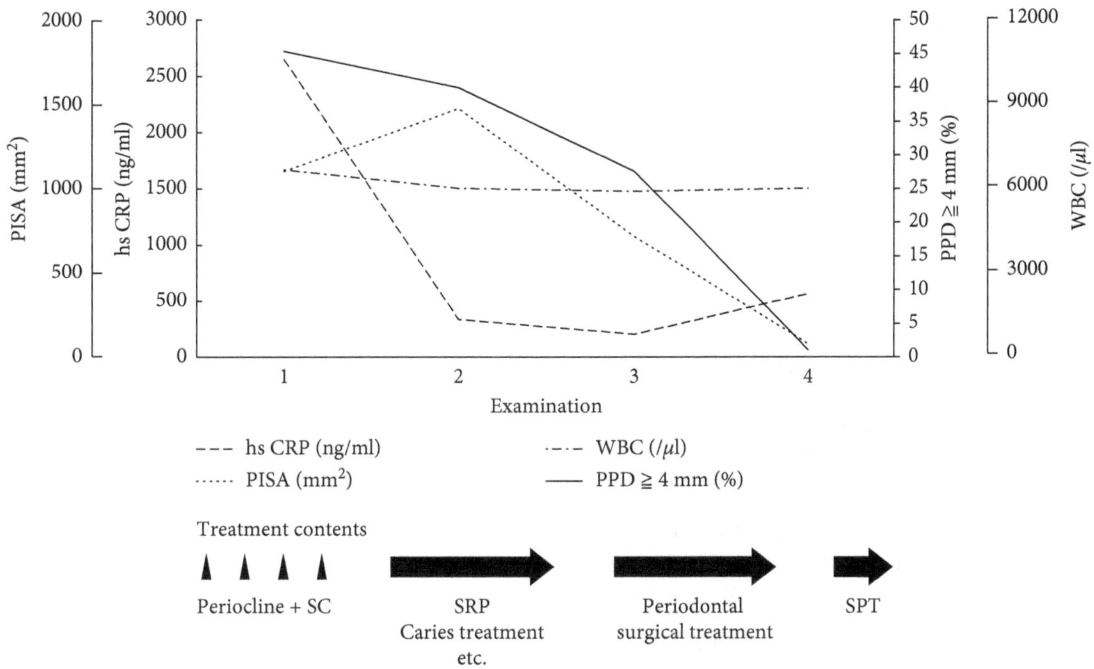

FIGURE 3: The course of dental treatment and the changes in hs-CRP levels, WBC, PISA value, and the ratio of PPD >4 mm. As periodontal treatment advanced, the value of inflammatory markers showed a decreased tendency.

Dental metals, focal infections, and low-grade inflammation are possible deteriorating factors that influence the pathology of PPP. In this case, the symptoms of PPP improved, even without the removal of dental metals. Therefore, intraoral focal infections and inflammation should be carefully considered. Removing oral infectious lesions may become first-line therapy in dental and medical treatment because controlling infections is much easier and more cost effective than replacing restorative materials. Some reports have indicated that intraoral and pharyngeal focal infections are closely related to the onset of PPP [5, 17]. In this regard, calculating PISA as an indicator of local intraoral inflammation and measuring hs-CRP as an indicator of low-grade systemic inflammation would be useful markers to assess the contribution of periodontitis to the deterioration of PPP.

In conclusion, this case highlights the importance of comprehensive dental examinations, including those for dental infections, such as periodontitis, dental abscesses, and other unrecognized sources of infections, dental treatment, and assessment of low-grade inflammatory markers as hs-CRP in the overall management of PPP.

Acknowledgments

This work was supported by the Japan Society for the Promotion of Science (JSPS) KAKENHI, Japan, Grant No. JP18K09578.

References

[1] E. Hagforsen, "The cutaneous non-neuronal cholinergic system and smoking related dermatoses: studies of the psoriasis variant palmoplantar pustulosis," *Life Sciences*, vol. 80, no. 24-25, pp. 2227–2234, 2007.

[2] T. Yamamoto, T. Hiraiwa, R. Tobita et al., "Characteristics of Japanese patients with pustulotic arthro-osteitis associated with palmoplantar pustulosis: a multicenter study," *International Journal of Dermatology*, vol. 59, no. 4, pp. 441–444, 2020.

[3] M. Kosugi, K. Ishihara, and K. Okuda, "Implication of responses to bacterial heat shock proteins, chronic microbial infections, and dental metal allergy in patients with pustulosis palmaris et plantaris," *The Bulletin of Tokyo Dental College* vol. 44, no. 3, pp. 149–158, 2003.

[4] K. Nakamura, S. Imakado, M. Takizawa et al., "Exacerbation of pustulosis palmaris et plantaris after topical application of metals accompanied by elevated levels of leukotriene B4 in pustules," *Journal of the American Academy of Dermatology* vol. 42, no. 6, pp. 1021–1025, 2000.

[5] N. Kikuchi and T. Yamamoto, "Dental infection as a triggering factor in palmoplantar pustulosis," *Acta Dermato-Venereologica*, vol. 93, no. 6, pp. 721-722, 2013.

[6] A. M. G. Brunasso and C. Massone, "Psoriasis and palmoplantar pustulosis: an endless debate?" *The Journal of the European Academy of Dermatology and Venereology*, vol. 31, no. 7, pp. e335–e337, 2017.

[7] H. Torii, H. Nakagawa, Y. Ishibashi, K. Tokunaga, and T. Juji, "Genetic polymorphisms in HLA-A, -B, -C and -DR antigens in Japanese patients with palmoplantar pustulosis," *Dermatology*, vol. 188, no. 4, pp. 290–292, 1994.

[8] P. Ungprasert, K. Wijarnpreecha, and D. A. Wetter, "Periodontitis and risk of psoriasis: a systematic review and meta-analysis," *Journal of the European Academy of Dermatology and Venereology*, vol. 31, no. 5, pp. 857–862, 2017.

[9] M. Kouno, A. Nishiyama, M. Minabe et al., "Retrospective analysis of the clinical response of palmoplantar pustulosis after dental infection control and dental metal removal," *The Journal of Dermatology*, vol. 44, no. 6, pp. 695–698, 2017.

[10] D. F. Kinane and I. G. Chestnutt, "Smoking and periodontal disease," *Critical Reviews in Oral Biology & Medicine*, vol. 11, no. 3, pp. 356–365, 2000.

[11] S. Sanada, M. Nishida, K. Ishii, T. Moriyama, I. Komuro, and K. Yamauchi-Takihara, "Smoking promotes subclinical atherosclerosis in apparently healthy men," *Circulation Journal*, vol. 76, no. 12, pp. 2884–2891, 2012.

[12] F. Nishimura, A. Taniguchi, Y. Iwamoto et al., "Porphyromonas gingivalis infection is associated with elevated C-reactive protein in nonobese Japanese type 2 diabetic subjects," *Diabetes Care*, vol. 25, no. 10, p. 1888, 2002.

[13] W. Nesse, F. Abbas, I. van der Ploeg, F. K. L. Spijkervet, P. U. Dijkstra, and A. Vissink, "Periodontal inflamed surface area: quantifying inflammatory burden," *Journal of Clinical Periodontology*, vol. 35, no. 8, pp. 668–673, 2008.

[14] B. S. McKenzie, R. A. Kastelein, and D. J. Cua, "Understanding the IL-23-IL-17 immune pathway," *Trends in Immunology*, vol. 27, no. 1, pp. 17–23, 2006.

[15] C. Zenobia and G. Hajishengallis, "Basic biology and role of interleukin-17 in immunity and inflammation," *Periodontology 2000*, vol. 69, no. 1, pp. 142–159, 2015.

[16] K. Bunte and T. Beikler, "Th17 cells and the IL-23/IL-17 axis in the pathogenesis of periodontitis and immune-mediated inflammatory diseases," *International Journal of Molecular Sciences*, vol. 20, no. 14, p. E3394, 2019.

[17] T. Yanagi, T. Shimizu, R. Abe, and H. Shimizu, "Zinc dental fillings and palmoplantar pustulosis," *The Lancet*, vol. 366, no. 9490, p. 1050, 2005.

25

Aeromonas hydrophila Survives the Treatment of Posttraumatic Cellulitis in the Shelter of an Obscured Fish-Bone Fragment

Areti Ganiatsa, [1] Constantina Gartzonika, [2] Georgios Gaitanis, [1] Paraskevi Voulgari, [3] Stamatina Levidiotou-Stefanou, [2] and Ioannis D. Bassukas [1]

[1] *Department of Skin and Venereal Diseases, Faculty of Medicine, School of Health Sciences, University of Ioannina, Ioannina, Greece*
[2] *Department of Microbiology, Faculty of Medicine, School of Health Sciences, University of Ioannina, Ioannina, Greece*
[3] *Rheumatology Clinic, Department of Internal Medicine, Faculty of Medicine, School of Health Sciences, University of Ioannina, Ioannina, Greece*

Correspondence should be addressed to Ioannis D. Bassukas; ibassuka@uoi.gr

Academic Editor: Sergio A. Cuevas Covarrubias

Fish bone and/or spine puncture injuries can result in infection of the upper extremities with aquatic bacterial pathogens. Additionally, in such injuries, the inoculation of foreign organic material is frequent and may further complicate the clinical presentation and course of the resulting infection. We describe the case of a 45-year-old female patient with a minimal fish rostrum puncture trauma acquired during preparation of fresh fish meal, which resulted in a galloping hand cellulitis. The alarming clinical presentation and the prompt response of the skin infection to clindamycin obscured the presence of inoculated fish rostrum remnants in the tissue that, three weeks later, gave rise to a foreign body granuloma, from which *Aeromonas hydrophila* was isolated. Final resolution was achieved with an additional two-week doxycycline treatment. In conclusion, the reported case highlights the potential of the accidentally implanted organic material, as are fish bones, not only to transfer uncommon pathogens but also to offer a sanctuary that favors microbial survival despite antibiotic therapy thus enabling latent or recurrent infections.

1. Introduction

Fish bone and/or spine puncture injuries can result in infection of the upper extremities with aquatic bacterial pathogens [1–3]. Additionally, in such injuries, the inoculation of a foreign organic material is frequent and may further complicate the clinical presentation and course of the resulting infection [1].

Herein, we describe a case of a fish rostrum puncture that resulted in a galloping hand cellulitis. The alarming clinical presentation obscured the presence of the fish rostrum remnants in the tissue that, three weeks later, gave rise to a foreign body granuloma, from which *Aeromonas hydrophila* was isolated. This case is a reminder that, in any fish bone injury, the insertion of a foreign body should always be considered and, if possible, localized and timely removed.

2. Case Report

An otherwise healthy, 45-year-old female presented with a painful, rapidly expanding erythematous edema of her right hand that developed within 5 hours after a puncture trauma during preparation of a swordfish for cooking. The edema involved the right hand and forearm and restricted hand function. No fever or palpable lymph nodes were present, and the puncture point was not visible. White blood cell counts, erythrocyte sedimentation rate, and C-reactive protein levels were within normal limits. No pathogens were isolated from superficial swab cultures. Cellulitis was diagnosed, tetanus prophylaxis with tetanus immunoglobulin (Tetagam®) was given, and the patient was treated with clindamycin (i.v. 600 mg t.i.d.) and ciprofloxacin (i.v. 400 mg b.i.d.). A three-day course of oral glucocorticosteroids

(32 mg methylprednisolone q.d.) was added to reduce the excessive edema. The clinical condition improved promptly with substantial reduction of the edema after the first 24 hours of treatment, and since no pathogens were isolated from the superficial lesional skin swabs, the treatment was not revised. The patient significantly improved during a 7-day hospitalization and was discharged with the instruction to continue treatment with oral clindamycin (300 mg t.i.d.) for additional 2 weeks.

Three weeks later, the patient returned with a tender, slow-growing, 8 mm large inflammatory nodule in the medial aspect of the first phalanx of the right middle finger (Figure 1(a)). The patient was otherwise healthy, and no further symptoms were reported. Subsequently, she was re-evaluated for nontuberculous mycobacteria infection and/or an evolving foreign body granuloma. Blood tests were within normal range, and the tuberculin skin reaction was negative. A tissue probe was transferred in anaerobic transport medium and cultured under aerobic and anaerobic conditions as well as in the solid and liquid medium for mycobacteria. The only pathogen isolated in tissue cultures was *A. hydrophila*. Identification and susceptibility testing were performed using conventional microbiological methods and the Vitek 2 system (bioMerieux, France). According to the susceptibility pattern, *A. hydrophila* was mainly sensitive to third-generation cephalosporins, aminoglycosides, and fluoroquinolones and to trimethoprim-sulfamethoxazole. Ultrasound and X-ray imaging of the area revealed the presence of a foreign body located at the site of the emerging granuloma, immediately beneath the skin (Figure 1(b)). The foreign body was removed; macroscopically, it was consistent with fish bone remnants. The patient was subsequently treated with oral ciprofloxacin for two weeks. The inflammation regressed quickly, and the patient had no evidence of infection at the 6-month follow-up examination.

3. Discussion

The rapidly progressing course of the present hand cellulitis coupled with the reported fish puncture injury raised the suspicion of a polymicrobial infection with the participation of marine pathogens, particularly *Vibrio vulnificus*, a species known to cause rapidly evolving skin and soft-tissue infections (SSTIs) [4–6]. However, the initial working diagnosis had to be modified after the development of a foreign body reaction and the following isolation of *A. hydrophila* from it. In retrospect, we suggest that *A. hydrophila*, if not the exclusive pathogen, was at least an important copathogen in a polymicrobial traumatic hand cellulitis. This hypothesis complies with the following clinical features of the present case: (1) Rapid response of the cellulitis to the initial combination treatment with intravenous ciprofloxacin and clindamycin. (2) Persistence of the microorganism in the relatively inaccessible to an antimicrobial sanctuary of the fish-bone fragments and its isolation after the development of the purulent granuloma. It is known that biofilm formation is facilitated by the presence of a foreign material and significantly increases the antibiotic resistance of microbes in the tissues [7]. The employment of the fish bone as a scaffold for the development of a biofilm was probably the main strategy of *A. hydrophila* to escape eradication during the first antibiotic course in this patient. (3) Unequivocal cure after the removal of the foreign body and an additional course of antibiotics. (4) *A. hydrophila* is frequently isolated from sites of polymicrobial hand infections, and most of the SSTIs with similar as the above clinical features are of polymicrobial nature [8, 9]. However, an accidental reinfestation of the patient with the same pathogen *A. hydrophila* cannot be fully excluded; this has been already described in the literature to explain some cases of hand infections due to *V. vulnificus* [4].

Aeromonas species are facultatively anaerobic, Gram-negative, rod-shaped bacteria that are ubiquitous in aquatic environments [3, 8]. They are frequently isolated from fresh or brackish water (rivers, lakes, ponds, and estuaries) including aquatic habitants, sewage, soil, and tap water, particularly during the warmer months of the year [3, 8]. In addition, different motile *Aeromonas* species, including *A. hydrophila*, are important fish pathogens [10]. In humans, they are opportunistic pathogens mostly implicated in gastroenteritis cases from the ingestion of inadequately processed contaminated food and SSTI [8, 11]. Skin trauma and exposure to environmental water appear to be the principal factors involved in the pathogenesis of SSTI due to *A. hydrophila* [3, 9]. In particular, *A. hydrophila* is regarded as the most common single cause of SSTI associated with fresh water injuries [12] that include simple abrasions and puncture wounds to less common yet exotic scenarios such as propeller accidents and alligator bites [3, 8]. Likewise, the resulting clinical spectrum ranges from cellulitis and localized skin and soft-tissue nodules and abscesses to alarming rapid spread of the pathogen into deeper layers of the skin and subcutaneous tissues [8, 11]. Therefore, the development of cellulitis with fulminant progression within a few hours and the anamnesis of an eliciting skin trauma in the aquatic environment or during handling fresh fish should alert the clinician for a possible *A. hydrophila* infection [8, 13]. In such cases, the prompt onset of antibiosis is essential in order to stop the invasive course of the infection, which may quickly progress into ecthyma gangrenosum, necrotizing fasciitis with severe myonecrosis of the adjacent muscles, osteomyelitis, and septicemia [3, 8, 9]. These latter, more severe complications are predominantly seen in patients with certain predisposing factors such as liver disease or malignancy [3, 9]. Surgical decompression with incision, drainage, and debridement may be required in order to prevent extensive tissue necrosis. In our present case, no surgical intervention was performed at initial presentation; the timely onset of a short systemic methylprednisolone course has probably induced the prompt reversion of the galloping edema. However, it may have also contributed to the initial masquerading of the presence of the foreign body [14].

The present case illustrates the persistence of the skin infection as the result of the omitted search for a foreign body during the initial patient's consultation. Therefore, the history of such a trauma should always raise concern of possible implantation of a slowly degradable organic

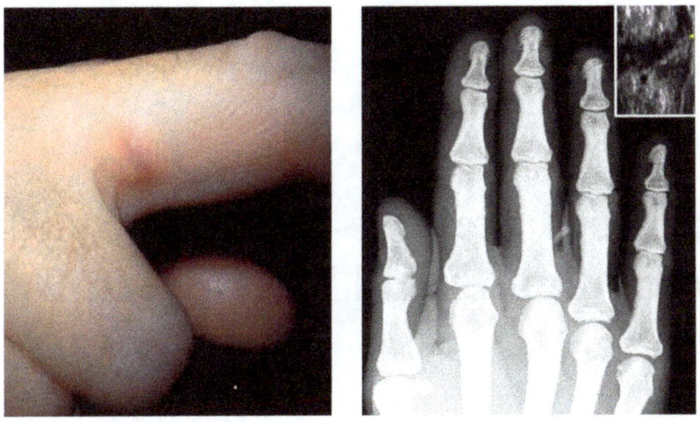

(a) (b)

FIGURE 1: (a) Skin lesion at the 2nd admission. (b) X-ray film of the right hand demonstrating a wedge-formed radio-opaque foreign body in the soft tissue of the lateral aspect of the 1st phalanx of the middle finger. Inset: ultrasound detail of the foreign body insertion site.

material that could favor the survival of inoculated pathogens and enable persistent or latent-recurrent infections [1]. However, it is worth noting that routine X-ray film examinations are not always reliable to detect inserted fish tissue fragments as their radiographic visibility decisively depends on the specific composition of the foreign material [15]. Using a soft-tissue technique will probably improve the efficacy of the latter study. Additional imaging studies, such as sonography or MRI, may be useful in cases of increased suspicion and negative radiologic findings.

In conclusion, community-acquired cellulitis following skin trauma in contact with environmental water or aquatic organisms should alert the clinician for the possibility of infection with uncommon marine pathogens including *A. hydrophila* [8, 16].

References

[1] D. A. Hudson and T. M. De Chalain, "Hand infections secondary to fish bone injuries," *Annals of the Royal College of Surgeons of England*, vol. 76, no. 2, pp. 99–101, 1994.

[2] R. Imberg, I. Potasman, Y. Weissman, and M. Grupper, "Hand infections following penetrating fish fins or bones injuries (FFBI): a large, hospital based, retrospective study," *Infection*, vol. 36, no. 6, pp. 565–569, 2008.

[3] C. M. Chao, C. C. Lai, H. J. Tang, W. C. Ko, and P.-R. Hsueh, "Skin and soft-tissue infections caused by Aeromonas species," *European Journal of Clinical Microbiology & Infectious Diseases*, vol. 32, no. 4, pp. 543–547, 2013.

[4] E. Calif and S. Shalom, "Hand infections caused by delayed inoculation of *Vibrio vulnificus*: does human skin serve as a potential reservoir of vibrios?" *Hand Surgery*, vol. 09, no. 01, pp. 39–44, 2004.

[5] J. D. Oliver, "Wound infections caused by *Vibrio vulnificus* and other marine bacteria," *Epidemiology and Infection*, vol. 133, no. 3, pp. 383–391, 2005.

[6] R. Finkelstein and I. Oren, "Soft tissue infections caused by marine bacterial pathogens: epidemiology, diagnosis, and management," *Current Infectious Disease Reports*, vol. 13, no. 5, pp. 470–477, 2011.

[7] H. Wu, C. Moser, H.-Z. Wang, N. Høiby, and Z.-J. Song, "Strategies for combating bacterial biofilm infections," *International Journal of Oral Science*, vol. 7, no. 1, pp. 1–7, 2014.

[8] J. M. Janda and S. L. Abbott, "The genus *Aeromonas*: taxonomy, pathogenicity, and infection," *Clinical Microbiology Reviews*, vol. 23, no. 1, pp. 35–73, 2010.

[9] W. L. Gold and I. E. Salit, "*Aeromonas hydrophila* infections of skin and soft tissue: report of 11 cases and review," *Clinical Infectious Diseases*, vol. 16, no. 1, pp. 69–74, 1993.

[10] R. L. Thune, L. A. Stanley, and R. K. Cooper, "Pathogenesis of Gram-negative bacterial infections in warmwater fish," *Annual Review of Fish Diseases*, vol. 3, pp. 37–68, 1993.

[11] J. L. Parker and J. G. Shaw, "*Aeromonas* spp. Clinical microbiology and disease," *Journal of Infection*, vol. 62, no. 2, pp. 109–118, 2011.

[12] S. Esposito, S. Noviello, and S. Leone, "Epidemiology and microbiology of skin and soft tissue infections," *Current Opinion in Infectious Diseases*, vol. 29, no. 2, pp. 109–115, 2016.

[13] C. A. Weber, S. J. Wertheimer, and A. Ognjan, "Aeromonas hydrophila-its implications in freshwater injuries," *The Journal of Foot and Ankle Surgery*, vol. 34, no. 5, pp. 442–446, 1995.

[14] J. Hoffman, "Extremely late presentation of catfish spine injury to the hand," *Wilderness & Environmental Medicine*, vol. 21, no. 4, p. 383, 2010.

[15] R. C. Russel, D. A. Williamson, J. W. Sullivan et al., "Detection of foreign bodies in the hand," *Journal of Hand Surgery*, vol. 13, pp. 254–259, 1988.

[16] V. Haddad, O. Lupi, J. P. Lonza, and S. K. Tyring, "Tropical dermatology: marine and aquatic dermatology," *Journal of the American Academy of Dermatology*, vol. 61, no. 5, pp. 733–750, 2009.

26

Carbamazepine Induced Stevens-Johnson Syndrome that Developed into Toxic Epidermal Necrolysis: Review of the Literature

Yousef S. Abuzneid,[1] Hussam I. A. Alzeerelhouseini,[1] Duha Rabi,[1] Ihab Hilail,[1] Hatem Rjoob,[1] Abdelrahman Rabee,[1] Naser Amro,[1] Qutaiba Qafisheh,[1] and Mohammad Kharraz[2]

[1]*Al-Quds University Faculty of Medicine, Jerusalem, State of Palestine*
[2]*An-Najah National University Hospital, Nablus, State of Palestine*

Correspondence should be addressed to Yousef S. Abuzneid; yo_usef97@hotmail.com

Academic Editor: Tak-Wah Wong

Background. Stevens-Johnson syndrome and toxic epidermal necrolysis are both skin diseases believed to be following the pattern of a type IV hypersensitivity mechanism, which can be triggered by infectious agents or administration of a variety of drugs as part of the spectrum of severe cutaneous adverse reactions (SCARs). Fever and blisters, that peel forming painful raw areas, are early symptoms of this condition, and complications such as dehydration, sepsis, pneumonia, and multiple organ failure are typically seen during the course of the disease. *Case Presentation.* We present a case of a 23-year-old female patient referred to our hospital after taking carbamazepine and developing high-grade fever and ulcers that appeared initially in her mouth and face but then progressed despite treatment, extending all over her body and involving about 90% of her BSA. *Conclusion.* The use of IVIG and plasmapheresis was a good management for our case, helping in our patient's well-being and recovery. Even if there is no stipulated guideline treatment for cases of SJS and TEN, we think that further investigations about IVIG and plasmapheresis should be investigated as a possible way to treat both conditions.

1. Introduction

Stevens-Johnson syndrome (SJS) and toxic epidermal necrolysis (TEN) are both rare skin reactions that are often triggered by particular medications and can be life-threatening. Antiepileptic drugs (AEDs), nonsteroidal anti-inflammatory drugs (NSAIDs), and certain antibiotics have been shown to trigger these reactions [1].

At the beginning, SJS and TEN were addressed as different conditions, but now they are considered as two forms of the same skin disease. SJS is defined as detachment of less than 10% of the total body surface area (BSA), while TEN is the detachment of greater than 30% of the total BSA [2].

Both conditions are characterized by full-thickness epidermal necrosis and severe mucous membrane inflammation leading to mucocutaneous sloughing and denudation [3].

It affects all age groups, affecting more those individuals that have HIV, autoimmune diseases, immunocompromised patients, and those who have an underlying malignancy. Also, it is thought to be an immune mediated drug reaction with higher rates in certain population (for example, carbamazepine associated SJS/TEN has been linked to Han Chinese and other Asian groups due to HLA-B*1502) [4].

The incidence of these reactions is estimated to be 1.5–8.3 cases per 1000000 person-year. The mortality from SJS is approximately 5%, whereas the mortality from TEN is approximately 30%. There are studies showing that even after one year of hospitalization, the mortality risk for those patients who suffer from SJS/TEN continues.

This condition appears to be more lethal in the early phase of the disease. Older age and the presence of comorbidities are two significant risk factors that can increase the mortality rate [1]. It has been reported that patients who survive SJS/TEN are at high risk of developing long-term complications involving the skin, eyes, mucosa, and respiratory, renal, and/or hepatic systems [1].

2. Case Presentation

We present a 23-year-old female patient from Gaza, with a history of medicated major depressive disorder. She was in her usual state of health until she started developing multiple painful ulcers over her face and oral cavity after 10 days of the addition of carbamazepine to her treatment regimen for her headaches and anxiety disorder. She sought immediate medical advice and was diagnosed with Stevens-Johnson syndrome and was put on hydrocortisone (100 mg × 2) with no improvement.

The rash rapidly progressed over her entire body, and she developed high-grade fever (41°C). Thus, antibiotics were added, and she was referred to our hospital.

When she arrived, the patient was confused and could not be aroused. She had ulcerations resembling burns covering her entire body with diffuse skin desquamation, sloughed skin, high-grade fever, and severe dehydration (Figure 1). Her vital signs showed a blood pressure of 80/40 and heart rate of 130 beats/min. WBC was 24×10^9/L and procalcitonin was 4 ng/mL, making septic shock clearer. The patient had more than 10% of body surface area involved, tachycardia, a serum glucose of 74 mg/dL (4.1 mmol/L), a serum urea of 39 mmol/L, and a serum bicarbonate of 12 mmol/L; so, her SCORTEN score (severity-of-illness score for toxic epidermal necrolysis) was calculated to be 4.

Furthermore, a central line was inserted in ER carefully because of extensive skin desquamation, and an IV normal saline and broad-spectrum antibiotics were started which included tigecycline, colistin, and fluconazole. Skin culture was done, showing heavy growth of Gram-negative bacteria bacilli that was later found to be a multidrug-resistant *Acinetobacter baumannii* strain. Thus, she remained on the same medication regimen.

Due to the extensive desquamation of almost 90% of her body, the patient's case was diagnosed as toxic epidermal necrolysis, which is known to have a high mortality rate. Our patient's situation was especially progressive and severe, necessitating a DNR order discussion with her family.

Pulse steroids with Solu-Medrol (methylprednisolone sodium succinate that was given 1 g × 1) were also initiated, and medical consultation was sought in order to start plasma exchange treatment and plastic surgery.

After 6 sessions of plasmapheresis in addition to IVIG, we noticed that the patient condition started to improve, the fever disappeared, and the desquamation of the skin started to heal.

Afterwards, an ophthalmologist consultation was required because the patient had developed a complication of closure of the left eye due to the necrosis of the periorbital skin which needed to be opened surgically.

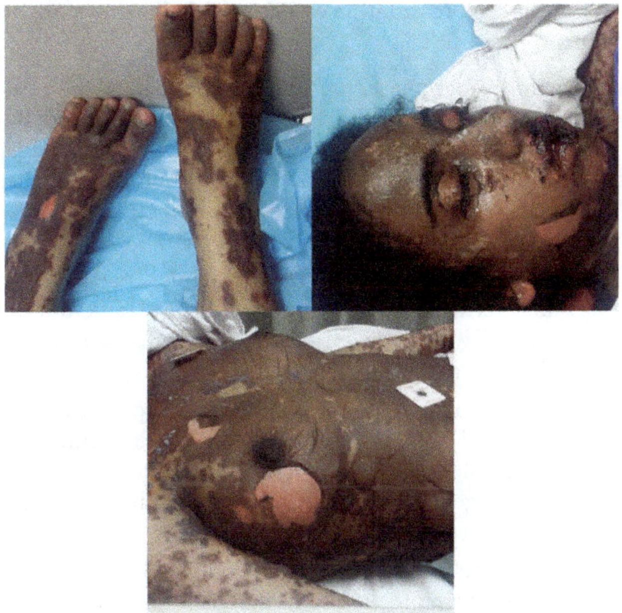

FIGURE 1: Diffuse skin desquamation resembling burns covering almost 90% of the patient's body.

The patient was discharged after 28 days and then had follow-up appointments by regular call phones (since people from Gaza need a special permit to come to the West Bank). She was advised not to take anticonvulsants because of their well-established side effects (including SJS and TEN). She was also recommended to take SNRIs (serotonin and norepinephrine reuptake inhibitors). After six months, she presented to our hospital in a good condition with excellent performance.

3. Discussion

The pathophysiology of the disease is not fully understood, but it is believed to be a delayed hypersensitivity reaction mediated by Th1 cells which is the cause of keratinocyte apoptosis by Fas (CD95) and FasL ligand (CD95L) interaction and the release of perforin and granzyme B pathways [5].

SJS and TEN have many causes, but drugs are the most common. Antiepileptics (lamotrigine, carbamazepine, phenytoin, and phenobarbital), allopurinol, oxicam, nonsteroidal anti-inflammatory drugs, and sulfa drugs are the most implicated. Other causes such as infection and malignancy were also reported, and the risk of developing the disease increases in immunocompromised and HIV-infected patients [6].

There is a strong association between some HLA alleles and drug-induced SJS/TEN. The most significant is HLA-B*15 : 02 with carbamazepine-induced SJS among the Asian population. Genetic screening for HLA-B*15:02 can be performed prior to the prescription of carbamazepine, especially in Southeast Asia, where the prevalence of this allele is high [3]. Unfortunately, in our case, we cannot confirm that the allele is the cause for TEN as a genetic test was not performed.

The clinical presentation of SJS and TEN mainly consists of three phases [2]:

(1) Prodromal phase: present 2-3 days before the acute phase and characterized by fever (100% of cases); flu-like symptoms such as cough, malaise, myalgia, arthralgia; and anorexia. Other symptoms may also present in this phase, such as conjunctivitis (32% of cases) and pharyngitis (25% of cases).

(2) Acute phase: characterized by tender, painful macular eruptions with nonblanching "targetoid lesions," which classically develop symmetrically on the face and trunk and spread to the extremities.

    Lesions may become bullous and rupture, leaving denuded skin susceptible to a secondary infection. Mucosal involvement can also occur, involving pharyngeal, tracheal, bronchial, gastrointestinal, and vaginal regions.

(3) Reepithelialization period: may take 3–6 weeks and secondary infection can increase the risk of scar formation.

Patients with TEN can develop multiorgan involvement resulting in renal, gastrointestinal, respiratory, and cardiovascular damages. However, sepsis from a secondary infection is the most common cause of death [6].

There are no specific laboratory tests (other than biopsy) that can definitively establish the diagnosis of SJS and TEN. Therefore, diagnosis is clinical, with emphasis on previous drug usage. CBC may reveal normal or nonspecific leukocytosis, but marked WBC elevation may indicate superimposed bacterial infection. So skin, urine, and blood cultures have been advocated because the incidence of serious bacterial bloodstream infections and sepsis significantly contribute to morbidity and mortality [5].

On skin biopsy, the disease is characterized by widespread necrotic keratinocytes, lymphocytic infiltration, and full-thickness epidermal necrosis with sloughing from the dermal-epidermal junction which is the cause of positive Nikolsky's sign (separation of epidermis at the subbasilar plane with gentle lateral pressure) [6]. Immunohistochemical studies revealed that CD8+ T lymphocytes predominate in the epidermis, whereas CD4+ T lymphocytes predominate in the dermis [2].

Management of patients with SJS or TEN mainly requires immediate withdrawal of the drug, which are the most important actions affecting significantly morbidity and mortality. Then, supportive and symptomatic treatment should be performed in intensive care units or burn centers, which include body temperature control, hydration, and electrolyte replacement, special attention to the airways, preventing secondary infection, pain control, maintenance of venous access distant from the affected areas, early oral nutrition or parenteral nutrition (if necessary), and anticoagulation [5].

Skin lesions are treated in the same manner of extensive burns treatment. Topical antiseptics can be used, but silver sulfadiazine should be avoided due to the association between SJS and sulfonamides [7].

Prophylactic antibiotic therapy is not recommended as it can increase microbial resistance. Some antibiotics can also trigger SJS/TEN, so their use should only be in cases of proven infection, a positive bacterial culture, the presence of high-grade fever, or significant leukocytosis [8]. In our case, the presence of high-grade fever increases the suspicion of infection, so a prophylactic antibiotic was given till the culture revealed multidrug-resistant *Acinetobacter baumannii* infection.

Active interventions specific to SJS and TEN are controversial. The low prevalence of the disease and its high mortality rate make it difficult to perform randomized clinical trials on SJS/TEN patients. Some reviews concluded that steroids do not shorten the duration of disease and may also increase the risk of sepsis and delay wound healing. Many authors do not recommend the routine use of systemic steroids in the treatment of SJS/TEN; however, some centers advocate an early pulse (first 48 hours) [7, 8].

Viard et al., in 1998, reported that commercial preparations of IVIG contained anti-Fas (anti-CD95) antibodies that blocked Fas-FasL interaction, thus intervening in disease the pathogenesis [9]. Successful treatment depends on the dose and its early use [10–12]. In our case, plasmapheresis and IVIG showed vast improvement in the patient's condition.

Mainly, the prognosis is significantly linked to early diagnosis with rapid identification of the causative drug and its discontinuation and appropriate treatment initiation. The prognosis does not seem to be affected by the type or the dose of the drug [5].

The SCORTEN score which was introduced in 2000 by Bastuji-Garin et al. [13] can be used to determine the prognosis and mortality rate in patients with SJS and TEN. Interestingly, one study published by some of the authors of the original SCORTEN paper found that the predictive value of the SCORTEN is most accurate when calculated on the 3rd day of hospitalization. Therefore, Guegan et al. [14] suggested that the SCORTEN score should be calculated not only on day 1 but also on day 3 of hospitalization [15]. Other factors associated with poor prognosis include late removal of the causative drug and delay in transfer of the patient to the burn unit [5].

4. Conclusion

In our case, treatment with plasmapheresis and intravenous immunoglobulin therapy were a successful management for the patient. Thus, we hope that our case will help other physicians in the treatment of toxic epidermal necrosis and Stevens-Johnson syndrome, since there is no stipulated and definitive treatment to both conditions, and they are both severe and life-threating diseases that need prompt management. Hence, we suggest more investigations regarding the management of these conditions hoping that in the future a specific treatment will be available.

Consent

Written informed consent was obtained from the patient itself for publication of this case report and accompanying images.

Authors' Contributions

Mohammad Kharraz conceptualized and designed the study. Yousef S. Abuzneid, Hussam I. A. Alzeerelhouseini, Duha Rabi, Ihab Hilail, Hatem Rjoob, Abdelrahman Rabee, Naser Amro, and Qutaiba Qafisheh wrote the manuscript. Yousef S. Abuzneid, Hussam I. A. Alzeerelhouseini. Yousef S. Abuzneid, and Hussam I. A reviewed and edited the manuscript. Alzeerelhouseini contributed equally to this work.

References

[1] E. P. Borrelli, E. Y. Lee, A. M. Descoteaux, S. J. Kogut, and A. R. Caffrey, "Stevens-johnson syndrome and toxic epidermal necrolysis with antiepileptic drugs: an analysis of the US food and drug administration adverse event reporting system," *Epilepsia*, vol. 59, no. 12, pp. 2318–2324, 2018.

[2] L.-Y. Huang, W.-C. Liao, C.-C. Chiou, J.-P. Lou, P. Hu, and F.-C. Ko, "Fatal toxic epidermal necrolysis induced by carbamazepine treatment in a patient who previously had carbamazepine-induced Stevens-Johnson syndrome," *Journal of the Formosan Medical Association*, vol. 106, no. 12, pp. 1032–1037, 2007.

[3] S. A. Nasir, H. L. Tan, H. J. Tan, H. M. Hussaini, and R. Ramli, "Stevens-johnson syndrome following failure of genetic screening prior to carbamazepine prescription," *Case Reports in Dentistry*, vol. 2017, Article ID 4201357, 5 pages, 2017.

[4] J. T. Masuka, S. Khoza, and D. Chibanda, "An interesting case of carbamazepine-induced stevens-johnson syndrome," *Drug Safety—Case Reports*, vol. 6, no. 1, p. 1, 2018.

[5] A. Wong, A. A. Malvestiti, and M. d F. S. Hafner, "Stevens-Johnson syndrome and toxic epidermal necrolysis: a review," *Revista da Associação Médica Brasileira (1992)*, vol. 62, no. 5, pp. 468–473, 2016.

[6] N. N. Ferguson, "Stevens-johnson syndrome/toxic epidermal necrolysis," in *Inpatient Dermatology*, M. Rosenbach, K. Wanat, R. Micheletti, and L. Taylor, Eds., Springer, Cham, Germany, 2018.

[7] R. A. Schwartz, P. H. McDonough, and B. W. Lee, "Toxic epidermal necrolysis," *Journal of the American Academy of Dermatology*, vol. 69, no. 2, p. 173.el, 2013.

[8] R. L. Hamm, "Drug-hypersensitivity syndrome: diagnosis and treatment," *Journal of the American College of Clinical Wound Specialists*, vol. 3, no. 4, pp. 77–81, 2011.

[9] I. Viard, P. Wehrli, R. Bullani et al., "Inhibition of toxic epidermal necrolysis by blockade of CD95 with human intravenous immunoglobulin," *Science*, vol. 282, no. 5388, pp. 490–493, 1998.

[10] S. L. Fernando, "The management of toxic epidermal necrolysis," *Australasian Journal of Dermatology*, vol. 53, no. 3, pp. 165–171, 2012.

[11] J. Cotliar, "Approach to the patient with a suspected drug eruption," *Seminars in Cutaneous Medicine and Surgery*, vol. 26, no. 3, pp. 147–154, 2007.

[12] P.-D. Ghislain and J.-C. Roujeau, "Treatment of severe drug reactions: Stevens-Johnson syndrome, toxic epidermal necrolysis and hypersensitivity syndrome," *Dermatology Online Journal*, vol. 8, no. 1, pp. 1087–1108, 2002.

[13] S. Bastuji-Garin, B. Rzany, R. S. Stern, N. H. Shear, L. Naldi, and J. C. Roujeau, "Clinical classification of cases of toxic epidermal necrolysis, Stevens-Johnson syndrome, and erythema multiforme," *Archives of Dermatology*, vol. 129, no. 1, pp. 92–96, 1993.

[14] S. Guégan, S. Bastuji-Garin, E. Poszepczynska-Guigné, J.-C. Roujeau, and J. Revuz, "Performance of the SCORTEN during the first five days of hospitalization to predict the prognosis of epidermal necrolysis," *Journal of Investigative Dermatology*, vol. 126, no. 2, pp. 272–276, 2006.

[15] J. A. Schneider and P. R. Cohen, "Stevens-johnson syndrome and toxic epidermal necrolysis: a concise review with a comprehensive summary of therapeutic interventions emphasizing supportive measures," *Advances in Therapy*, vol. 34, no. 6, pp. 1235–1244, 2017.

27

Syringocystadenocarcinoma Papilliferum in a Fifteen-Year-Old Girl: A Case Report and Review of the Literature

Jordan N. Halsey,[1] Esteban Fernandez Faith,[2,3] Suzanna J. Logan,[3,4] Archana Shenoy,[3,4] Kathleen M. Schieffer,[5] Catherine E. Cottrell,[3,5] Anna P. Lillis,[6] Jennifer H. Aldrink,[3,7] Bhuvana A. Setty,[8] and Gregory D. Pearson[1,3]

[1]*Department of Plastic Surgery, Nationwide Children's Hospital, Columbus, OH, USA*
[2]*Division of Dermatology, Department of Pediatrics, Nationwide Children's Hospital, Columbus, OH, USA*
[3]*The Ohio State University College of Medicine, Columbus, OH, USA*
[4]*Department of Pathology and Laboratory Medicine, Nationwide Children's Hospital, Columbus, OH, USA*
[5]*The Steve and Cindy Rasmussen Institute for Genomic Medicine, Nationwide Children's Hospital, Columbus, OH, USA*
[6]*Department of Radiology, Nationwide Children's Hospital, Columbus, OH, USA*
[7]*Department of Surgery, Division of Pediatric Surgery, Nationwide Children's Hospital, Columbus, OH, USA*
[8]*Division of Hematology/Oncology/BMT, Nationwide Children's Hospital, Columbus, OH, USA*

Correspondence should be addressed to Jordan N. Halsey; jordanhalseymd@gmail.com

Academic Editor: Alireza Firooz

Syringocystadenocarcinoma papilliferum (SCACP) is a rare malignant neoplasm arising from adnexal tissues and is the malignant complement to the benign neoplasm syringocystadenoma papilliferum (SCAP). SCACP lesions appear as raised nodules or inflammatory plaques and can be associated with SCAP or nevus sebaceous. There have been fewer than 100 described cases of this neoplasm in the literature, and all previously published cases have been described in adults, with the majority occurring in the elderly. We present a case of an adolescent female with a syringocystadenocarcinoma papilliferum arising from a large thigh mass harboring an in-frame alteration in *MAP2K1* along with a brief review of the literature.

1. Case Report

A fifteen-year-old female presented to our institution with a large pedunculated posterior thigh mass. According to the patient's mother, the lesion initially appeared as "three small cuts" at birth and grew proportionally with the patient, now appearing hypervascular and measuring $11.5 \times 6 \times 2$ cm in size (Figure 1). There were no reports of pain or bleeding from the lesion, and a review of systems confirmed constitutional symptoms were negative.

There was no prior imaging. An ultrasonographic examination demonstrated two hypoechoic masses with Doppler flow showing arterial and venous enhancement. A subsequent MRI showed the extent of the masses to be $11.9\text{ cm} \times 6.3\text{ cm} \times 1.8\text{ cm}$, extending down to muscle fascia with robust perfusion supplied by perforators of the deep femoral artery (Figure 2). The patient's overall presentation and imaging was discussed at an interdisciplinary vascular malformations conference; the leading diagnosis at that time was syringocystadenoma papilliferum (SCAP). Surgical excision to grossly negative margins was performed with primary wound closure.

Microscopic examination revealed an exophytic, papillary lesion with an abrupt transition from the skin surface, overlying a tubular and cystic component diffusely involving the dermis (Figure 3(a)). Papillae were lined by a florid epithelial proliferation forming tufts and maze-like intraepithelial spaces along the lesional surface, with complex glandular spaces within expanded papillary cores (Figure 3(b)). Outer epithelial cells exhibited crowding and

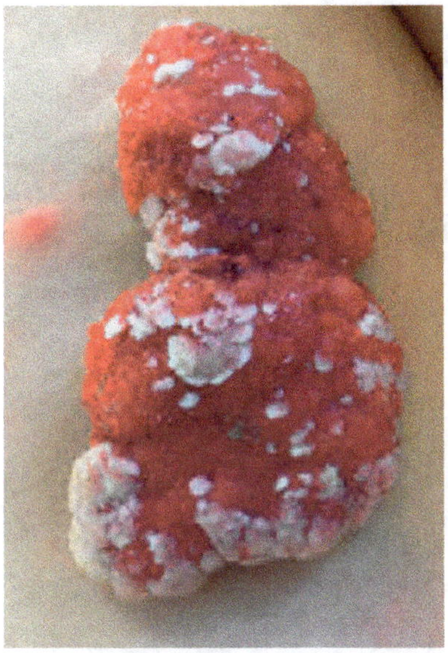

FIGURE 1: Left posterior thigh pedunculated mass.

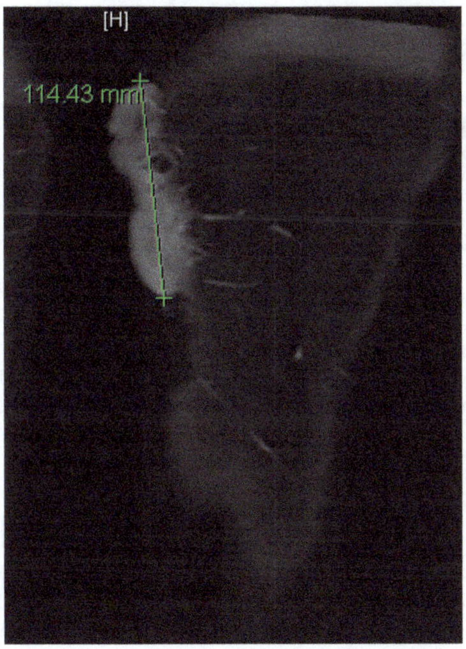

FIGURE 2: MRI imaging of the left thigh showing posteromedial mass, with arterial blood supply from branches of the deep femoral artery.

disarray and were delimited by a distinct basal cell layer (Figure 3(c)). These lesional cells possessed an eosinophilic cytoplasm, atypical nuclei, fine to optically clear chromatin, and prominent nucleoli (Figure 3(c)). Stromal plasma cell clusters were readily identified within the papillary cores. The deep component extended throughout the dermis and into the subcutaneous tissue, extending to margins of resection. This component was characterized by small tubules lined by a multilayered epithelium with the surface resembling large, dilated glands consistent with an apocrine tubular adenoma component (Figure 3(d)).

Focally, tubules and glands contained intraluminal proteinaceous material with single necrotic cells. Mitotic figures up to 3 per mm^2 were present throughout the lesion. CK7 immunohistochemistry was diffusely positive in the epithelial cells of the exophytic component and luminal epithelial cells in the dermal component (Figure 3(e)). Based on the florid epithelial proliferation, increased nuclear atypia, and mitotic activity, final diagnosis was SCACP, arising in an SCAP. P63 immunohistochemistry was performed on different blocks and demonstrated basal cells at the periphery of lesional glands and tubules throughout the dermis (Figure 3(f)) as well as in the exophytic component, indicating an *in situ* carcinoma.

In response to the SCACP diagnosis, diagnostic imaging of the chest, abdomen, and pelvis with computed tomography (CT) (chest) and magnetic resonance imaging (MRI) (abdomen/pelvis), as well as a full-body PET scan, were obtained. No distant metastases were identified. To complete staging, a left inguinal sentinel lymph node biopsy was performed in conjunction with wide reresection using 2 cm margins. Reresection included all subcutaneous tissue to the level of the semimembranosus muscle fascia in order to ensure complete resection. A skin graft was required to close the large defect on the posterior thigh, which healed well without complication (Figure 4). Although residual SCACP was identified within subcutaneous tissue, surgical margins and sentinel lymph nodes were negative. The patient is now doing well and will be closely followed up for recurrence with routine surveillance.

Given the rare diagnosis of SCACP, the patient was enrolled on an institutional translational research protocol (see the supplementary materials (available here)). Paired comparator germline and disease-involved enhanced exome sequencing was performed to evaluate for single-nucleotide variants (SNVs), small insertion-deletions (indels), and copy number alterations (CNAs). RNA sequencing of disease-involved tissue was performed to assess for gene fusions, complex structural rearrangements, and outlier gene expression. We did not identify any clearly medically meaningful variation in cancer or other disease-associated genes in the comparator germline. Furthermore, no somatic CNAs, gene fusions, or complex structural rearrangements were identified. The tumor tissue harbored a complex indel in exon 3 of *MAP2K1* (NM_002755.4, encoding MEK1) resulting in an in-frame deletion of codons Leu101-Lys104 (ΔLEIK), replaced with two amino acids (Asn and Ser) (c.301_311delinsAATTC:p.Leu101_Lys104delinsAsnSer) (Figure 5(a)). This in-frame complex indel was confirmed by Sanger sequencing (Figure 5(b)). Although this particular alteration has not been described in the literature, deletions of amino acids encompassed within this alteration, specifically p.Glu102_Ile103del, are described in cancer databases, such as cBioPortal (Figure 5(c)). In-frame deletions constituting part of the $\beta3$-αC loop within the kinase domain (encoded by amino acids 98–104) encompass a class of MAP2K1 variants that demonstrate RAF-independent

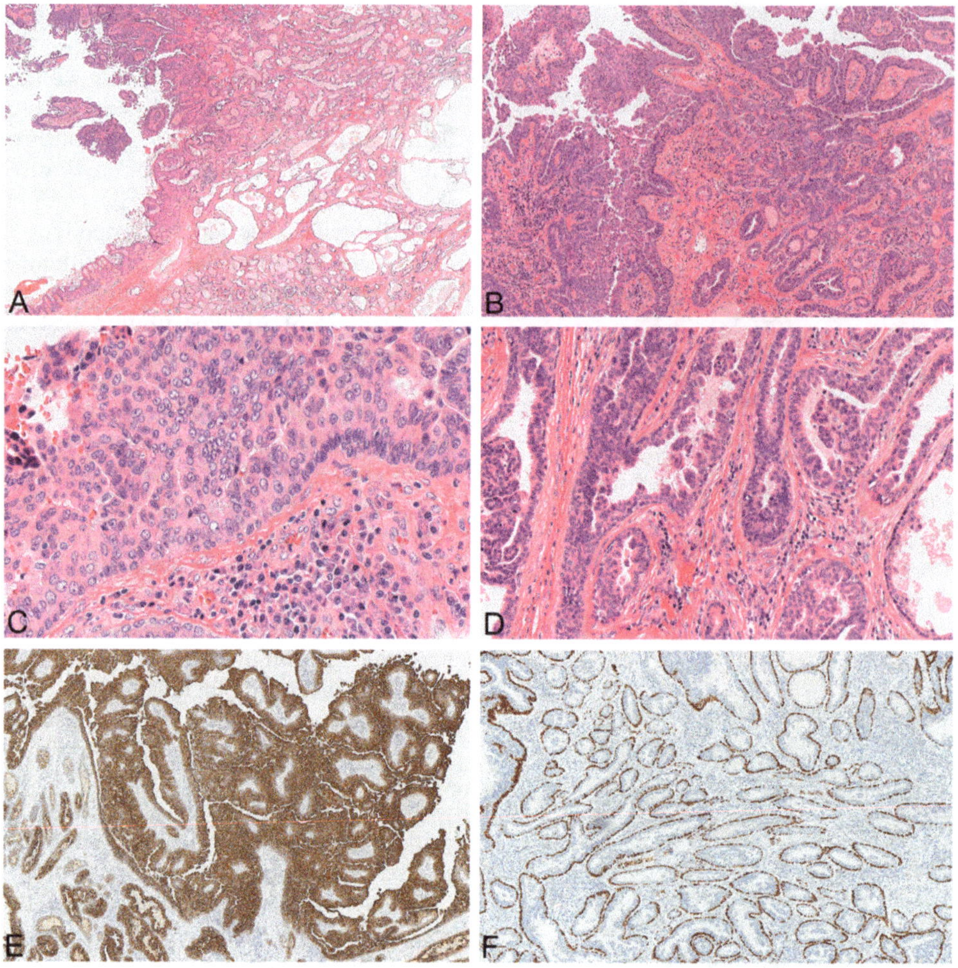

Figure 3: The tumor was composed of both exophytic and underlying infiltrative components, the former showing a papillary pattern similar to syringocystadenoma papilliferum and the latter showing closely spaced tubular glands similar to tubular apocrine adenoma (a). Florid overgrowth of the outer epithelial cells produced complex, maze-like spaces between epithelial cells and cellular tufts off the surface of the tumor (b). The outer epithelial cells showed crowded, overlapping, atypical nuclei with prominent nucleoli with mitotic activity (c). The inner luminal cells of the dermal glands demonstrated bulbous, micropapillary projections (d). CK7 was diffusely expressed by both outer epithelial cells of the papillae and inner luminal cells of the dermal glands (e). P63-positive basal cells bordered the papillae and glands (f).

constitutive signaling due to receptor homodimerization and transphosphorylation.

This patient is the youngest described case of SCACP in the literature, which reports the median age of SCACP to be 63.6 years (reported range 22–93) [1]. These lesions are known to arise from existing SCAP lesions or nevus sebaceous and commonly occur within the head and neck [2, 3]. SCACP often presents as a fleshy or vascular-appearing exophytic tumor with overlying crusting due to the exudative nature of the apocrine glands [4]. These masses can also ulcerate and become painful [5].

Wide local excision is the treatment of choice for SCACP, though there have been cases where SCACP was treated effectively with chemotherapy and radiation in patients with inoperable tumors or who are poor surgical candidates [6]. Specific recommendations regarding surgical margins have not been established. In evaluating data from 49 patients with SCACP, locoregional lymph node metastasis was reported in 22% of patients and distant metastasis in 6% of patients. All patients with disseminated disease in this case series expired from sequelae related to their SCACP diagnosis [1]. Local recurrence with and without distant metastasis has been described [1, 3]. Although SCACP has been traditionally thought to be a low-grade malignancy with a favorable prognosis [7], more recent studies suggest close follow-up is warranted.

Pathologic examination of SCACP resembles SCAP. In both variants, the epithelium is typically composed of an inner columnar cell layer and an outer cuboidal layer. The stroma of the tumor often contains plasma cells and other inflammatory cells [8]. In SCACP, the tumors can extend into underlying tissues and exhibit a high nuclear-to-cytoplasmic ratio, coarse chromatin, and increased mitotic activity [9]. Several of these characteristics were noted in our patient's tumor.

Histologically, SCACP can vary widely in presentation, ranging from an adenocarcinoma-like appearance to having features more consistent with invasive squamous cell carcinoma [10]. This histologic variability can make differentiation of SCACP from other neoplasms arising from

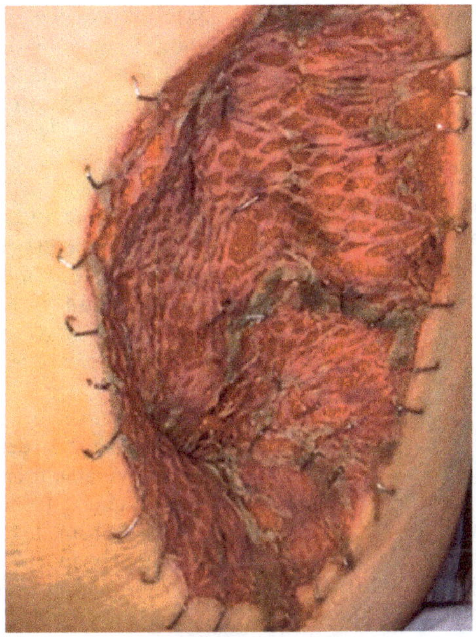

FIGURE 4: Postoperative image following reresection with margins and skin graft placement.

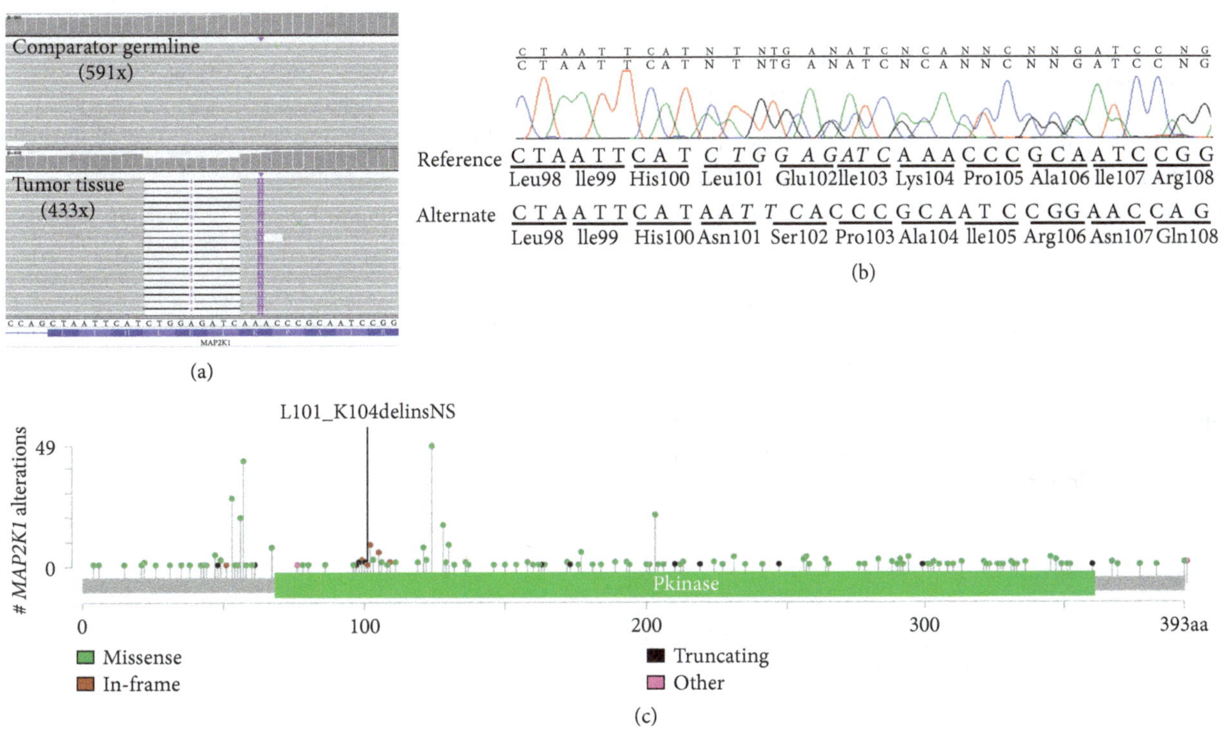

FIGURE 5: (a) Integrative genomics viewer image of aligned sequencing reads for exon 3 of MAP2K1 derived from enhanced exome sequencing. The top panel shows the comparator germline (peripheral blood) with the absence of the complex indel at an average of 591*x* depth for this region. The bottom panel shows the tumor tissue demonstrating an in-frame complex indel with an average of 433*x* depth for this region. (b) Sanger sequencing chromatogram of the in-frame *MAP2K1* (NM_002755.4) complex indel (c.301_311delinsAATTC: p.Leu101_Lys104delinsAsnSer). The corresponding amino acid sequence is described below the genomic sequence. Italicized reference sequence in red indicates the deletion, and the italicized alternate sequence in blue indicates the insertion. (c) Lollipop plot of *MAP2K1* variants deposited in cBioPortal. The p.Leu101_Lys104delinsAsnSer described in this report has not been previously reported.

adnexal structures challenging [11]. Moreover, distant metastasis from other primary adenocarcinomas can also resemble SCACP [5]. Characteristics that can aid in the diagnosis of SCACP include the continuity with the epidermis and visualization of areas of residual SCAP or sebaceous nevus [10]. Histologic staining, especially with p63 stains and GCDFP-15, can also be useful to aid in diagnosis [11].

The genetic landscape of SCACP is poorly characterized; however, aberrant signaling of the RAS-MAPK pathway has been associated with benign precursors, including nevus sebaceous and SCAP. Mosaicism for *HRAS* p.Gly13Arg and *KRAS* p.Gly12Asp was first described in nevus sebaceous, prompting additional study in secondary tumors arising from this lesion. *BRAF* p.Val600Glu was later identified in a subset of SCAP. In this case report, we expand the genomic landscape to include activating alterations within the *MAP2K1* gene, as the *MAP2K1* p.Leu101_Lys104delinsAsnSer is predicted to activate RAS-MAPK signaling. Given the clinical utility of MEK inhibitors in tumors with described RAS-MAPK pathway activation and ongoing clinical trials, the utility for targeted inhibition in patients with in-frame MEK1 β3-αC loop alterations has been explored. Notably, allosteric MEK inhibitors (MEKi), such as trametinib, are ATP noncompetitive kinase inhibitors that bind and stabilize an inactive conformation of MEK1. *MAP2K1* missense and in-frame deletions occurring outside of the β3-αC loop (amino acids 98–104) demonstrate full or partial dependence on RAF activation and exhibit sensitivity to allosteric MEKi. However, in-frame deletions within the β3-αC loop, such as described in this report, result in RAF-independent stability of the inactive MEK conformation and resistance to allosteric MEKi. A selective ATP-competitive MEKi, MAP855, has shown promising results through inhibition of pERK across all *MAP2K1* alterations and may be of future benefit to patients with tumor harboring in-frame β3-αC loop deletions.

In conclusion, SCACP is a rare malignancy often arising within an existing nevus sebaceous or SCAP in adults. Our case report demonstrates that SCACP can also rarely affect pediatric patients. Awareness of such atypical presentations can facilitate timely diagnosis. Standard clinical management guidelines for surgical management and surveillance are lacking, and future studies outlining strategies for clinical management are desired.

Disclosure

This research was performed by physicians employed at Nationwide Children's Hospital in Columbus, Ohio.

References

[1] K. G. Lee, W. Choi, J. S. Lim, H. J. Hahn, K. B. Myung, and S. H. Cheong, "Syringocystadenocarcinoma papilliferum: a case report and review of the literature," *Annals of Dermatology*, vol. 31, no. 5, pp. 559–562, 2019.

[2] R. Bondi and C. Urso, "Syringocystadenocarcinoma papilliferum," *Histopathology*, vol. 28, no. 5, pp. 475–477, 1996.

[3] L. Castillo, A. Moreno, and J. C. Tardío, "Syringocystadenocarcinoma papilliferum in situ: report of a case with late recurrence," *The American Journal of Dermatopathology*, vol. 36, no. 4, pp. 348–352, 2014.

[4] D. V. Kazakov, L. Requena, H. Kutzner et al., "Morphologic diversity of syringocystadenocarcinoma papilliferum based on a clinicopathologic study of 6 cases and review of the literature," *The American Journal of Dermatopathology*, vol. 32, no. 4, pp. 340–347, 2010.

[5] Y. Zhang, Y.-Y. Kong, X. Cai, X.-X. Shen, and J.-C. Kong, "Syringocystadenocarcinoma papilliferum: clinicopathologic analysis of 10 cases," *Journal of Cutaneous Pathology*, vol. 44, no. 6, pp. 538–543, 2017.

[6] P. B. Rao, S. Ghosh, M. Mohapatra et al., "Chemoradiotherapy in a case of malignant syringocystadenocarcinoma papilliferum of vulva with loco-regional failure," *Case Reports in Oncological Medicine*, vol. 2015, Article ID 638294, 4 pages, 2015.

[7] J. Peterson, K. Tefft, J. Blackmon, A. Rajpara, and G. Fraga, "Syringocystadenocarcinoma papilliferum: a rare tumor with a favorable prognosis," *Dermatology Online Journal*, vol. 19, Article ID 19620, 2013.

[8] M. S. Kim, J. H. Lee, W.-M. Lee, and S.-J. Son, "A case of tubular apocrine adenoma with syringocystadenoma papilliferum that developed in a nevus sebaceus," *Annals of Dermatology*, vol. 22, no. 3, pp. 319–322, 2010.

[9] J. Chen, M. Beg, and S. Chen, "Syringocystadenocarcinoma papilliferum in situ, a variant of cutaneous adenocarcinoma in situ: a case report with literature review," *The American Journal of Dermatopathology*, vol. 38, no. 10, pp. 762–765, 2016.

[10] N. Leeborg, M. Thompson, S. Rossmiller, N. Gross, C. White, and K. Gatter, "Diagnostic pitfalls in syringocystadenocarcinoma papilliferum: case report and review of the literature," *Archives of Pathology & Laboratory Medicine*, vol. 134, no. 8, pp. 1205–1209, 2010.

[11] A. Ishida-Yamamoto, K. Sato, T. Wada, H. Takahashi, and H. Iizuka, "Syringo-cystadenocarcinoma papilliferum: case report and immunohistochemical comparison with its benign counterpart," *Journal of the American Academy of Dermatology*, vol. 45, no. 5, pp. 755–759, 2001.

28

Acquired Acrodermatitis Enteropathica in a 28-Year-Old Male with Type 1 Diabetes

Owen Ngalamika[1,2] **Wencilaus M. P. Selvaraj,**[1] **Fatima K. Yikona,**[3] **and Chibamba Mumba**[2,4]

[1]*Dermatology and Venereology Division, University Teaching Hospital, Lusaka, Zambia*
[2]*University of Zambia School of Medicine, Lusaka, Zambia*
[3]*Chelston Level One Hospital, Lusaka, Zambia*
[4]*Pathology and Microbiology Department, University Teaching Hospital, Lusaka, Zambia*

Correspondence should be addressed to Owen Ngalamika; owen_ngalamika@yahoo.com

Academic Editor: Sergio A. Cuevas Covarrubias

Acrodermatitis enteropathica (AE) is a rare disorder arising from inherited or acquired zinc deficiency. It is mainly characterized by acral dermatitis, periorificial dermatitis, alopecia, and gastrointestinal symptoms in the form of diarrhea. There are many complications of AE including local and systemic infections that may develop as a result of untreated AE. In addition, due to the role of zinc in glucose metabolism, chronic zinc deficiency may pose a challenge in the control of blood glucose levels in diabetics. We report the case of a 28-year-old male with type 1 diabetes who presented with signs and symptoms of AE.

1. Introduction

Acrodermatitis enteropathica (AE) is a rare disorder that is a result of a defect in zinc absorption. The primary form of AE is an autosomal recessive disorder due to mutations in the *SLC39A4* gene encoding a transmembrane zinc transporter protein [1]. The acquired form of AE may be due to inadequate zinc intake, conditions such as inflammatory bowel syndrome that may reduce zinc absorption, and excessive zinc excretion [2]. Classical clinical manifestations of AE include inflammation and/or blistering of the skin in the acral areas and around the mouth, hair loss, and diarrhea.

Zinc is an essential trace element that has many physiological functions including regulation of the immune system, wound healing, and growth [3, 4]. Zinc deficiency is associated with many conditions including diarrhea disease, lung and gastrointestinal infections, and poor wound healing [5, 6]. Here, we present the case of a young adult male who presented with signs and symptoms of AE.

2. Case Presentation

A 28-year-old male was referred from a primary-level hospital to the University Teaching Hospital (a tertiary-level hospital located in the city of Lusaka, Zambia) for adult onset of malnutrition. The patient had a history of generalized body swelling for 6 months. He also had loss of appetite and watery diarrhea (five times a day) for a duration of 5 months. The patient also gave a history of developing blisters in the lower limbs, upper limbs, and abdomen which later ruptured and peeled off resulting in hyperpigmentation of the affected areas. The lesions started on the lower limbs and then moved upwards to involve the trunk and upper limbs. He also gave a history of hair loss and discoloration. He denied other symptoms such as cough, fever, paroxysmal nocturnal dyspnea, or joint pains. Despite treatment at the local clinic, the condition continued to deteriorate, and therefore, he was referred to our tertiary institution for further management. The patient was a type 1 diabetic and was on insulin for 3 years prior to admission. He was said to be in good health before this illness. He gave a history of smoking and was a heavy alcohol drinker until he became unwell a few months before admission.

On admission to the University Teaching Hospital, the patient underwent a full clinical assessment including laboratory investigations. On examination, the patient was lethargic and was unable to sit without support. His blood pressure was 93/60 mmHg, body temperature was 35.7°C, radial pulse rate was 89 beats per minute, respiratory rate was 24 breaths per minute, and peripheral oxygen saturation was 100%. He had conjunctival and palmar pallor with no signs of jaundice. He was noted to have generalized body swelling mostly involving the periorbital area, hands, and abdomen (ascites). His tongue was glossy and beefy red, and he had gingivitis and angular cheilitis. On local examination of the skin, he was noted to have hyperpigmented patches and erosions with some intact bullae on both the upper and lower limbs and the abdomen. The patient was also noted to have sparse hair with brownish discoloration (Figure 1). On examination of the genitalia, he was noted to have extensive skin erosions and scrotal swelling. Examination of the respiratory and cardiovascular systems was significant for a resting tachycardia and bibasal posterior crepitations. He had mild pedal edema on the lower limbs, feet, and hands. In addition, he had an infected ulcer on the left antecubital fossa.

A number of laboratory investigations were conducted which included a complete blood count which showed severe anemia, liver function test which revealed a hypoalbuminemia, and kidney function tests which were normal (Table 1). A pus swab for microscopy and culture collected from the infected ulcer located on the left antecubital fossa showed the presence of *Staphylococcus aureus* and Acinetobacter species. Blood culture initially showed *Staphylococcus aureus*, and a repeat blood culture performed two weeks later showed the presence of yeast cells and Gram-negative bacilli. Other organisms identified on the same culture were *Candida* and *Klebsiella pneumoniae* species. A skin biopsy of an intact lesion was performed, and it showed features consistent with AE including spongiosis with epidermal pallor, parakeratosis, and keratinocyte necrolysis (Figure 2). Upper gastrointestinal endoscopy was performed and showed villous blunting, and biopsies of the duodenum and ilium were also performed and showed blunting of the villi (Figure 3).

A diagnosis of acquired AE with sepsis was made based on the clinical findings. The differential diagnosis was pemphigus foliaceous. The patient was initiated on oral zinc sulphate at 50 mg three times a day with hematinics (folic acid and ferrous sulphate) and antibiotics. A few days after initiation of zinc, the patient showed remarkable improvement in the skin lesions including a reduction in the edema, resolution of diarrhea, and improvement in appetite (Figure 4). Measurement of plasma zinc levels was performed several days after the patient had been commenced on zinc sulphate and showed high zinc levels. On admission, he also received a blood transfusion for the anemia.

Despite improvement in the skin lesions and diarrhea, the patient's general condition continued to deteriorate. His sugar levels were fluctuating with episodes of hyper- and hypoglycemia, and he continued to have signs and symptoms of sepsis. The patient eventually died after 25 days of admission.

3. Discussion

AE is a rare disorder resulting from zinc deficiency. Primary AE is commonly diagnosed in childhood and has a strong genetic basis [7]. Acquired AE on the other hand is commonly a secondary manifestation of malabsorption syndromes [8]. While it is relatively easy to make a diagnosis of primary AE, secondary AE usually requires an exclusion of other possible disorders and also diagnosing other conditions that may predispose to zinc deficiency. Laboratory diagnostic tests for acquired AE are neither sensitive nor specific, and therefore, clinicians mostly depend on how the patient responds to zinc therapy [9].

Our patient had classical signs and symptoms of AE including perioral dermatitis, bullous eruptions in the acral areas and extremities, alopecia, and diarrhea. In addition, he also had other signs that were highly suggestive of AE including glossitis, anemia, and infections. His age at initial presentation was suggestive of the acquired instead of the primary form of AE. In addition, his history of heavy alcohol intake also supported a diagnosis of acquired AE as previously reported [8].

Individuals with zinc deficiency are susceptible to inflammatory dermatoses, which may include bullous eruptions, perioral dermatitis, and glossitis, as seen in our patient. Zinc is important in keratinocyte proliferation and differentiation [10]. Thus, zinc deficiency results in keratinocyte apoptosis [11] and poor differentiation [12], which were evident in our patient both clinically (bullae) and on pathology (parakeratosis).

Our patient had a skin infection and sepsis. Zinc is important in both innate and adaptive immune responses [13]. Zinc deficiency can result in an impaired innate immune system including reduced natural killer cell activity, impaired chemotaxis, phagocytosis, and microbicidal activity of neutrophils and monocytes/macrophages [5]. Zinc deficiency can also lead to a defective adaptive immune system by impairing the development and function of T cells [14]. Low levels of zinc in plasma are associated with an increased incidence of infections in the elderly [15]. Persistently low levels of serum zinc have also been associated with recurrent sepsis in critically ill patients [16]. In addition, zinc oxide nanoparticles have been observed to have antibacterial activity against infections by multiple organisms including methicillin-resistant *Staphylococcus aureus* [17]. Zinc deficiency may have been the predominant predisposing factor to the cutaneous infection and sepsis observed in our patient.

Our patient also had diarrhea, a common feature in AE. Zinc plays a key role in promoting growth and differentiation of enterocytes and inhibiting the excessive secretion of fluids and ions caused by some organisms including *Vibrio cholerae* and *Shigella* [18]. In addition, zinc is important in development and function of the innate and adaptive immune responses [18]. In particular, zinc has been shown to

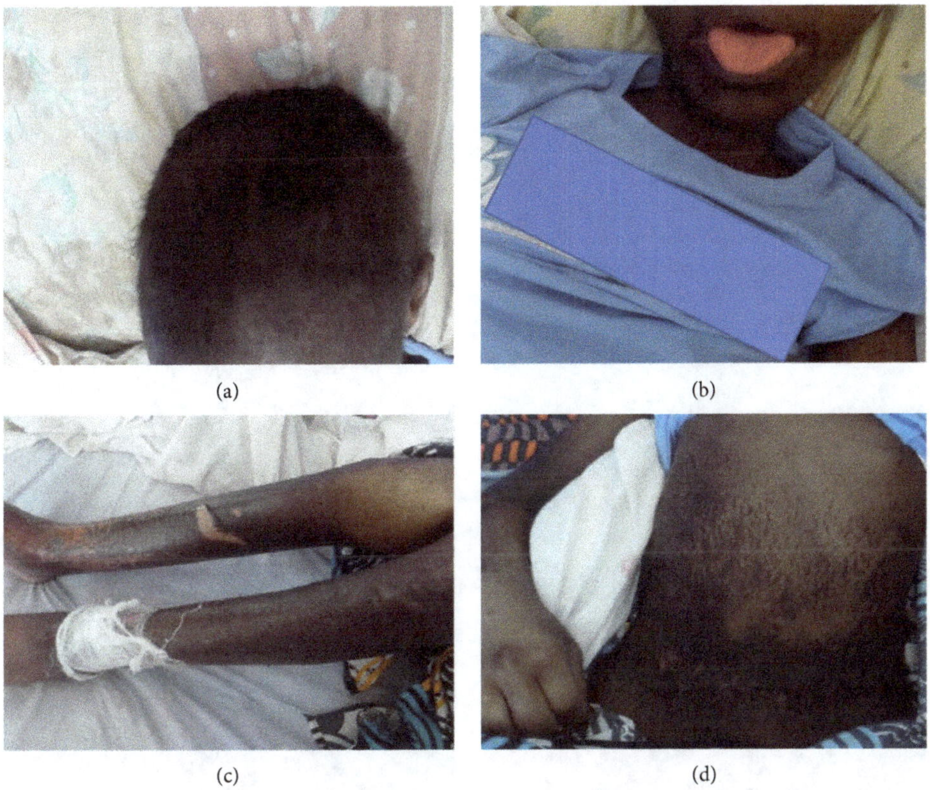

Figure 1: Dermatological manifestations on admission showing (a) hair dyspigmentation and alopecia; (b) perioral dermatitis and glossitis; and (c), (d) bullae and erosions.

Table 1: Laboratory investigations conducted.

	On admission	After admission	Reference range
Complete blood count*			
White cell count ($\times 10^9$/l)	6.30	7.20	4.00–10.00
Hemoglobin (g/dl)	6.5	8.5	13.0–17.00
Mean cell volume (fl)	82.3	82.9	83.0–101.0
Mean cell hemoglobin (pg)	26.7	25.7	27.0–32.0
Platelet count ($\times 10^9$/l)	155	123	150–410
Liver function tests			
Albumin (g/l)	10.6		35.0–52.0
Total protein (g/l)	36.6		60.0–78.0
Serum calcium (mg/dl)	1.48		2.15–2.50
Bilirubin (μmol/l)	5.4		2.0–21.0
Alanine transaminase (u/l)	37.7		0.0–45.0
Aspartate transaminase (u/l)	23.1		0.0–35.0
Kidney function tests			
Urea (mmol/l)	1.74		2.80–7.10
Creatinine (μmol/l)	55.9		59.0–104.0
Other tests			
Random blood sugar*	4.8	9.4	<11.0
Serum zinc (μmol/l)#	Unknown	22.4	10.7–18.4

*Repeat complete blood count and random blood sugar determined 2 days after admission; #serum zinc determined after 11 days of admission.

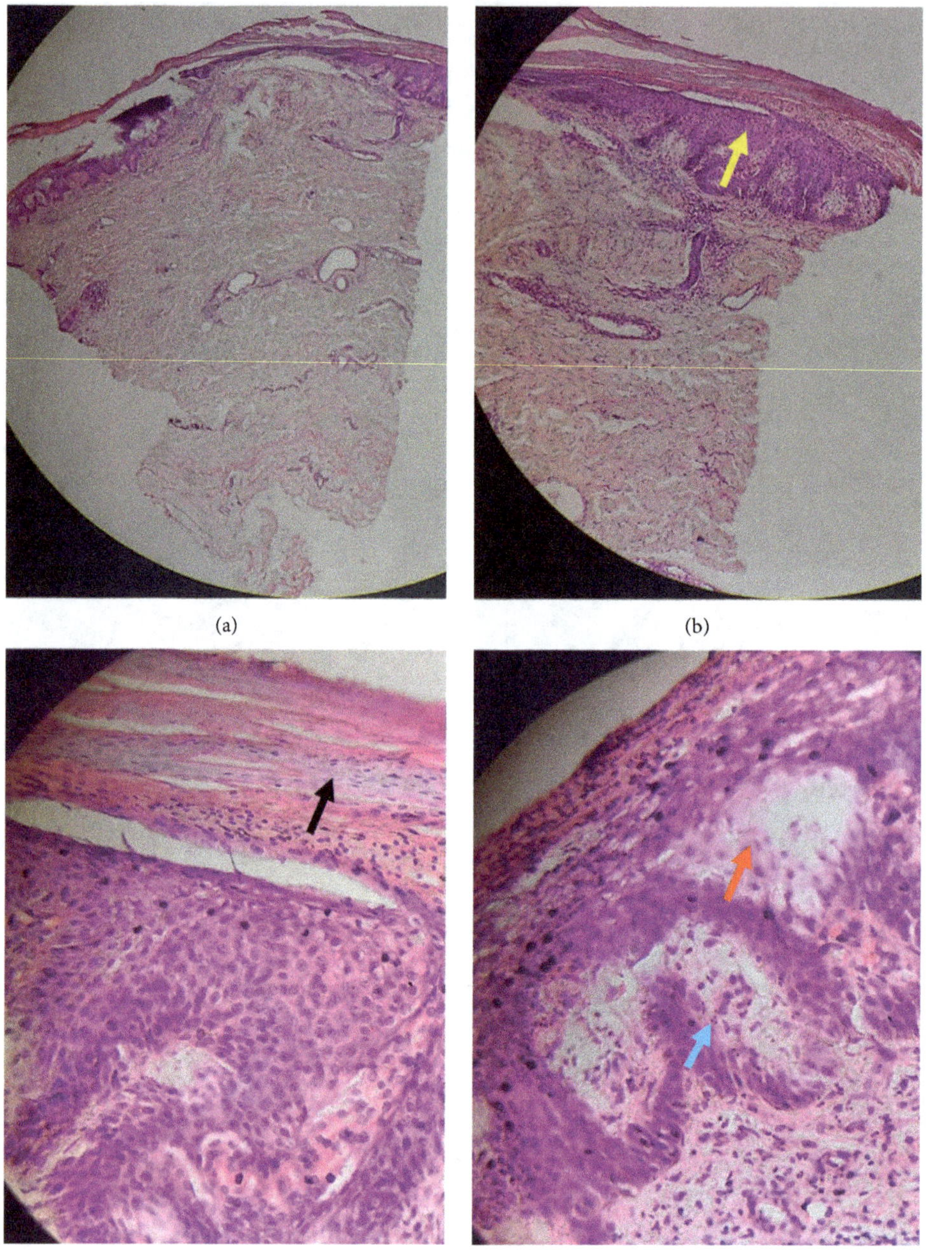

(a) (b) (c) (d)

Figure 2: Hematoxylin-and-eosin-stained skin biopsy showing (a) the epidermis and dermis; (b) acanthosis (yellow arrow); (c) parakeratosis (black arrow); and (d) neutrophilic epithelial infiltrate (blue arrow) and spongiosis (red arrow). (a) ×100, (b) ×200, and (c) and (d) ×400 magnification.

enhance innate immunity against enterotoxigenic *Escherichia coli* [19]. Both the skin and gastrointestinal infections could have been responsible for the sepsis observed in our patient, and zinc deficiency was most likely a significant predisposing factor for these infections.

Our patient was also a type 1 diabetic. Low serum zinc levels have been associated with poor glycemic control in both type 1 and 2 diabetics [20, 21]. Zinc is a cofactor in the synthesis, storage, and secretion of insulin [20]. In addition, since zinc is essential in the formation and function of antioxidant enzymes, zinc deficiency may result in an increase in intracellular oxidants and free radicals in diabetics [22]. The poor control of blood sugar levels in our patient could be attributed to the chronic hypozincemia.

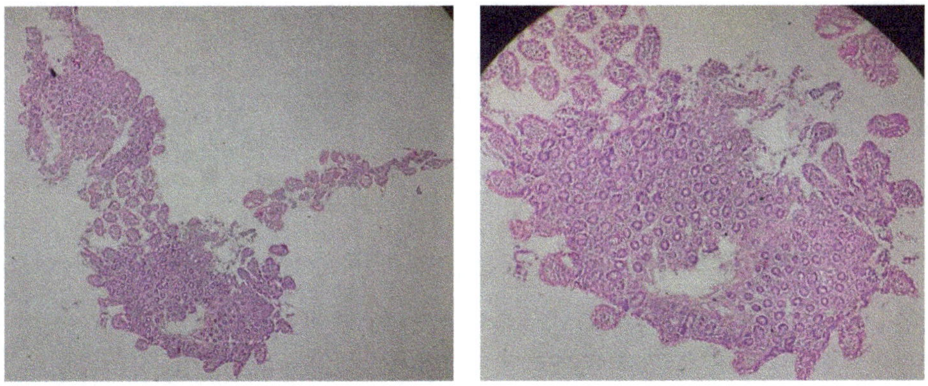

(a) (b)

FIGURE 3: Hematoxylin-and-eosin-stained ileal biopsy showing mild focal loss and blunting of the villi.

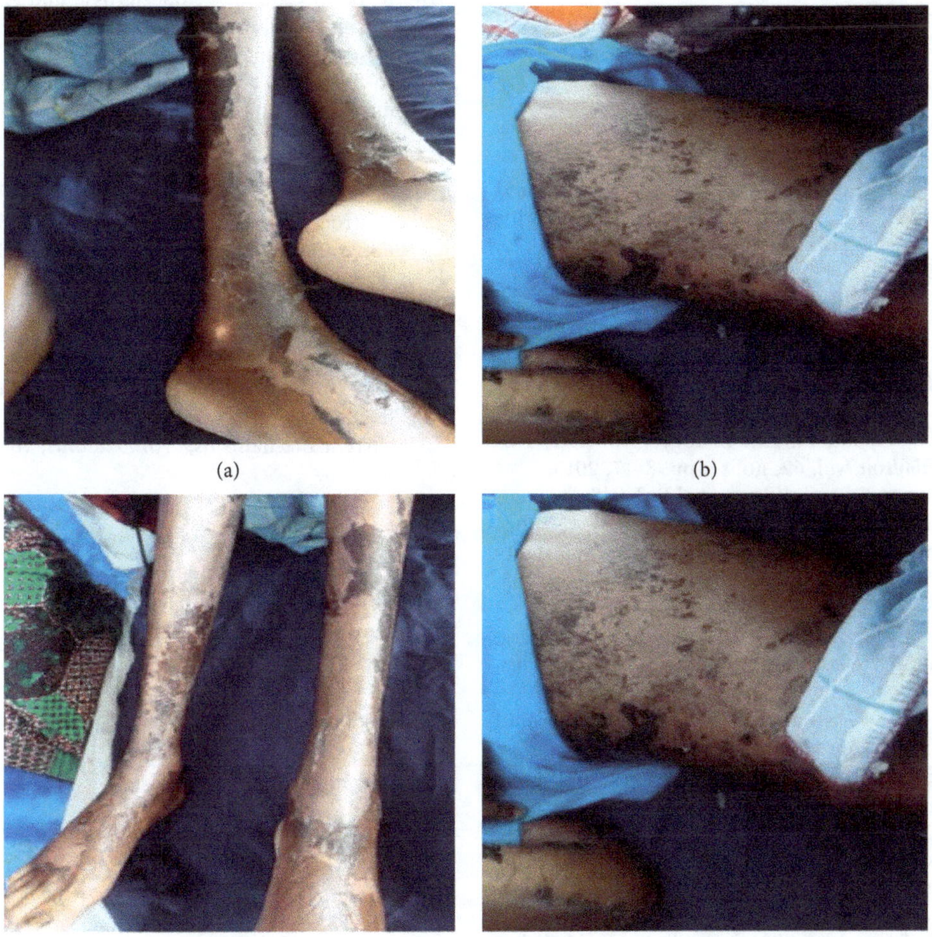

(a) (b) (c) (d)

FIGURE 4: Skin changes after zinc replacement with evident re-epithelialization after about a week of zinc supplementation.

4. Conclusions

Zinc deficiency in the form of AE is an uncommon condition that may lead to life-threatening complications if left untreated. Clinicians should have a high index of suspicion for possible zinc deficiency so as to treat the condition early and prevent the complications that may arise from it.

Consent

The authors obtained written informed consent from the patient for publication of this case report and accompanying images.

Acknowledgments

The authors are very grateful to the patient for consenting to publish this case while he was under our care.

References

[1] A. Nakano, H. Nakano, Y. Toyomaki, K. Hanada, and K. Nomura, "Novel SLC39A4 mutations in acrodermatitis enteropathica," *Journal of Investigative Dermatology*, vol. 120, no. 6, pp. 963–966, 2003.

[2] J. Uaariyapanichkul, P. Saengpanit, P. Damrongphol, K. Suphapeetiporn, and S. Chomtho, "Skin lesions associated with nutritional management of maple syrup urine disease," *Case Reports in Dermatological Medicine*, vol. 2017, Article ID 3905658, 2017.

[3] N. W. Solomons, "Update on zinc biology," *Annals of Nutrition and Metabolism*, vol. 62, no. s1, pp. 8–17, 2013.

[4] M. E. Penny, "Zinc supplementation in public health," *Annals of Nutrition and Metabolism*, vol. 62, no. s1, pp. 31–42, 2013.

[5] R. E. Black, "Zinc deficiency, infectious disease and mortality in the developing world," *The Journal of Nutrition*, vol. 133, no. 5, pp. 1485S–1489S, 2003.

[6] P. H. Lin, M. Sermersheim, H. Li, P. H. U. Lee, S. M. Steinberg, and J. Ma, "Zinc in wound healing modulation," *Nutrients*, vol. 10, no. 1, 2017.

[7] I. R. L. D. Ciampo, R. Sawamura, L. A. D. Ciampo, and M. I. M. Fernandes, "Acrodermatite enteropática: manifestações clínicas E diagnóstico pediátrico," *Revista Paulista de Pediatria*, vol. 36, no. 2, pp. 238–241, 2018.

[8] A. A. Chaudhry, M. M. Warthan, R. J. Pariser, and A. F. Hood, "Acquired acrodermatitis enteropathica secondary to alcoholism," *Cutis*, vol. 82, no. 1, pp. 60–62, 2008.

[9] N. Nistor, L. Ciontu, O.-E. Frasinariu, V. V. Lupu, A. Ignat, and V. Streanga, "Acrodermatitis enteropathica," *Medicine*, vol. 95, no. 20, Article ID e3553, 2016.

[10] Y. Ogawa, M. Kinoshita, S. Shimada, and T. Kawamura, "Zinc and skin disorders," *Nutrients*, vol. 10, no. 2, 2018.

[11] D. Wilson, G. Varigos, and M. L. Ackland, "Apoptosis may underlie the pathology of zinc-deficient skin," *Immunology & Cell Biology*, vol. 84, no. 1, pp. 28–37, 2006.

[12] B.-H. Bin, J. Bhin, N.-H. Kim et al., "An acrodermatitis enteropathica-associated Zn transporter, ZIP4, regulates human epidermal homeostasis," *Journal of Investigative Dermatology*, vol. 137, no. 4, pp. 874–883, 2017.

[13] W. Alker and H. Haase, "Zinc and sepsis," *Nutrients*, vol. 10, no. 8, 2018.

[14] H. Haase and L. Rink, "Zinc signals and immune function," *Biofactors*, vol. 40, no. 1, pp. 27–40, 2014.

[15] A. S. Prasad, F. W. Beck, B. Bao et al., "Zinc supplementation decreases incidence of infections in the elderly: effect of zinc on generation of cytokines and oxidative stress," *The American Journal of Clinical Nutrition*, vol. 85, no. 3, pp. 837–844, 2007.

[16] J. Hoeger, T.-P. Simon, T. Beeker, G. Marx, H. Haase, and T. Schuerholz, "Persistent low serum zinc is associated with recurrent sepsis in critically ill patients - a pilot study," *PLoS One*, vol. 12, no. 5, Article ID e0176069, 2017.

[17] U. Kadiyala, E. S. Turali-Emre, J. H. Bahng, N. A. Kotov, and J. S. VanEpps, "Unexpected insights into antibacterial activity of zinc oxide nanoparticles against methicillin resistant Staphylococcus aureus (MRSA)," *Nanoscale*, vol. 10, no. 10, pp. 4927–4939, 2018.

[18] R. Berni Canani, V. Buccigrossi, and A. Passariello, "Mechanisms of action of zinc in acute diarrhea," *Current Opinion in Gastroenterology*, vol. 27, no. 1, pp. 8–12, 2011.

[19] A. Sheikh, S. Shamsuzzaman, S. M. Ahmad et al., "Zinc influences innate immune responses in children with enterotoxigenic Escherichia coli-induced diarrhea," *The Journal of Nutrition*, vol. 140, no. 5, pp. 1049–1056, 2010.

[20] M. Farooq, "Zinc deficiency is associated with poor glycemic control," *Journal of the College of Physicians and Surgeons Pakistan*, vol. 29, no. 3, pp. 253–257, 2019.

[21] P. Ranasinghe, S. Pigera, P. Galappatthy, P. Katulanda, and G. R. Constantine, "Zinc and diabetes mellitus: understanding molecular mechanisms and clinical implications," *Daru*, vol. 23, p. 44, 2015.

[22] D. D. Marreiro, K. J. Cruz, J. B. Morais, J. B. Beserra, J. S. Severo, and A. R. de Oliveira, "Zinc and oxidative stress: current mechanisms," *Antioxidants*, vol. 6, no. 2, 2017.

29

Erythema Multiforme Induced by a "Milker's Nodule" Pseudocowpox Infection: A Case Report and Review of Literature

Kyle Wu, Sara de Menezes, and Aaron Robinson

Department of Dermatology, St Vincent's Hospital Melbourne, 41 Victoria Parade, Fitzroy VIC 3065, Melbourne, Australia

Correspondence should be addressed to Kyle Wu; kyle.a.wu@gmail.com

Academic Editor: Alireza Firooz

Milker's nodule is caused by the pseudocowpox virus following inoculation from infected cattle. We report the case of erythema multiforme induced by pseudocowpox infection in an 18-year-old female from regional Australia. While erythema multiforme has been described as a complication of orf, it is rare as a sequela of pseudocowpox infection. Greater clinical knowledge of this disease and potential complications aid in guiding appropriate management of this phenomenon.

1. Introduction

Milker's nodule is a disease caused by pseudocowpox virus of the genus *Parapoxvirus* that is prevalent in non-metropolitan areas. The infection is of bovine source, typically involving infected teats and mouth of cattle. The disease typically manifests as localised erythematous-violaceous nodules at the site of inoculation after a brief incubation period of 5–15 days [1, 2]. Erythema multiforme (EM) is a hypersensitivity reaction of the skin or mucosa against specific antigens with ninety percent of cases induced by infections [3]. It is most commonly associated with herpetic infections, but scant reports have described EM reaction as a rare complication of pseudocowpox virus. We herein describe a case of pseudocowpox virus presenting with secondary erythema multiforme.

2. Case Description

An 18-year-old female from rural Australia with no medical history, presented to the emergency department with a three-day history of spreading, papulovesicular, pruritic eruption on bilateral knees, hands with preferential involvement of the right hand, as well as a superficial crusting of the lips. She reported being bitten on the right hand by her pet calf 2 weeks prior. She remained systemically well and denied constitutional symptoms including fevers or arthralgias. She denied any new or regular medications or preceding illness. She denied exposure to sheep, goats, gardening, or fish tanks.

On examination, there was a violaceous, eroded nodule on the dorsal aspect of her right middle finger with an associated erythematous-yellow papulovesicular eruption (Figure 1). Erythematous papules and nodules were present on the dorsal and palmar surfaces of her left hand (Figure 2) and on bilateral knees with no pustules (Figure 3). Superficial yellow crusting was present on the lips (Figure 4). There were no bullae observed and no lymphadenopathy.

Skin biopsy was non-specific, showing inflammatory material and keratin debris with no microorganisms noted on PAS, Grocott, Ziehl–Neelsen, and Wade Fite stains. PCR was positive for parapoxviruses. In combination with the history and examination findings, the patient was diagnosed with milker's nodule on the right hand with secondary erythema multiforme-like reaction involving bilateral upper and lower limbs with mucous membrane involvement. She was managed with betamethasone dipropionate ointment for pruritus; she was counselled on the use of gloves to reduce potential risk of transmission. On follow-up in one week's time, the eruption had completely resolved.

3. Discussion

Pseudocowpox, caused by zoonotic parapoxvirus, is generally transmitted by direct contact with infected lesions of

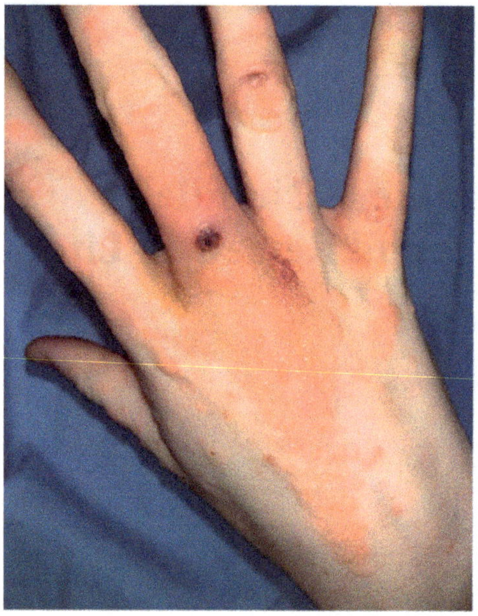

FIGURE 1: Dorsum of the right hand.

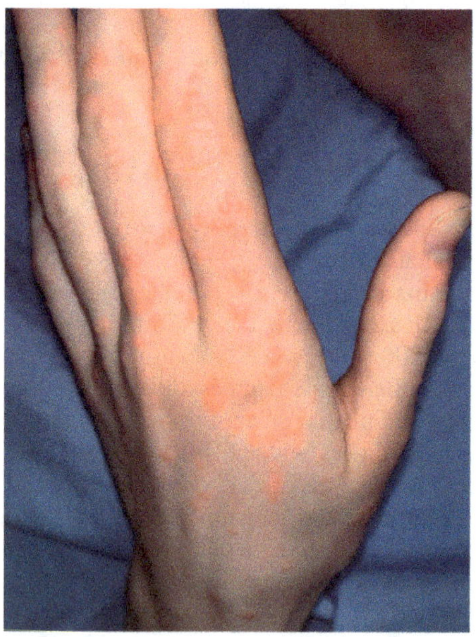

FIGURE 2: Dorsum of the left hand.

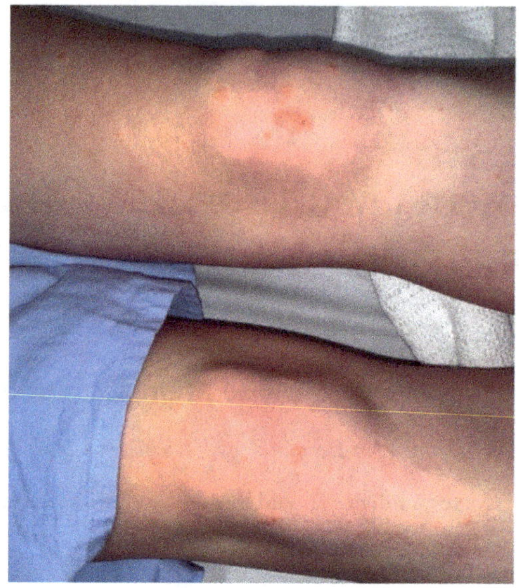

FIGURE 3: Bilateral knees.

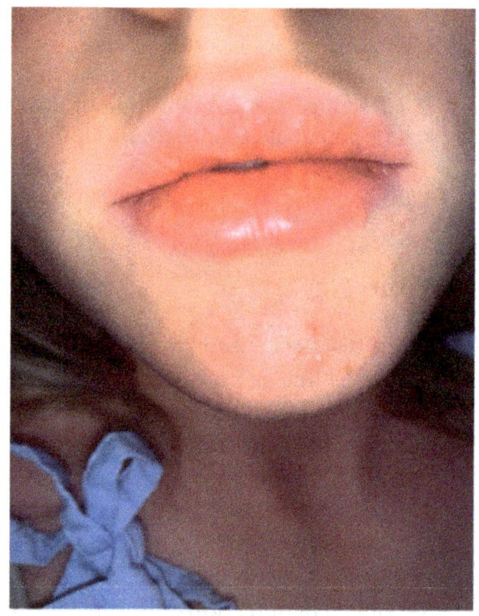

FIGURE 4: Superficial lip crusting.

cows, typically manifesting on patient's fingers and hands as milker's nodule. Erythema multiforme (EM) reaction, as presented in this case, is a rare complication of parapoxvirus infections. More common complications of milker's nodule include systemic symptoms of fever, lymphadenopathy, as well as possible bacterial superinfection. Bullous pemphigoid-like eruption has been reported as a rare sequela of orf and other parapoxviruses [4].

Despite similar clinical presentation, milker's nodule is a distinct entity from orf, the primary hosts of orf being sheep and goats rather than cattle [1, 5]. Other differential diagnoses aside from orf and other occupational zoonotic diseases include anthrax, atypical mycobacteriosis, tularaemia, and pyogenic granuloma [5]. Current PCR assays are unable to distinguish between pseudocowpox and orf with only subtle differences on tissue culturing [1]. Thus, the clinical history of suspected infection source and exposures is key to accurate diagnosis. Overall, milker's nodule and orf are notoriously underreported due to the typically self-limited natural history as well as common awareness amongst rural communities where it is most prevalent. Medical advice is often only sought once potential complications occur including EM [6].

The pathogenesis of EM is not completely understood, but hypothesized to be a cell-mediated immune reaction against specific antigens. In viral-associated EM, viral fragments are phagocytosed by Langerhans cells and transferred to epidermal keratinocytes, triggering the recruitment of CD4+ Th1 cells. Proinflammatory mediators such as IFN-γ are upregulated and induce an inflammatory cascade that promotes lysis of the infected keratinocytes and epidermal damage [4].

Viral triggers of EM include herpes simplex virus, Epstein–Barr virus, adenoviruses, enteroviruses, hepatitis viruses, influenza, and parapoxviruses [3]. While it is most commonly related to herpes simplex virus type 1, there are only scant reports describing EM reactions in pseudocowpox virus or milker's nodule [4, 7]. Within the *Parapoxvirus* genus, EM is again most commonly associated with orf infection rather than milker's nodule [4]. There are approximately 30 cases of orf-induced EM reported in the literature with reports of up to 18% of orf cases complicated by EM [8]. A Finish report from 1974 described an epidemic of milker's nodule with 7 out of 44 cases having secondary exanthem [9]. To our understanding, there has only been one other case of milker's nodule-associated EM reported in the English literature in an immunosuppressed patient triggered by graft-versus-host disease [6].

The paucity of literature also relates to the management of patients with secondary complications relating to milker's nodule. Systemic steroids have been demonstrated to be effective in treatment of patients with orf-associated EM [10]. Large lesions in immunocompromised patients have benefited from the use of cidofovir, an antiviral with broad-spectrum activity against DNA viruses [11]. In our case, no active treatment was necessary despite the complication of EM, with a complete resolution of disease within 3 weeks of initial inoculation. Supportive management and counselling still remain mainstays of treatment. It is important to emphasize the use of nonpermeable gloves when handling infected cattle to reduce risk of further infections. Misdiagnosis can lead to overtreatment including reported surgical excision of nodules and inappropriate antibiotic use [11]. Appropriate management is made possible with increased awareness and clinical knowledge of disease and its complications.

Milker's nodule is an underreported infection caused by the pseudocowpox virus of the *Parapoxvirus* genus, acquired from a bovine source. Targeted history taking and recognition of both common and rarer complications are critical in the diagnosis of milker's nodule. In addition to the classic local presentation, this case report illustrates the potential for secondary complications as a presenting complaint, including a rare systemic EM reaction. Accurate diagnosis of milker's nodule can help prevent exposing patients to unnecessary treatment.

References

[1] R. W. Groves, E. Wilson-Jones, and D. M. MacDonald, "Human orf and milkers' nodule: a clinicopathologic study," *Journal of the American Academy of Dermatology*, vol. 25, no. 4, pp. 706–711, 1991.

[2] A. R. Adriano, C. D. Quiroz, M. L. Acosta, T. Jeunon, and F. Bonini, "Milker's nodule—case report," *Anais brasileiros de dermatologia*, vol. 90, no. 3, pp. 407–410, 2015.

[3] O. Sokumbi and D. A. Wetter, "Clinical features, diagnosis, and treatment of erythema multiforme: a review for the practicing dermatologist," *International Journal of Dermatology*, vol. 51, no. 8, pp. 889–902, 2012.

[4] M. Ilkit, M. Durdu, and M. Karakaş, "Cutaneous id reactions: a comprehensive review of clinical manifestations, epidemiology, etiology, and management," *Critical Reviews in Microbiology*, vol. 38, no. 3, pp. 191–202, 2012.

[5] A. E. Werchniak, O. P. Herfort, T. J. Farrell, K. S. Connolly, and R. D. Baughman, "Milker's nodule in a healthy young woman," *Journal of the American Academy of Dermatology*, vol. 49, no. 5, pp. 910-911, 2003.

[6] W. R. Slattery, M. Juckett, W. A. Agger, C. A. Radi, T. Mitchell, and R. Striker, "Milkers' nodules complicated by erythema multiforme and graft-versus-host disease after allogeneic hematopoietic stem cell transplantation for multiple myeloma," *Clinical Infectious Diseases*, vol. 40, no. 7, pp. e63–e66, 2005.

[7] A. Batalla, M. E. Álvarez-Argüelles, M. B. González-Martínez, and J. R. Curto, "Nódulo de los ordeñadores complicado con eritema multiforme," *Medicina Clínica*, vol. 141, no. 3, p. e5, 2013.

[8] R. H. Joseph, F. A. Haddad, A. L. Matthews, A. Maroufi, B. Monroe, and M. Reynolds, "Erythema multiforme after orf virus infection: a report of two cases and literature review," *Epidemiology and Infection*, vol. 143, no. 2, pp. 385–390, 2015.

[9] K. Kuokkanen, J. Launis, and A. Mörttinen, "Erythema nodosum and erythema multiforme associated with milker's nodules," *Acta Dermato-Venereologica*, vol. 56, no. 1, pp. 69–72, 1976.

[10] S. Alian, F. Ahangarkani, and S. Arabsheybani, "A case of orf disease complicated with erythema multiforme and bullous pemphigoid-like eruptions," *Case Reports in Infectious Diseases*, vol. 2015, Article ID 105484, 4 pages, 2015.

[11] K. Geerinck, G. Lukito, R. Snoeck et al., "A case of human orf in an immunocompromised patient treated successfully with cidofovir cream," *Journal of Medical Virology*, vol. 64, no. 4, pp. 543–549, 2001.

30

Multiple Bluish Nodules in a 20-Year-Old Female with Similar Lesions in her Father

Punyawee Ongsri and Supenya Varothai

Department of Dermatology, Faculty of Medicine Siriraj Hospital, Mahidol University, Bangkok, Thailand

Correspondence should be addressed to Punyawee Ongsri; punyawee.ongsri@gmail.com

Academic Editor: Hristo Dobrev

Glomuvenous malformations are congenital, benign, vascular malformations classified as subtypes of glomus tumors with predominant blood vessels, usually present at birth or childhood with multiple, bluish, soft papules and nodules or plaque-like cutaneous lesions. Later present with pronounced segmental lesions, superimposed on the primary lesions, suggesting type 2 segmental mosaicism. We present a rare case of familial glomuvenous malformations, a healthy young female presented with multiple bluish papules since birth which later developed dissemination later in her adolescence. Moreover, her father also had similar skin lesions on his left lower back.

1. Introduction

Glomuvenous malformations (GVMs) or previously termed glomangiomas are congenital, benign, vascular malformations, classified as a histological subtype of glomus tumors with predominant blood vessels [1, 2].

Glomus tumors are benign tumors or hamartomas of the perivascular structure, arise from modified smooth muscle cells, called glomus cells, located in the walls of the Sucquet-Hoyer canal, a specialized arteriovenous anastomosis central to thermoregulation [1, 2].

There are two forms of glomus tumor, solitary variant (90% of the cases) and multiple variant (10%) [3], while the solitary variant is usually painful and located in subungual area, the latter is mostly present in children with similar lesions in their family members, which is thought to be inherited in autosomal dominant fashion [1, 2].

Glomuvenous malformations usually present at birth as multiple, bluish, less than 1 cm in diameter, soft papules and nodules or plaque-like cutaneous lesions that are typically painful on compression. They slowly grow in size and number with age, involving in dermis and subcutis, with hyperkeratotic and cobblestone appearance, affecting predominantly extremities.

Histologically, GVMs appear as distended vein-like malformed vascular channels surrounded by one or more layers of glomus cells; uniform blue cuboidal cells with plump nuclei and eosinophilic cytoplasm [4]. These glomus cells demonstrated smooth muscle characteristics which are stained positively for vimentin and α-smooth muscle actin and negatively for desmin [5].

2. Case Presentation

A 20-year-old Thai female from Chonburi, presented with multiple bluish papules on left thigh since birth. She noticed some new lesions later developed on her right lower back ten years ago. The lesions were asymptomatic until the last 2 months, they became painful on palpation (Figure 1). She was otherwise healthy. Her father also had similar skin lesions on his left lower back (Figure 2). He did not recognize the exact onset but they became more apparent in his childhood. Unlike his daughter, his lesions were asymptomatic and did not grow bigger in size or numbers.

Physical examination revealed multiple discrete soft, noncompressible painful bluish papules and nodules on her right lower back and left inner thigh. She denied episodes of bleeding from the cutaneous lesions or gastrointestinal tract.

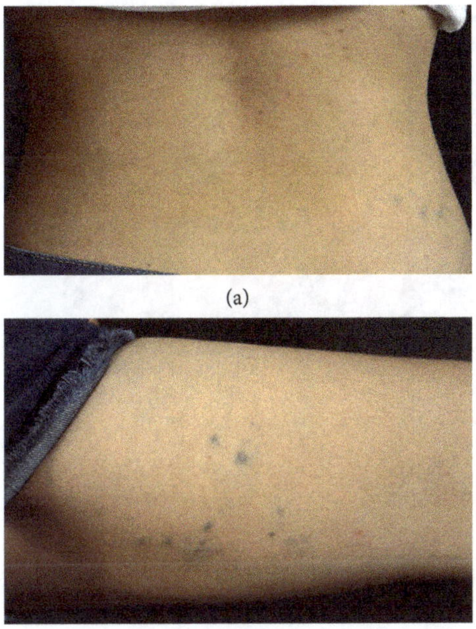

(a)

(b)

FIGURE 1: Clinical presentation of a 20-year-old female with multiple discrete soft, non-compressible painful bluish papules and nodules on her right lower back (a) and left inner thigh (b).

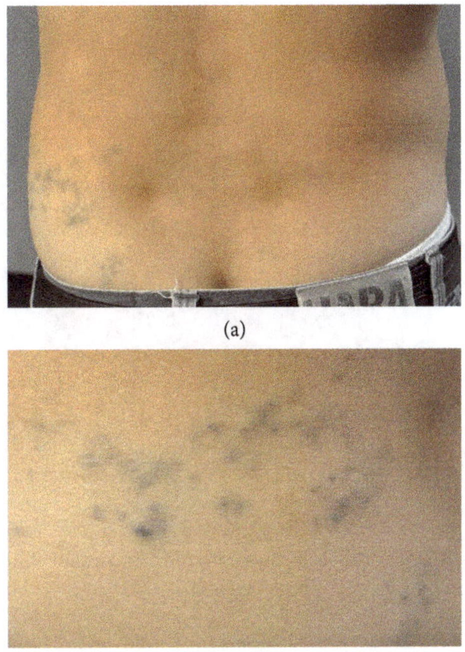

(a)

(b)

FIGURE 2: Her father also had similar skin lesions on his left lower back (a) and flank (b).

Computed tomography angiography (CTA) of lower abdomen and left thigh revealed multiple discrete small cutaneous and subcutaneous enhancing nodules at the anteromedial aspect of left upper thigh, size up to 1 cm, and no evidence of vascular malformations. The excisional skin biopsy was done on her left thigh and sent for pathology. Histological examination revealed large dilated, blood-filled vascular channels, surrounded by layers of glomus cells in the dermis (Figure 3).

Laboratory tests revealed normal complete blood count and coagulation. Her blood chemistry tests are otherwise within normal limits.

After the diagnosis was made, the prognosis and treatment options were informed to the patient. She does not have a cosmetic concern and seeks no further treatment.

3. Discussion

Glomuvenous malformations (GVMs) mostly present since infancy or childhood without gender predilection [4], multiple lesions usually develop and disseminate later in lives in different sites from the initial lesions. They are often asymptomatic, but some lesions may be tender upon compression. Unlike, glomus tumors which are usually solitary benign vascular lesions predilected for a subungual area with predominance on the ring finger, present in adulthood and almost always painful and sensitive to changes in temperature [6].

GVMs are caused by loss of function mutations in the glomulin gene (GLMN, at chromosome 1p21p22) which encodes glomulin protein [7]; a component of a multiprotein complex utilized in vascular morphogenesis. Despite somatic mutations in sporadic cases, familial GVMs were reported with an autosomal dominant transmission with incomplete penetrance and variable expressivity [5]; penetrance varies from 80% at 20 to about 100% at age 30 years [8]. In addition, somatic second-hit mutations can alter the size and number of the lesions [9].

Some patients with familial or congenital multiple GVMs may later present with pronounced segmental lesions, arranged in a flag-like pattern, superimposed on the ordinary, non-segmental phenotype, suggesting type 2 segmental mosaicism (T2SM). Like our case, we present an otherwise healthy young female presented with GMV lesions since birth which later developed dissemination later in her adolescence. There have been less than 15 cases of congenital multiple GVM with type 2 segmental manifestation reported to date [10, 11].

In the past, GVM was considered a subtype of venous malformations (VMs) but recently proposed as a distinct entity according to its different clinical characteristic, histopathological findings, prognosis and treatment responses. Other clinical differential diagnosis includes blue rubber bleb nevus syndrome, Mafucci syndrome and congenital plaque-like blue nevi [3, 5]. While eccrine spiradenoma, leiomyoma, and angiolipoma are also in differential diagnosis but they usually occur later in life [12].

Venous malformations (VM) are compressible, bluish lesions that affect deeper tissue. They shrink when externally compressed or subjected to an antigravitational posture. Phleboliths and stasis can be associated with pain. Unlike GVMs, which are less compressible and painful under compression. D-dimer elevation can also be found more commonly in VM [13]. Magnetic resonance imaging (MRI) was the best investigation to determine the extent of the GVM lesions and their relationship to other anatomic structures [14]. Doppler ultrasound may demonstrate the slow-flow

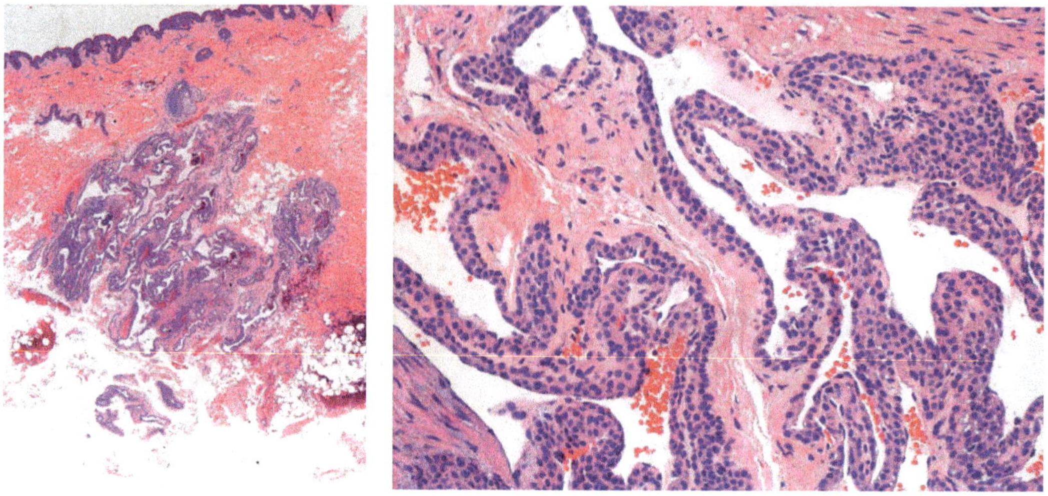

FIGURE 3: Histological study (hematoxylin and eosin staining) demonstrated large dilated, blood-filled vascular channels in the dermis (a), surrounded by layers of glomus cells (b).

nature of GVMs, and the higher cellularity and weaker compressibility compared with VM [15]. However, histological examination is crucial to distinguish GVMs from ordinary VMs, despite distinctive clinical features [4].

Blue rubber bleb nevus syndrome (BRBNS) is a rare congenital disorder associated with double (cis) somatic activating TEK mutations [4, 16, 17], characterized by multifocal cutaneous and visceral venous malformations. Multiple easily compressible cutaneous rubbery blue nodules since birth are the characteristic presentation, whereas gastrointestinal bleeding resulting in iron deficiency anemia is an extracutaneous complication associated with significant morbidity and mortality [5].

Mafucci syndrome is an extremely rare, sporadic, and nonhereditary disease characterized by multiple enchondromas and subcutaneous hemangio-endotheliomas localized on extremities especially on fingers and toes [5]. These lesions can cause fractures, deformities, pain, and undergo malignant transformation. Association with heterozygous mutations in *IDH1* (NADP(+)-dependent isocitrate dehydrogenase 1 gene) has been identified, with the same mutation found in enchondromas and spindle cell hemangiomas [4, 16, 18].

The goals of treatment in GVMs are mainly aesthetic considerations, pain relief, functional improvement and prevention of complications. Current treatment options include surgical excision, sclerotherapy, and laser.

Unlike VM, GVMs, especially plaque-type, responded poorly to sclerotherapy or embolization. Surgical excision is less appropriate due to their extensive and multifocal nature, additionally, it could result in disfiguring scars and demonstrated 10% of recurrence rate [19].

Many case reports and studies demonstrated satisfying efficacy using laser treatments on GVM lesions. Dual-wavelength Pulsed Dye Laser and Neodynium-doped Yttrium Aluminium Garnet laser (PDL-Nd:YAG) showed the most promising results in 60% of size reduction and improvement in color with safety profile [20], the youngest patient successfully treated was reported of a 6-month-old girl, with less cutaneous adverse effects compared to Nd:YAG alone, the latter more frequently resulted in ulceration and scarring, especially in children [21].

The mechanism of its effectiveness is that the laser system provides deeper penetration of the tissue to the lesions of GVMs, of which affect both the dermis and hypodermis. PDL allows greater absorption of the Nd:YAG laser due to the production of methemoglobin via hemoglobin, requiring less fluencies of the latter and therefore a decreased risk of adverse effects [19]. Focal GVM lesions showed better clinical outcome than plaque-like lesions treating with this laser system, while the latter had a greater risk of ulceration and atrophic scarring [20].

References

[1] C. Fletcher, "Tumors of blood vessels and lymphatics," in *Diagnostic Histopathology of Tumors*, C. Fletcher, Ed., pp. 75–76, Churchil Livingstine, Edinburgh, 2000.

[2] J. S. Chatterjee, A. H. Youssef, R. M. Brown, and H. Nishikawa, "Congenital nodular multiple glomangioma: a case report," *Journal of Clinical Pathology*, vol. 58, no. 1, pp. 102–103, 2005.

[3] V. O. Carvalho, K. Taniguchi, and S. Giraldi, "Congenital plaquelike glomus tumor in a child," *Pediatric Dermatology*, vol. 18, pp. 223–226, 2001.

[4] E. Paula, "Vascular Neoplasms and Neoplastic-Like Proliferations," in *Dermatology*, J. L. Bolognia, J. L. Jorizzo, and J. V. Schaffer, Eds., pp. 2044–2046, Elsevier, Saunder, 4th edition, 2018.

[5] C. Solovan, C. Elena, B. Doina, Z. Sabina, and B. Flavia, "Multiple disseminated glomuvenous malfonations: do we know enough?" *Romanian Journal of Morphology and Embryology*, vol. 53, no. 4, pp. 1077–1080, 2012.

[6] K. Hufschmidt, R. Foissac, O. Camuzard, N. Cardot-Leccia, B. Chignon-Sicard, and T. Balaguer, "Glomus tumors of the upper limb: single-center retrospective study of clinical and

functional outcomes," *Hand Surgery and Rehabilitation*, vol. 36, no. 4, pp. 290–295, 2017.

[7] P. Brouillard, L. M. Boon, N. Revencu et al., "Genotypes and phenotypes of 162 families with a glomulin mutation," *Molecular Syndromology*, vol. 4, no. 4, pp. 157–164, 2013.

[8] B. Riccardo, G. Sara, D. Marta, G. Maurizia, and A. Elosia, "Incomplete penetrance of GLMN gene c.395-1G>C mutation in a family with glomuvenous malformations," *International Journal of Dermatology*, vol. 53, pp. 1362–1364, 2014.

[9] M. Amyere, V. Aerts, P. Brouillard et al., "Somatic uniparental isodisomy explains multifocality of glomuvenous malformations," *The American Journal of Human Genetics*, vol. 92, no. 2, pp. 188–196, 2013.

[10] R. Hoekzema, I. M. Zonnevald, and A. C. van der Wal, "Type 2 segmental glomangiomas," *Dermatology*, vol. 16, no. 1, p. 8, 2010.

[11] R. C. Camila, L. M. Julliene, and C. F. T. Ana, "Type 2 segmental glomangioma - case report," *Anais Brasileiros de Dermatologia*, vol. 90, no. 3, pp. S97–S100, 2015.

[12] C. Eduardo and B. Thomas, "Vascular tumors: tumors and tumor-like conditions of blood vessels and lymphatics," in *Lever's Histopathology of the Skin*, E. E. David, Ed., Wolters Kluwer, Philadephia, USA, 11th edition, 2015.

[13] L. M. Boon, J. B. Mulliken, O. Enjolras, and M. Vikkula, "Glomuvenous malformation (glomangioma) and venous malformation: distinct clinicopathologic and genetic entities," *Archives of Dermatology*, vol. 140, no. 8, pp. 971–976, 2004.

[14] C. Mounayer, M. Wassef, O. Enjolras, M. Boukobza, and J. B. Mulliken, "Facial, glomangiomas: large facial venous malformations with glomus cells," *Journal of the American Academy of Dermatology*, vol. 45, no. 2, pp. 239–245, 2001.

[15] A. Dompmartin, N. Revencu, L. M. Boon, and M. Vikkula, "Disorders Affecting Cutaneous Vasculature," in *Rook's Textbook of Dermatology*, C. Griffths, J. Barker, T. Bleiker, R. Chalmer, and D. Creamer, Eds., pp. 13–14, 9th edition, 2016.

[16] B. Eulalia, "Vascular malformations," in *Dermatology*, J. L. Blognia, J. L. Jorizzo, and J. V. Schaffer, Eds., pp. 1805–1826, Elsevier, Saunder, 4th edition, 2018.

[17] J. Soblet, J. Kangas, M. Natynki et al., "Blue rubber bleb nevus syndrome is caused by somatic tek (tie2) mutations," *Journal of Investigative Dermatology*, vol. 137, no. 1, pp. 207–216, 2017.

[18] T. C. Pansuriya, R. van Eijk, P. d'Adamo et al., "Somatic mosaic IDH1 and IDH2 mutations are associated with enchondroma and spindle cell hemangioma in Ollier disease and Maffucci syndrome," *Nature Genetics*, vol. 43, no. 12, pp. 1256–1261, 2011.

[19] E. Grillo, B. Pablo, P. John, V. Sergio, C. Rosario, and J. Pedro, "Congenital plaque-like glomangioma treated successfully with dual wavelength pulsed-dye and neodymium:yttrium-aluminum-garnet laser," *Photodermatology, Photoimmunology & Photomedicine*, vol. 29, pp. 212–214, 2013.

[20] O. M. Moreno-Arrones, N. Jimenez, A. Alegre-Sanchez, P. Fonda, and P. Boixeda, "Glomuvenous malformations: dual PDL-Nd:YAG laser approach," *Lasers in Medical Science*, vol. 33, no. 9, pp. 2007–2010, 2018.

[21] V. N. Tien, M. B. Emily, and A. M. William, "Plaque-type glomuvenous malformations successfully treated using combined pulsed dye laser and neodymium-doped yttrium aluminium garnet laser," *Dermatologic Surgery*, vol. 40, no. 1, pp. 89–91, 2014.

31

New-Onset Bullous Pemphigoid in a COVID-19 Patient

Natalie Olson[1], **David Eckhardt**[1] **and Angela Delano**[2]

[1]*Rocky Vista University, Parker, CO 80134, USA*
[2]*St. Anthony North Family Medicine Residency Program, Denver, CO 80208, USA*

Correspondence should be addressed to Natalie Olson; natalie.anne1207@gmail.com

Academic Editor: Sergio A. Cuevas Covarrubias

This manuscript presents a report of bullous pemphigoid rash associated with COVID-19 for the first time. The objective of this manuscript is to present a unique dermatological case in the setting of a COVID-19-positive infection to further recognize the virus symptomatology. A 37-year-old female with a past medical history of class III obesity, type II diabetes mellitus, and hypertension presented to the emergency department in September 2020 with inpatient and outpatient follow-up through to November 2020. The patient denied any personal or family history of skin disorders. The patient tested positive for COVID-19 prior to hospitalization and presented to the hospital with severe, persistent, pruritic rash meeting dermatopathological, serologic, and clinical criteria for bullous pemphigoid diagnosis. Histopathology H&E punch biopsy from her left flexor wrist demonstrated epidermal keratinocyte necrosis, subepidermal vesiculation with eosinophils, gossamer stranding of the papillary dermis, and subepidermal edema. Direct immunofluorescence punch biopsy from her left flexor wrist demonstrated strong linear IgG staining at the dermoepidermal junction, with weaker and focal linear C3 staining. Antigen-specific serology was consistent with bullous pemphigoid. There was no previously reported cutaneous association of COVID-19 infection with bullous pemphigoid making this case an important addition to the body of evidence helping to identify bullous pemphigoid in the setting of viral infection.

1. Introduction

In 2019, a (Novel) coronavirus emerged in Wuhan, China. The virus has been found to cause severe pneumonia and has affected 35 million people, resulting in 1.5 million deaths worldwide since its emergence. Severe acute respiratory syndrome coronavirus 2 (SARS-CoV-2) is a single-stranded RNA virus that spreads via aerosolized droplets and enters host cells through the angiotensin-converting enzyme 2 (ACE2) receptor [1]. It is widely accepted that high ACE2 expression has been found in the type II alveolar cells and secretory cells of the lungs; however, it has also been suggested that ACE2 receptors are found in the small intestinal epithelium, oral epithelial cells, endothelial cells, and keratinocytes in the skin [1]. Though most symptomatic patients who contract the virus present with flu-like symptoms including fever, cough, fatigue, and malaise, recent evidence suggests that some patients have also experienced cutaneous manifestations of the disease. It is important to consider the dermatologic manifestations of SARS-CoV-2 as they may help to guide practitioners towards the diagnosis of COVID-19 among other respiratory viruses. Here, we present a report on a unique dermatological presentation of bullous pemphigoid (BP) in a known COVID-19-positive patient.

2. Case Report

Our patient is a 37-year-old female with a past medical history of type II diabetes mellitus, hypertension, and class III obesity who presented to the emergency department in September 2020 with a worsening rash. On the day of admission, she noted the development of red, raised lesions on her arms over the course of the last week. The lesions were mildly pruritic and nontender. The following day, she began experiencing typical COVID-19 symptoms (fever, shortness of breath, and muscle aches) and tested positive for COVID-19 on day 3 of her symptoms. She had no personal or family history of dermatologic or autoimmune conditions. No recent changes in the environment, detergent, soaps, or lotions were reported. No recent immunizations or changes in medications were reported. Medications included lisinopril 20 mg QD since February 2020 for hypertension and metformin 500 mg BID since February 2020 for type II diabetes mellitus.

The rash spread to her lower extremities, torso, and ultimately onto her neck and chin over the ten days before she presented to the ED. The lesions became larger, and some started to blister. The severity of the pruritus and discomfort motivated her to come to the emergency department. She was found to be tachypneic but oxygenated well on room air. Supplemental oxygen was given at 1-2 L by using a nasal cannula to relieve tachypnea with no hypoxia noted during hospitalization.

On examination, the patient reported negative Nikolsky sign, blanching, blisters tense and tender to palpation, and scaly lesions nontender to palpation. No mucosal involvement was observed on physical exam (Figure 1).

Hematologic studies for the patient were found to be normal. On admission, she did demonstrate mild hypokalemia (which resolved during her hospital stay), elevated blood glucose (serum ranged from 134 mg/dL to 146 mg/dL and HbA1C 5.8%), hypoalbuminemia, and elevated liver enzymes (ALT and AST). A D-dimer and C-reactive protein were also ordered and found to be elevated. Figures 2(a)–2(e) demonstrate the laboratory results for the patient at the time of admission, including abnormal values highlighted in yellow.

Table 1 lists the results of skin biopsy, direct immunofluorescence, and antigen-specific serologic testing for the patient. Pathology images were not available.

Differential diagnoses were erythema multiforme, chemical burn or exposure, leukocytoclastic vasculitis, drug reaction, granulomatosis with polyangiitis, urticarial vasculitis, and other viral exanthems.

She was treated with oral diphenhydramine, topical diphenhydramine, triamcinolone 0.5% cream, and IV dexamethasone 6 mg. Her home medications (metformin and lisinopril) were held during her hospital stay, and the patient was placed on sliding-scale correctional insulin for persistently elevated blood glucose values. Lisinopril was withheld due to the association with bullous pemphigoid, though the patient had been taking it without issues for years. She was discharged on oral dexamethasone 6 mg to complete a 10-day course in addition to topical diphenhydramine and triamcinolone. Since discharge, she has repeated multiple steroid courses due to the persistent discomfort associated with the rash as it improves with steroids and then flares back up upon completion of steroid courses. She has also been taking nicotinamide to help with her rash. Her dyspnea, body aches, and fever resolved shortly after discharge, and the rash was her only remaining symptom.

The patient has completed multiple steroid courses with continued exacerbations of the rash. At the end of November 2020, she was starting her third prednisone taper since discharge in addition to doxycycline. At the time of publication, immune-modulating therapies were under consideration but not yet initiated.

Pathological disease course since initial admission is as follows:

(i) First clinic visit on 11/17/2020: the patient was started on doxycycline 100 mg BID and nicotinamide 500 mg TID, and prednisone taper was initiated. She initially declined immunosuppressive agents given the COVID-19 pandemic.

(ii) Telehealth visit on 12/9/2020: the patient stopped doxycycline and nicotinamide as per the provider's recommendation.

(iii) The patient was admitted on 12/11–12/14 for bullous pemphigoid flare requiring hospitalization for pain control and wound care.

(iv) Office visit on 12/29/2020: the patient noted worsening with the painful blister formation on the face, arms, groin, legs, and back, with interference with the ability to sleep and work.

(v) The patient received two rituximab infusions on 1/11/2021 and 1/25/2021. She continued hydroxyzine 25–50 mg nightly QHS for pruritus.

(vi) Pt was seen at dermatology clinic on 3/23 and is doing very well after the second rituximab infusion. Has no blisters and is down to 7.5 mg prednisone. Will continue to slowly decrease dose. Patient to follow up in 4 weeks.

Verbal consent for the use of images and the case report was obtained from the patient. No written consent has been obtained from the patient as there are no identifiable data included in this case report.

3. Discussion

This submission presents a review of the current literature related to cutaneous manifestations of SARS-CoV-2 and the case of a woman who tested positive for COVID-19 after she noticed an annular, bullous, pruritic rash on her extremities two days prior to her diagnosis. The clinical picture of her rash was consistent with bullous pemphigoid, a condition which, to date, has not been associated with COVID-19.

In a recent literature review, Gisondi et al. reported on novel cutaneous manifestations of COVID-19 and discovered several dermatological presentations. These included exanthems (varicella-like, papulovesicular, and morbilliform rash), vascular (chilblain-like, purpuric/petechial, and livedoid lesions), urticarial, and acropapular eruption [2]. Our patient, who presented with a bullous, pruritic rash, does not quite fit into any of these reported categories, making her case especially unique as there are no published data on bullous dermatological patterns in COVID-19 patients to date. Perhaps, the most similar reported presentation is the varicella-like manifestation, which was recently found to be a possible early and quite specific manifestation of COVID-19 [2].

A popular opinion among cutaneous involvement of COVID-19 is that patients experience varying types of vasculitis, one being its effect on the dermal/epidermal

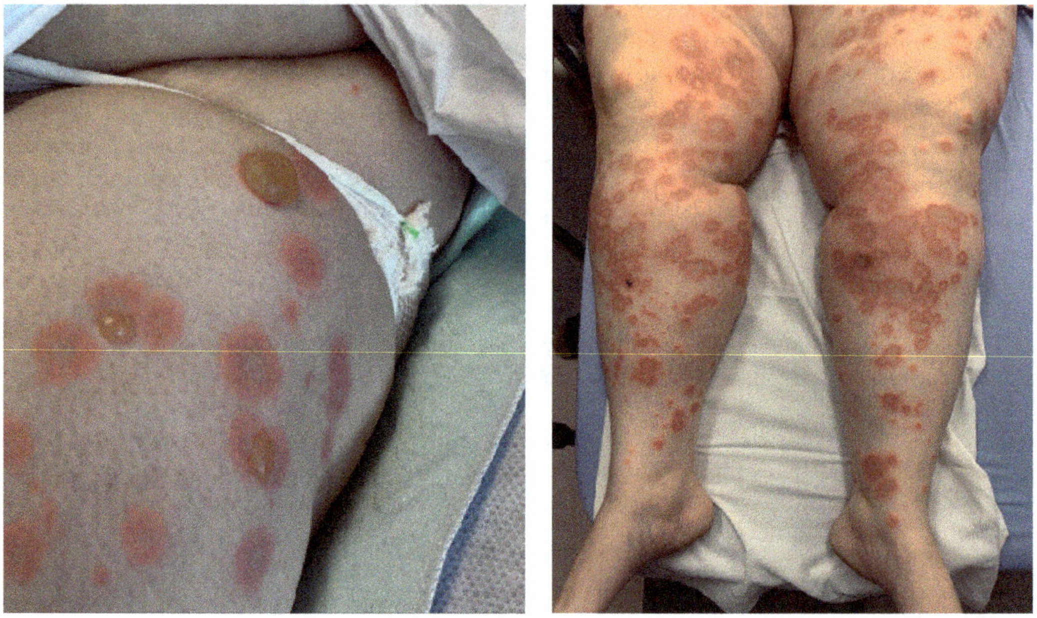

(a) (b)

Figure 1: (a) Left hip with blanching and tense blisters that are tender to palpation. (b) Bilateral lower extremities with erythematous, scaly annular lesions which are pruritic and at varying stages of the disease.

Component	Latest Ref Rng & Units	9/19/2020	9/20/2020	9/21/2020	9/22/2020
WBC White Blood Count	3.7 - 11.1 10*3/µL	8.6	6.7	6.4	8.1
RBC Red Blood Count	4.11 - 5.63 10*6/µL	4.85	4.44	4.26	4.52
HGB Hemoglobin	11.9 - 16.3 g/dL	14.4	13.2	12.7	13.3
HCT Hematocrit	37.0 - 47.7 %	44.4	40.5	39.1	41.4
MCV Mean Cell Volume	81 - 97 fL	92	91	92	92
MCH Mean Cell Hemoglobin	26.7 - 33.1 pg	29.7	29.7	29.8	29.4
MCHC Mean Cell Hgb Conc	31.1 - 35.3 g/dL	32.4	32.6	32.5	32.1
RDW-CV	12.3 - 15.9 %	13.6	13.6	13.6	13.3
RDW-SD	37.1 - 49.6 fL	46.8	46.3	46.4	45.2
PLT Platelet Count	150 - 400 10*3/µL	239	225	229	272
MPV Mean Platelet Volume	fL	10.2	10.1	10.0	10.3
Neutrophils %	%	75	64	55	76
Immature Granulocytes % (Auto)	%	0.3	0.6	0.5	0.7
Lymphocytes %	%	16	23	30	18
Monocytes %	%	4	5	6	5
Eosinophils %	%	4	6	8	1
Basophils %	%	0	0	0	1
Neutrophils Absolute	1.70 - 7.10 10*3/uL	6.45	4.31	3.52	6.13
Immature Granulocytes Absolute	<0.1 10*3/µL	0.03	0.04	0.03	0.06
Lymphocytes Absolute	1.1 - 3.7 10*3/uL	1.4	1.6	1.9	1.4
Monocytes Absolute	0.3 - 0.9 10*3/uL	0.4	0.4	0.4	0.4
Eosinophils Absolute	0.0 - 0.5 10*3/uL	0.4	0.4	0.5	0.1
Basophils Absolute	0.0 - 0.1 10*3/uL	0.0	0.0	0.0	0.0
Nucleated RBC	0 /100 WBCs	0	0	0	0

(a)

Component	Latest Ref Rng & Units	9/19/2020	9/20/2020	9/21/2020	9/21/2020	9/22/2020
				4:44 AM	4:44 AM	
Sodium	136 - 145 mmol/L	137			140	139
Potassium	3.5 - 5.1 mmol/L	2.9 (L)			3.5	3.5
Chloride	96 - 111 mmol/L	101			103	104
CO2 Carbon Dioxide	20 - 30 mmol/L	26			25	23
BUN Urea Nitrogen	6 - 24 mg/dL	9			12	10
Creatinine, Ser	0.53 - 1.26 mg/dL	0.88			0.85	0.64
BUN:Creatinine Ratio	6 - 25	10			14	16
Glucose	70 - 99 mg/dL	134 (H)			99	146 (H)
Calcium	8.3 - 10.1 mg/dL	8.3			8.3	8.5
Anion Gap	6 - 18	13			16	16
Albumin	3.4 - 5.3 g/dL	2.9 (L)	2.6 (L)	2.6 (L)	2.6 (L)	2.7 (L)
Globulin	2.2 - 4.2 g/dL	4.4 (H)	3.9	4.0	4.0	4.4 (H)
Albumin:Globulin Ratio	0.8 - 2.0	0.7 (L)	0.7 (L)	0.7 (L)	0.7 (L)	0.6 (L)
Protein Total	6.4 - 8.2 g/dL	7.3	6.5	6.6	6.6	7.1
Bilirubin Total	0.2 - 1.2 mg/dL	0.6	0.6	0.4	0.4	0.3
Alkaline Phosphatase	20 - 125 U/L	91	80	75	78	89
ALT Alanine Aminotransferase	12 - 78 U/L	202 (H)	150 (H)	137 (H)	137 (H)	113 (H)
AST Aspartate Amino Transferase	7 - 37 U/L	110 (H)	72 (H)	71 (H)	82 (H)	42 (H)
GFR Glomerular Filtration Rate	>60.0 mL/min	84.2			87.8	114.4

(b)

Component	Latest Ref Rng & Units	9/19/2020
D-dimer	<=0.49 mg/L FEU	5.85 (H)

(c)

Component	Latest Ref Rng & Units	9/19/2020
CRP C-Reactive Protein	0.00 - 2.99 mg/L	102.60 (H)

(d)

Component	Latest Ref Rng & Units	9/21/2020
Hemoglobin A1C	4.0 - 5.6 %	5.8 (H)
eAG Estimated Ave Glucose	mg/dL	120

(e)

Figure 2: Laboratory results. (a) Complete blood count. (b) Complete metabolic panel. (c) D-dimer. (d) C-reactive protein. (e) Hemoglobin A1C.

junction of the skin. Becker examined the effects of COVID-19 on the circulatory system and found multiple case reports in which urticarial vasculitis was implicated [3]. Upon histopathologic examination of biopsy-derived material, dermatitis and vascular degeneration of the basal epidermal layer were evident. Endotheliitis within lymphocytic infiltration of the dermal vesicles and arterioles and microthrombosis of papillary dermal capillaries are also common findings [3].

There have also been numerous case studies that have described dermatologic conditions associated with COVID-19,

Table 1: Patient lab results.

Diagnostic	Location/type	Result	Normal value
Biopsy	Left flexor wrist	Epidermal keratinocyte necrosis, subepidermal vesiculation with eosinophils, gossamer stranding of the papillary dermis, subepidermal edema	<20 RU/mL (negative)
Direct immunofluorescence	Left flexor wrist	Strong linear IgG staining at the dermoepidermal junction, with weaker and focal linear C3 staining	≥20 RU/mL (positive)
Antigen-specific serologic testing	Bullous pemphigoid 180 IgG Abs	211.4 RU/mL	<20 RU/mL (negative)
	Bullous pemphigoid 230 IgG Abs	<1.0 RU/mL	≥20 RU/mL (positive)

which do not necessarily fall under the category of vasculitis. Due to the difficulty in accessing dermatology consultation during the pandemic, skin manifestations of the disease may be underrecognized, and it is important to study them further.

While COVID-19-related dermatologic conditions have been relatively well documented in the literature, our patient's presentation of bullous pemphigoid has not previously been associated with COVID-19 infection. Bullous pemphigoid is an uncommon intraepidermal blistering disease caused by autoantibodies to adhesion molecules expressed in the skin and mucous membranes. The bullae appear spontaneously and are painful when they rupture. Bullous pemphigoid is a relatively benign pruritic disease characterized by tense blisters most commonly seen in flexural areas, with a course characterized by exacerbations and remissions [4]. The disease most often presents in patients who are 40–60 years old and with prodromal symptoms including pruritus, dermatitis, or urticaria. Lesions may occur anywhere on the skin surface in a localized or diffuse manner but are most frequently found on the flexural surfaces of the arms, axillae, legs, groin, and lower abdomen [5]. Our patient's presentation seems to fit this clinical picture with multiple exacerbations of her rash after initial treatment and the location of her rash being on the arms, groin, legs, and back.

Bullous pemphigoid flares are associated with the binding of autoantibodies to the proteins of hemidesmosomes triggering an inflammatory pathophysiological process ultimately leading to dermal-epidermal junction cleavage and blister formation [6]. It is thought that both inflammatory infiltrating cells and skin-resident cells, including keratinocytes, fibroblasts, and endothelial cells, produce cytokines and chemokines which contribute to the pathophysiologic process of bullous pemphigoid [6]. Interestingly, in many patients who have suffered severe cases of COVID-19, one of the main causes of multiorgan failure is thought to be related to a cytokine storm in which excessive amounts of inflammatory cells lead to organ damage in the lungs and liver. According to an article published in the *Mediators of Inflammation* journal, cytokines associated with COVID-19 included IL-1B, IL-17, and TNF-α, which have also been implicated in patients with bullous pemphigoid [6]. This finding could be related to some form of cytokine crossover in patients who present with cutaneous manifestations of the disease and should be studied further to gain a deeper understanding of the mechanism related to the inflammatory response of COVID-19. Lab values for our patient demonstrated an elevation in alanine aminotransferase (ALT) and aspartate aminotransferase (AST), which may indicate damage to the liver, as well as elevations in C-reactive protein, a marker for acute inflammation. Interleukin values were not measured at the time of admission, and as the patient was afebrile throughout her hospital stay, we did not believe that the patient was experiencing the systemic inflammation related to cytokine storm seen in some patients with COVID-19.

It is well understood that the underlying cause of bullous pemphigoid is due to autoantibodies that are directed at adherence proteins within the skin; however, little evidence exists that discusses the triggering factors for the development of such autoantibodies [7]. Patel et al. proposed that the etiology of bullous pemphigoid is likely multifactorial in nature, with components of environmental triggers, genetic predisposition, and a potential role of complement deposition due to evidence of complement seen within the blister fluid [7].

There have been case reports of patients developing bullous pemphigoid following vaccine administration and viral infection [8]. A popular theory is that introduction of a vaccine or virus leads to cellular activation of IL-17 and ultimately the release of proinflammatory cytokines and proteolytic enzymes, which may result in disruption to hemidesmosomes and blister formation [8].

Though recent literature reports a strong correlation between viral infections and the development of BP, it is prudent to consider that most patients diagnosed with pemphigus rashes have a genetic predisposition to the development of autoantibodies directed towards the dermal proteins BP180 and BP230, which play a critical role in maintaining epidermal adhesion [7, 9]. It is important to recognize that individuals with a genetic predisposition who are exposed to certain medications may develop drug-induced BP, including DPV inhibitors such as vildagliptin and linagliptin and certain diuretic medications such as furosemide and spironolactone, as well as certain antipsychotic medications and checkpoint inhibitors [10]. The second class of drugs that has been associated with bullous pemphigoid is angiotensin-converting enzyme inhibitors, or ACE-Is, specifically losartan, valsartan, and lisinopril [11]. Interestingly, our patient had been taking lisinopril. Although a pemphigus reaction to lisinopril is rare, this medication was stopped upon the patient's first admission. It is unlikely that her symptoms were secondary to her medications as the symptoms usually resolve upon discontinuing the medication, which is not the case here. It is also less likely as the patient had been taking the medication without issues for nearly 20 years.

Recent studies have reported that nearly all patients who develop pemphigoid rash have an increased frequency of the DQB1 * 0301 allele with some studies showing that the BP180-specific Th1 and Th2 cells are restricted to HLA-DQB1 * 0301 [7, 9, 12–14]. Of note, the BP180 and BP230 antibodies were detected in our patient. Though we did not perform genetic testing on our patient, it is important to recognize that her genome could have contributed to the development of her rash.

The role of complement deposits found within the blister fluid is also an important consideration in the etiology of BP, especially in our patient who was newly diagnosed with COVID-19. Romeijn et al. cited that complement deposits are found in the blister fluid of 83.1% of the skin biopsies of patients diagnosed with bullous pemphigoid [15]. This is important to consider based on Java et al.'s report on the coronavirus ability to activate complement pathways and their potential involvement in the severity of the disease [16]. It would be interesting to understand more thoroughly the involvement of complement pathways in both BP and COVID-19 and their correlation with one another.

It is important to note that it is entirely possible that our patient had developed both conditions simultaneously without one precipitating the other. It would be prudent to consider the possibility that the two disease processes were unrelated conditions in this patient. Further investigation for a causative relationship between COVID-19 and BP is warranted.

4. Conclusion

This case presents a unique dermatologic presentation of COVID-19 and recent literature on potential pathophysiology of BP in COVID-19-positive patients. SARS-CoV-2 enters the host cell through the ACE2 receptor, which is found on multiple cell types including dermatological cells. Once it enters into a host cell, the virus activates complement, and, in turn, inflammatory cells are recruited to the cell eliciting a response [16]. There has been speculation as to the contributing etiology of bullous pemphigoid, and this case brings to light new evidence of COVID-19 as a potential triggering event in patients with BP and should be studied further.

This research is important for medical practitioners to continue to understand COVID-19 and associated dermatological manifestations. The pathogenesis of both COVID-19 and bullous pemphigoid is complex. Perhaps, their relation to one another as in this case will allow for a deeper understanding of each disease and the mechanisms by which they evolve and progress.

4.1. Patient Perspective. "It's been really horrible and difficult. The itching and the pain have been difficult to deal with. The outcome of having bullous pemphigoid so young makes me worried. It's supposed to take years to fully go away and usually happens to older people. It's embarrassing when the blisters are on my arms and people can see them. If it is from COVID, then people should really listen when they tell us not to attend group gatherings.

I experience worsening symptoms whenever I take less than 30 mg of prednisone.

It's difficult to sleep at night because the blisters on my back are so itchy and it's hard to lay on them. Insurance only pays for a small amount of topical creams and I need to use so much over my whole body, so it doesn't really work as an option. Hot showers sometimes help the itching, but I still don't sleep well. It's just so difficult and I hope it gets better."

Acknowledgments

The authors wish to thank Kelsey Sherman, Bradley Brown, Jonathan Dill, Kimberly Insel, Trevor Harrington, Tom Califf, and Zoey Thompson for providing care for their patient and for informative discussions which helped shape this manuscript. Images were provided by Tom Califf and Angela Delano.

References

[1] X. Xue, Z. Mi, Z. Wang, Z. Pang, H. Liu, and F. Zhang, "High expression of ACE2 on keratinocytes reveals skin as a potential target for SARS-CoV-2," *Journal of Investigative Dermatology*, vol. 141, no. 1, pp. 206–209, 2021.

[2] P. Gisondi, S. PIaserico, C. Bordin, M. Alaibac, G. Girolomoni, and L. Naldi, "Cutaneous manifestations of SARS-CoV-2 infection: a clinical update," *Journal of the European Academy of Dermatology and Venereology*, vol. 34, no. 11, pp. 2499–2504, 2020.

[3] R. C. Becker, "COVID-19-associated vasculitis and vasculopathy," *Journal of Thrombosis and Thrombolysis*, vol. 50, no. 3, pp. 499–511, 2020.

[4] M. A. Papadakis and S. J. McPhee, "Chapter 6 dermatologic disorders," in *Fifty-Sixth Current Medical Diagnosis and Treatment*, pp. 139-140, McGraw Hill Education, New York, NY, USA, 2017.

[5] Distinguishing pemphigus and pemphigoid for the non-dermatologist. Consultant 360. Accessed October 17, 2020. https://www.consultant360.com/articles/distinguishing-pemphigus-and-pemphigoid-non-dermatologist.

[6] M. Riani, S. Le Jan, J. Plée et al., "Bullous pemphigoid outcome is associated with CXCL10-induced matrix metalloproteinase 9 secretion from monocytes and neutrophils but not lymphocytes," *Journal of Allergy and Clinical Immunology*, vol. 139, no. 3, pp. 863–872, 2017.

[7] F. Patel, R. Wilken, F. B. Patel et al., "Pathophysiology of autoimmune bullous diseases: nature versus nurture," *Indian Journal of Dermatology*, vol. 62, no. 3, pp. 262–267, 2017.

[8] L. Baroero, P. Coppo, L. Bertolino, S. Maccario, and F. Savino, "Three case reports of post immunization and post viral Bullous Pemphigoid: looking for the right trigger," *BMC Pediatrics*, vol. 17, no. 1, p. 60, 2017.

[9] G. Genovese, G. Di Zenzo, E. Cozzani, E. Berti, M. Cugno, and A. V. Marzano, "New insights into the pathogenesis of bullous pemphigoid: 2019 update," *Frontiers in Immunology*, vol. 10, 2019.

[10] D. Miyamoto, C. G. Santi, V. Aoki, and C. W. Maruta, "Bullous pemphigoid," *Anais Brasileiros de Dermatologia*, vol. 94, no. 2, pp. 133–146, 2019.

[11] R. A. Ballout, U. Musharrafieh, and J. Khattar, "Lisinopril-associated bullous pemphigoid in an elderly woman: a case report of a rare adverse drug reaction," *British Journal of Clinical Pharmacology*, vol. 84, no. 11, pp. 2678–2682, 2018.

[12] A. Lo Schiavo, E. Ruocco, G. Brancaccio, S. Caccavale, V. Ruocco, and R. Wolf, "Bullous pemphigoid: etiology, pathogenesis, and inducing factors: facts and controversies," *Clinics in Dermatology*, vol. 31, no. 4, pp. 391–399, 2013.

[13] M. Hertl, R. Eming, and C. Veldman, "T cell control in autoimmune bullous skin disorders," *Journal of Clinical Investigation*, vol. 116, no. 5, pp. 1159–1166, 2006.

[14] C. Haase, L. Büdinger, L. Borradori et al., "Detection of IgG autoantibodies in the sera of patients with bullous and gestational pemphigoid: ELISA studies utilizing a baculovirus-encoded form of bullous pemphigoid antigen 2," *Journal of Investigative Dermatology*, vol. 110, no. 3, pp. 282–286, 1998.

[15] T. R. Romeijn, M. F. Jonkman, C. Knoppers, H. H. Pas, and G. F. H. Diercks, "Complement in bullous pemphigoid: results from a large observational study," *British Journal of Dermatology*, vol. 176, no. 2, pp. 517–519, 2017.

[16] A. Java, A. J. Apicelli, M. K. Liszewski et al., "The complement system in COVID-19: friend and foe?" *JCI Insight*, vol. 5, no. 15, 2020.

32

Carbamazepine-Induced Toxic Epidermal Necrolysis Managed by Mobile Teledermatology in COVID-19 Pandemic in Rural Nepal

Vikash Paudel[1] **and Deepa Chudal**[2]

[1]*National Medical College, Birgunj, Parsa, Nepal*
[2]*Nepal Police Hospital, Kathmandu, Nepal*

Correspondence should be addressed to Vikash Paudel; vikashpoudel@iom.edu.np

Academic Editor: Jacek Cezary Szepietowski

Toxic epidermal necrolysis is a life-threatening dermatological emergency with high mortality if not treated in time. Here we report a case of toxic epidermal necrolysis due to carbamazepine in rural Nepal in COVID-19 pandemic who was successfully treated with the help of mobile teledermatology. The clinical impression of toxic epidermal necrolysis was made from "WhatsApp" video calls using a smart phone. The supportive features were the history of starting of carbamazepine 2 weeks prior for seizure disorder, clinical findings in serial photographs of skin with 40 percent body surface area involvement of necrotic skin lesions and bulla, and involvement of oral mucosa and eyes. The patient was immediately asked to stop carbamazepine and was treated with intravenous fluids and systemic steroids along with symptomatic management. As the whole world was suffering from lockdown due to COVID-19 crisis, it was impossible for the rural area patient to visit a dermatologist. Thus, with the help of paramedics staff in a community health center and mobile teledermatology, the patient was diagnosed as carbamazepine-induced toxic epidermal necrolysis and treated successfully with good outcome.

1. Introduction

Toxic epidermal necrolysis (TEN), also known as Lyell's syndrome [1], is a potentially life-threatening dermatological emergency with high mortality [2]. Though TEN is less common in dermatological practice, carbamazepine is one of the commonest culprits among all the drugs [3]. Here, we present a case of carbamazepine induced toxic epidermal necrolysis in a young female from rural Nepal, who was successfully treated using simple mobile teledermatology in COVID-19 pandemic.

2. Case Report

This is a story of a 12-year-old female from rural Nepal who developed rapidly progressive generalized rash along with mild fever and headache. She was diagnosed with seizure disorder 2 weeks prior to the current illness and was prescribed carbamazepine at the dose of 200 mg daily. On the 14th day of carbamazepine, she developed those rashes which were purpuric, some of which later turned to blisters, dusky colored, itchy to start with which later were tender, and covered almost 40% of body surface area covering trunk and face with involvement of oral mucosa and eye. It was associated with swelling of the face and mild fever.

As the whole country was under lockdown due to COVID-19 pandemic, it was impossible for the rural patient to visit the dermatologist. For this, she went to a nearby community health center, from where mobile teleconsultation was made with the help of a community health worker (health assistant).

On assisted physical examination with the help of the health worker, it was found that the patient was febrile with areas of blistering and peeling of the skin involving face, trunk, and extremities with crusting seen over lips and eyes (Figures 1 and 2). The Nikolsky sign was positive. The erythematous rash was covered almost all over the trunk with epidermal detachment of 40% body surface area.

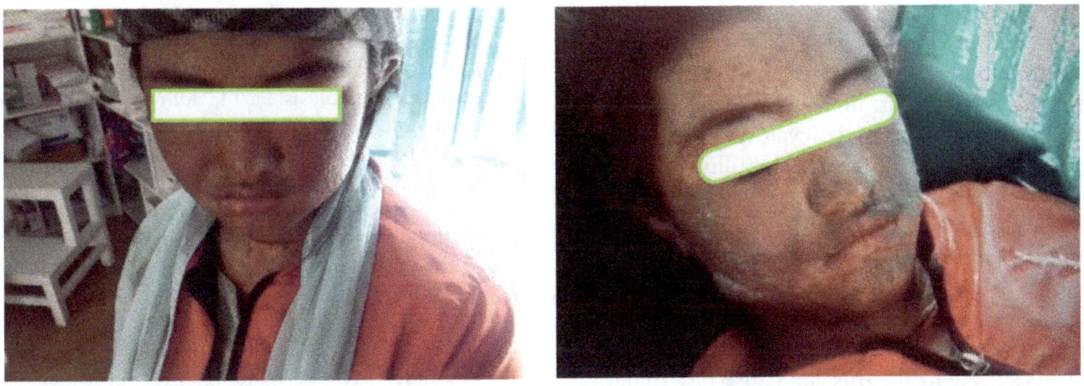

(a) (b)

FIGURE 1: (a, b) Erythema and vesicobullous lesions involving the face and neck.

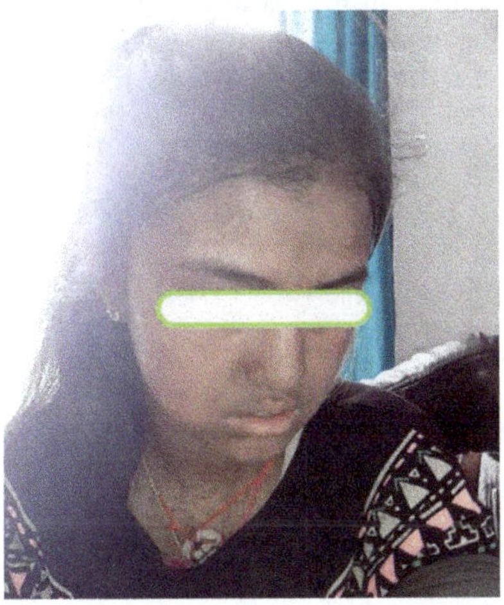

FIGURE 2: Patient during discharge from the health center at 2 weeks.

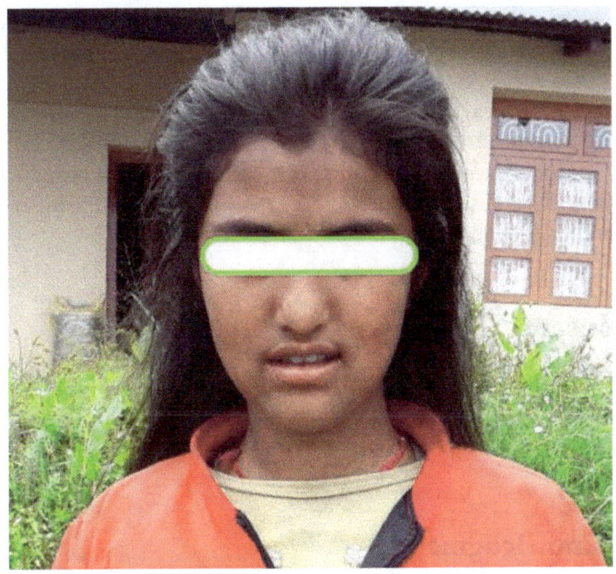

FIGURE 3: Patient on follow-up at 4 weeks.

The clinical impression of toxic epidermal necrolysis due to carbamazepine was made after taking detail history and serial clinical findings in video calls and photos sent in the mobile device.

Regarding the management of the patient in rural setting, carbamazepine was stopped immediately. She was supplemented with a rapidly tapering dose of intravenous hydrocortisone along with fexofenadine, mupirocin ointment, and moisturizer. The erosions were smeared with mupirocin and paraffin gauges. Supportive treatment given included parenteral analgesics for pain management and intravenous fluids. The patient was advised for better nutrition for healing of the wound by giving adequate carbohydrate, high-protein diet, and vitamin supplements. She was switched over to oral prednisolone once the lesions started healing after five days. Later on, prednisolone was slowly tapered slowly over two weeks. The lesions healed with postinflammatory hyperpigmentation (Figures 2 and 3).

3. Discussion

TEN is a severe cutaneous adverse drug reaction and life-threatening dermatological emergency [1]. The common causes are mostly drugs like sulphonamides, nonsteroidal anti-inflammatory drugs (NSAIDs), beta-lactum antibiotics, quinolones, nevirapine, antitubercular drugs, allopurinol, and aromatic antiepileptics like carbamazepine, phenobarbital, and phenytoin [3]. The time duration of TEN after initiating carbamazepine is usually less than 3 weeks. Our patient presented with generalized erythema and peeling of the skin with mucosal erosions two weeks after initiating carbamazepine.

Recently, carbamazepine was found to be a common drug causing TEN [4]. The pathogenesis of TEN is cytotoxic destruction and apoptosis of keratinocytes. The proapoptotic molecules like TNF-α, interferon-γ, and inducible nitric oxide synthase may link drug-induced immune responses to keratinocyte damage [3, 5]. Soluble Fas ligands, perforin, granzyme, and, recently, granulysin have been implicated in death of keratinocyte [6]. Drug metabolites also act as haptens, and defect in the detoxification system of clearing those haptens may be the cause of severe drug reactions [3].

As the patient was from a very rural area without proper healthcare, even without a medical doctor, the access to dermatologist was unimaginable. However, the mobile teledermatology assisted with proper diagnosis and management of the case. The foremost part in the management of such severe drug reaction was to stop the culprit drug. The specific treatment modalities in management are high dose of corticosteroid (though debated), cyclosporine, plasmapheresis, and intravenous immunoglobulins [7]. We abruptly stopped carbamazepine. As the patient had only access to systemic steroid and thus was advised to administer intravenous hydrocortisone which was later switched to oral prednisolone.

Teledermatology is increasingly being used worldwide in these pandemics situations than ever, and mobile teledermatology is its simple form. This could also be a dynamic tool for the remote areas where a dermatologist is not available, even in post-COVID era as well [8]. They could be life-saving, timesaving, and economical at times like our scenario [9].

Carbamazepine-induced TEN was successfully managed at the outreach center with the help of mobile teledermatology. Awareness about the drugs implicated in severe drug reactions would help to prevent these life-threatening drug reactions. Besides, the use of teledermatology would help the healthcare workers and medical officers with less exposure of dermatology in identifying and managing skin diseases.

Consent

Written informed consent was obtained from the guardian of the patient, as she was a minor, for the publication of this case report and the accompanying images.

Acknowledgments

The authors would like to thank to the team of Nepal Help Community Health Centre and Mr. Prem Deuba, Health Assistant, for helping us managing the life-threatening case selflessly and successfully.

References

[1] A. Lyell, "Toxic epidermal necrolysis: an eruption resembling scalding of the skin," *British Journal of Dermatology*, vol. 68, no. 11, pp. 355–361, 1956.

[2] T. Bettuzzi, L. Penso, N. De Prost et al., "Trends in mortality rates for Stevens-Johnson syndrome and toxic epidermal necrolysis: experience of a single centre in France between 1997 and 2017," *British Journal of Dermatology*, vol. 182, no. 1, pp. 247-248, 2020.

[3] V. Harris, C. Jackson, and A. Cooper, "Review of toxic epidermal necrolysis," *International Journal of Molecular Sciences*, vol. 17, no. 12, p. 2135, 2016.

[4] M.-S. Yang, J. Y. Lee, J. Kim et al., "Searching for the culprit drugs for stevens-johnson syndrome and toxic epidermal necrolysis from a nationwide claim database in Korea," *The Journal of Allergy and Clinical Immunology: In Practice*, vol. 8, no. 2, pp. 690–695, 2020.

[5] R. A. Schwartz, P. H. McDonagh, and B. W. Lee, "Toxic epidermal necrolysis. Part I," *Journal of the American Academy Dermatology*, vol. 69, no. 2, pp. 173.E1–173.E13, 2013.

[6] I. Viard-Leveugle, O. Gaide, D. Jankovic et al., "TNF-alpha and IFN-gamma are potential inducers of Fas-mediated keratinocyte apoptosis through activation of inducible nitric oxide synthase in toxic epidermal necrolysis," *The Journal of Investigative Dermatology*, vol. 133, no. 2, pp. 489–498, 2013.

[7] Y. Kinoshita and H. Saeki, "A review of the active treatments for toxic epidermal necrolysis," *Journal of Nippon Medical School*, vol. 84, no. 3, pp. 110–117, 2017.

[8] V. Paudel, "Tele-dermatology in clinical management of suspected cutaneous leishmaniasis in COVID-19 pandemic," *Nepal Journal of Dermatology, Venereology & Leprology*, vol. 18, no. 1, pp. 91-92, 2020.

[9] S. Perkins, J. M. Cohen, C. A. Nelson, and C. G. Bunick, "Teledermatology in the era of COVID-19: experience of an academic department of dermatology," *Journal of the American Academy of Dermatology*, vol. 83, no. 1, pp. E43–E44, 2020.

33

Diagnosis of Woolly Hair using Trichoscopy

Mahesh Mathur, Prakash Acharya, Alina Karki, Nisha KC, and Jyoti Shah

Department of Dermatology, College of Medical Sciences, Bharatpur 44200, Nepal

Correspondence should be addressed to Prakash Acharya; prakashacharya888@gmail.com

Academic Editor: Hristo Dobrev

Hair shaft abnormalities including woolly hair are traditionally diagnosed by clinical examination and light microscopy which involves plucking of multiple hairs for examination. This is usually an inconvenient procedure especially in children. Trichoscopy may be a useful tool allowing close visualization of multiple hairs without causing discomfort to the patients. Trichoscopic findings of woolly hair have been described only in few reports. We report all of the trichoscopic findings of this rare disorder in one case which have only been reported separately in previous reports.

1. Introduction

Woolly hair (WH) is a rare congenital hair structure abnormality characterized by strongly coiled hair localized to a site or involving the whole scalp in non-black people [1]. Hair growth rate is usually normal, but the truncated anagen phase results in shorter hair. Kink formation, elliptical cross-section, and axial rotation are noted in the hair shafts [2]. Diagnosis is clinical and aided by light microscopic examination of multiple hairs. Videodermoscopy of hair and scalp (trichoscopy) allows visualization of hair shafts in vivo in high magnification without the need of pulling hair for microscopic examination [3]. The trichoscopic patterns of this disorder have been reported separately in previous studies [4–6]. We are reporting this case because of its rarity and all the trichoscopic findings seen in a single case.

2. Case Report

A 6-year-old Asian girl presented with short, sparse hair over the scalp noticed since birth (Figure 1). The hair never grew longer than the current length. There were no similar complaints in the family members. Examination revealed tightly coiled and curled light colored hairs thinly distributed over the scalp. Skin, palms, soles, nails, and teeth showed no abnormalities. There were no signs and symptoms suggestive of cardiac abnormalities or any other systemic involvement. Based on these findings, a diagnosis of woolly hair was made. Hematological and biochemical investigations were within normal limits.

Trichoscopy was performed using Firefly DE300 Polarizing Handheld USB Digital Dermoscope (Firefly Global, MA, USA) and photographs were captured by MacBook Pro 2013. Trichoscopy revealed "crawling snake" appearance, with short wave cycles (Figure 2(a)) and trichoptilosis (Figure 2(b)). Trichoscopy guided plucking of hair was done and a single strand was examined, which revealed kinking of the hair shaft and variation in shaft diameter (Figure 2(c)). After a complete workup, genetic counseling was done to the mother of the patient.

3. Discussion

Woolly hair is a rare congenital abnormality of hair which was first described by Gossage in 1907 in a European family characterized by an extremely curly hair with average curl diameter of 0.5 cm [7].

The presence of woolly hair in non-blacks is extremely rare [1]. Inherited woolly hair usually involves the entire scalp and can occur either in the absence of other physical findings or in association with other syndromes [8]. The reported syndromes which can be associated with woolly hair are the Naxos syndrome, the Carvajal-Huerta syndrome, the ectodermal dysplasia-skin fragility, the wooly hair/hypotrichosis, and the trichohepatoenteric syndrome [1]. Ramot and Zlotogorski [1] in 2015 proposed an algorithm

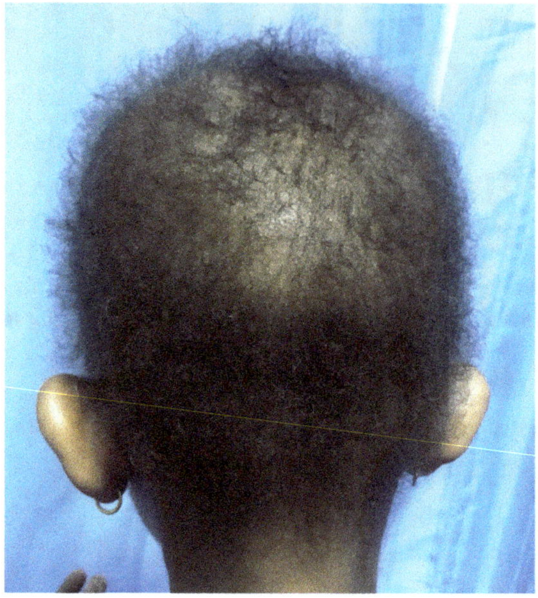

FIGURE 1: Short and sparse hair over the scalp.

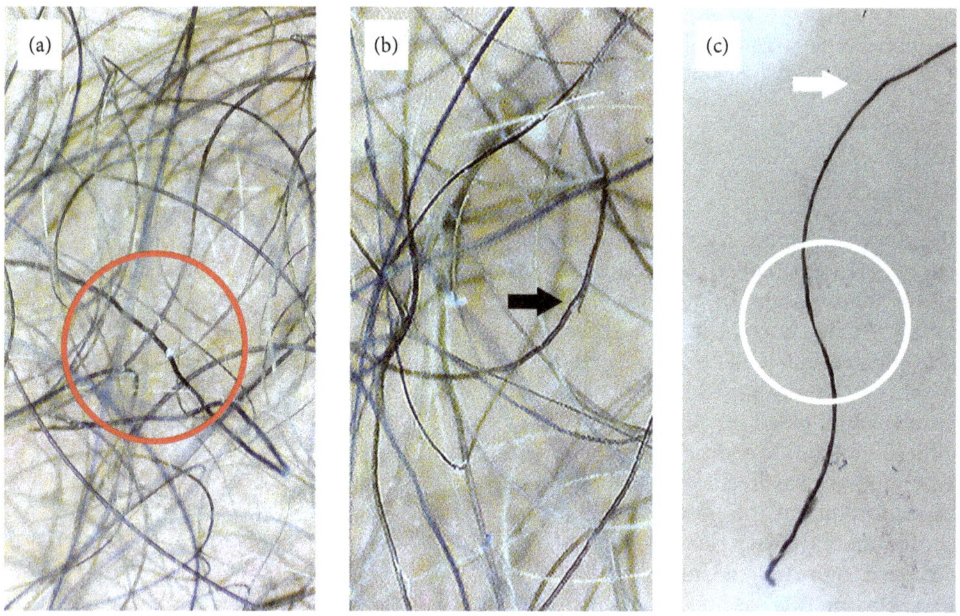

(a) (b) (c)

FIGURE 2: Trichoscopy (20x) showing (a) "crawling snake" appearance (red circle), (b) trichoptilosis (black arrow), and (c) variation in shaft diameter (white circle) and kinking of hair shaft (white arrow).

for the workup and diagnosis of woolly hair by classifying the condition into localized versus diffuse and syndromic versus nonsyndromic. They stated that although a definite diagnosis of woolly hair requires genetic testing, the proper history and examination can actually lead to the right diagnosis. The same study stated that the diffuse involvement of scalp present since birth or childhood should be determined as syndromic or nonsyndromic. Presence of palmoplantar keratoderma in a diffuse type of woolly hair should raise the suspicion of keratoderma with woolly hair types I-III requiring complete cardiac workup to rule out fatal cardiomyopathy [1]. Similarly, woolly hair associated with intractable diarrhea should be evaluated for inflammatory skin lesions, facial dysmorphism, and immune deficiency [1]. Cases of woolly hair along with keratosis pilaris and dental abnormalities have also been reported [2, 9]. Our patient was non-black with no systemic involvement and other associated features of various abovementioned syndromes.

Hutchinson et al. [10] classified woolly hair into three variants: hereditary woolly hair (autosomal dominant), familial woolly hair (autosomal recessive), and woolly hair nevus. Since there was no similar complaint in any member of the family, our patient could be a case of autosomal recessive variant without systemic involvement, similar to the case reported by Naveen et al. [6].

Light microscopy of the hair shafts in woolly hair revealed ovoid cross sections, 180-degree longitudinal twisting, trichorrhexis nodosa, and pili annulati [4].

Trichoscopy is a newer method which allows visualization of hair shafts in vivo in high magnification without the need of pulling hair for microscopic examination [6]. Currently, only a few studies have reported the trichoscopic findings of woolly hair which include variation in the thickness of hair shafts, "crawling snake" appearance, kinking of the hair shaft, and irregularity of shaft diameter [4–6]. These findings have been reported in separate cases previously highlighting the uniqueness of our case as all of these patterns were present. Trichoptilosis, a feature of hair shaft trauma seen in light microscopy of woolly hair as reported by Swami et al. [11], was also seen on trichoscopy in our case. Genetic testing could not be performed in our case due to economic constraints.

4. Conclusions

We are reporting this case because of its rarity and highlight the use of trichoscopy as a convenient diagnostic tool. Trichoscopy allows a simple, quick, and noninvasive examination of a single hair or multiple hairs in vivo which is not possible with a light microscope.

Consent

Informed consent was taken from the mother of the patient.

References

[1] Y. Ramot and A. Zlotogorski, "The twisting tale of woolly hair: A trait with many causes," *Journal of Medical Genetics*, vol. 52, no. 4, pp. 217–223, 2015.

[2] B. Vasudevan, R. Verma, A. Badad, and V. Pragasam, "A rare case of woolly hair with unusual associations," *Indian Dermatology Online Journal*, vol. 4, no. 3, p. 222, 2013.

[3] M. Olszewska, L. Rudnicka, A. Rakowska, E. Kowalska-Oledzka, and M. Slowinska, "Trichoscopy," *JAMA Dermatology* vol. 144, no. 8, p. 1007, 2008.

[4] A. Rakowska, M. Slowinska, E. Kowalska-Oledzka, and L. Rudnicka, "Trichoscopy in genetic hair shaft abnormalities," *Journal of Dermatological Case Reports*, vol. 2, pp. 14–20, 2008.,

[5] S. Patil, M. Marwah, N. Nadkarni, M. Gautam, and K. Godse, "The medusa head: Dermoscopic diagnosis of woolly hair syndrome," *International Journal of Trichology*, vol. 4, no. 3, pp. 184-185, 2012.

[6] K. N. Naveen, S. R. Shetty, H. Radha, S. B. Athaniker, and M. R. Gundannanavar, "Woolly hair with trichoscopic features," *Indian Journal of Paediatric Dermatology*, vol. 17, no. 1, pp. 56-57, 2016.

[7] A. M. Gossage, "The inheritance of certain human abnormalities," *The Quarterly Journal of Medicine*, vol. 1, pp. 331–347, 1907.

[8] A. J. Chien, M. C. Valentine, and V. P. Sybert, "Hereditary woolly hair and keratosis pilaris," *Journal of the American Academy of Dermatology*, vol. 54, no. 2, pp. S35–S39, 2006.

[9] F. Lacarrubba, F. Dall'Oglio, A. Rossi, R. A. Schwartz, and G. Micali, "Familial keratosis follicularis spinulosa decalvans associated with woolly hair," *International Journal of Dermatology*, vol. 46, no. 8, pp. 840–843, 2007.

[10] P. E. Hutchison, R. J. Cairns, and R. S. Wells, "Woolly hair," *Transactions of the St. John's Hospital Dermatological Society*, vol. 60, pp. 160–176, 1974.

[11] S. Swamy, B. Ravikumar, K. Vinay, D. Yashovardhana, and A. Aggarwal, "Uncombable hair syndrome with a woolly hair nevus," *Indian Journal of Dermatology, Venereology and Leprology*, vol. 83, no. 1, pp. 87-88, 2017.

34

A Case of Terbinafine-Resistant Tinea Cruris Caused by *Trichophyton tonsurans*

Alireza Firooz,[1] **Ensieh Lotfali**,[2] **Mahsa Fattahi**,[1] **Maryam Fattahi**,[3] **Akram Miramin Mohammadi**,[1] **and Mahshid Shahrzad Kavkani**[4]

[1]*Center for Research and Training in Skin Diseases and Leprosy, Tehran University of Medical Sciences, Tehran, Iran*
[2]*Department of Medical Parasitology and Mycology, School of Medicine, Shahid Beheshti University of Medical Sciences, Tehran, Iran*
[3]*Emergency Medicine Management Research Center, Iran University of Medical Sciences, Tehran, Iran*
[4]*Department of Microbial Biotechnology, Islamic Azad University, Damghan, Iran*

Correspondence should be addressed to Mahsa Fattahi; afattahi@sina.tums.ac.ir

Academic Editor: Hristo Dobrev

A 26-year-old male patient referred to our center with a history of extremely itchy crusted skin lesions in his groins for one year. Moreover, his friend, a 25-year-old male, also developed similar lesions in the groin after using the shared pool, whose condition also did not improve with similar treatment. A regular mycology test (direct and culture test) was performed, as well as molecular examination. The antifungal susceptibility assay to terbinafine, itraconazole, posaconazole, fluconazole, and voriconazole was conducted according to the Clinical and Laboratory Standards Institute M38 third ed. The sequencing study identified *T. tonsurans* as the causative organism in both patients. The abovementioned organism isolated from both patients displayed resistance against terbinafine and fluconazole (MIC $\geq 4\,\mu$g/ml and MIC $\geq 8\,\mu$g/ml, respectively). Moreover, the susceptibility of both subjects to posaconazole (0.313 μg/ml), voriconazole (0.25–0.0625 μg/ml), and (1 μg/ml) itraconazole increased. The present report aimed to emphasize the increase in antifungal resistance and a demand for antifungal stewardship, to control this public health threat.

1. Introduction

Dermatophytosis is known as the most common type of skin disease in the world which is caused by dermathophytes. It is approximated that dermatophytosis affects more than 20–25% of the world's population [1, 2].

2. Case Presentation

A 26-year-old male patient referred to our center with a history of extremely itchy crusted skin lesions in his groins for one year (shown in Figure 1(a)). Terbinafine tablet (250 mg/day) for 4 weeks and then fluconazole capsule (150 mg/day) for 6 weeks, clotrimazole cream, and antifungal shampoos were prescribed for him. Nevertheless, they were not able to improve his situation and his symptoms worsened. Moreover, his friend, a 25-year-old male, also developed similar lesions in the groin after using the shared pool, whose condition also did not improve with similar treatment (shown in Figure 1(b)). A regular mycology test (direct and culture test) was performed, and dermatophytosis caused by *Trichophyton* was confirmed. We isolated genomic DNA from a seven-day colony cultivated on Mycosel Agar (Merck, Germany) at 28°C using a genomic DNA extraction kit (Roche Life Science, Germany). Then, we amplified the ITS1/ITS2 area and sequenced the PCR products. Afterward, we made a comparison between the sequences and the reference data of the GenBank database via the BLAST program (http://www.ncbi.nlm.nih.gov/BLAST).

We also performed an antifungal susceptibility test to help us choose a proper treatment. We bought the antifungals from Sigma-Aldrich, USA. The *in vitro* activities of

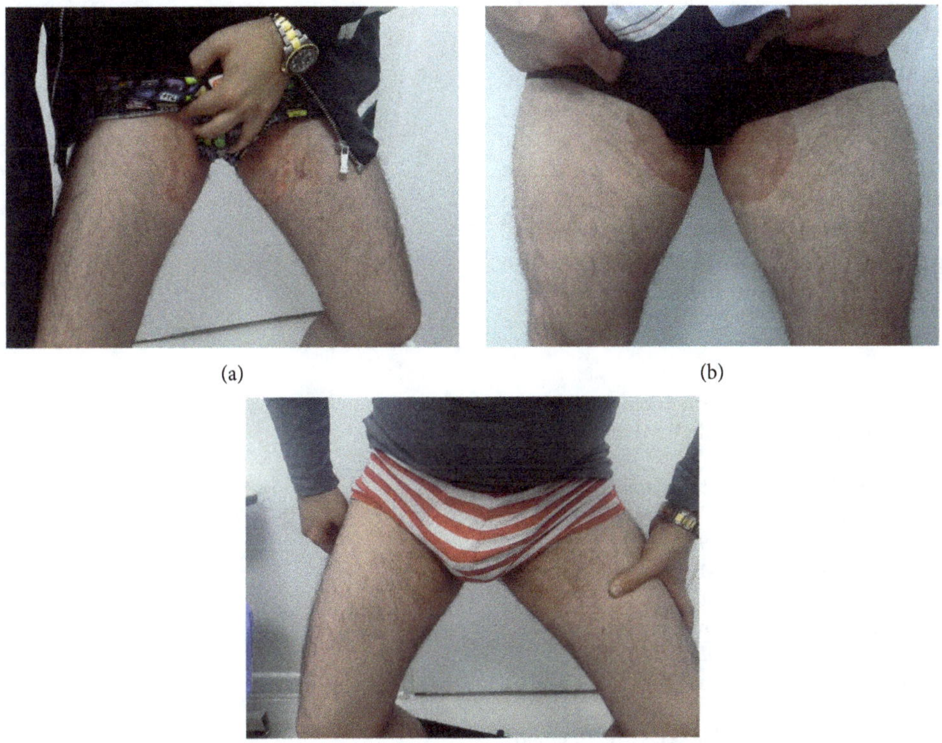

(a) (b) (c)

Figure 1: (a, b) Two patients with groin dermatophytosis which showed resistance to terbinafine; (c) sample of the same patients after treatment with voriconazole.

antifungal agents, including terbinafine, itraconazole, posaconazole, fluconazole, and voriconazole, were assessed by the broth microdilution protocol that was recommended by the Clinical and Laboratory Standards Institute M38 third ed. We selected *Candida parapsilosis* ATCC 22019 as the quality control strain in all the runs.

The sequencing study identified *T. tonsurans* as the causative organism in both patients and deposited in the GenBank OK479141. The abovementioned organism isolated from both patients displayed resistance against terbinafine and fluconazole (MIC ≥ 4 μg/ml, MIC ≥ 8 μg/ml, respectively). Moreover, the susceptibility of both subjects to posaconazole (0.313 μg/ml), voriconazole (0.25–0.0625 μg/ml), and itraconazole (1 μg/ml) increased.

They were treated for 3 months with itraconazole 100 mg for 3 months, but did not show favorable response. So, they were treated with voriconazole tablets 200 mg/day for two months which cleared the lesions (shown in Figure 1(c)). Then, the patients continued maintenance therapy with itraconazole (100 mg/day) for a month. They were followed up for 3 months and did not show any sign of recurrence. The patients were also given topical clotrimazole cream with both voriconazole and itraconazole.

3. Discussion

Treatment-resistant dermatophytosis is a public health issue that has recently become common. Nevertheless, the resistance of *T. tonsurans* to terbinafine is rare. The first case of resistant *T. tonsurans* was discovered *in vitro* [3]. Chen et al. reported a 62-year-old man who had Darier disease complicated by terbinafine-resistant *T. rubrum*. He was treated successfully with itraconazole [4]. We did not find any report of resistant cases to both terbinafine and fluconazole in the literature.

Long exposure to subinhibitory concentrations of antifungals is mentioned as a possible reason for drug resistance [5]. Resistance of *T. tonsurans* against terbinafine could be due to the changes in the squalene epoxidase gene [6, 7] that was implied in patients with *Trichophyton interdigitale* as well. It must be noted that the treatment of resistant *T. tonsurans* is difficult. Considering that these cases showed resistance to terbinafine and fluconazole, we had to prescribe voriconazole, which is an antifungal typically used for the treatment of severe fungal infections in immunocompromised cases. The symptoms and rash disappeared two months after the daily consumption of voriconazole 200 mg.

4. Conclusions

The present report aimed to emphasize the increase in antifungal resistance and a demand for antifungal stewardship, to control this public health threat.

Authors' Contributions

Alireza Firooz was involved in treatment consultation and physical examination and critical revision. Ensieh Lotfali performed antifungal susceptibility tests and drafted the manuscript. Akram Miramin Mohammadi performed molecular tests. Mahsa Fattahi conceptualized the study and drafted and critically revised the manuscript. Mahshid Sharzad Kavkani performed molecular tests, and Maryam Fattahi was involved in physical examination.

References

[1] B. Havlickova, V. A. Czaika, and M. Friedrich, "Epidemiological trends in skin mycoses worldwide," *Mycoses*, vol. 51, pp. 2–15, 2008.

[2] M.-P. Hayette and R. Sacheli, "Dermatophytosis, trends in epidemiology and diagnostic approach," *Current Fungal Infection Reports*, vol. 9, no. 3, pp. 164–179, 2015.

[3] Z. Salehi, M. Shams-Ghahfarokhi, and M. Razzaghi-Abyaneh, "Antifungal drug susceptibility profile of clinically important dermatophytes and determination of point mutations in terbinafine-resistant isolates," *European Journal of Clinical Microbiology & Infectious Diseases*, vol. 37, no. 10, pp. 1841–1846, 2018.

[4] E. Chen, M. Ghannoum, and B. E. Elewski, "Treatment-resistant tinea corporis, a potential public health issue," *British Journal of Dermatology*, vol. 184, no. 1, pp. 164-165, 2021.

[5] A. Fattahi, "Multidrug-resistant Trichophyton mentagrophytes genotype VIII in an Iranian family with generalized dermatophytosis: report of four cases and review of literature," *International Journal of Dermatology*, vol. 60, no. 6, 2020.

[6] A. Hsieh, S. Quenan, A. Riat, L. Toutous-Trellu, and L. Fontao, "A new mutation in the SQLE gene of Trichophyton mentagrophytes associated to terbinafine resistance in a couple with disseminated tinea corporis," *Journal de Mycologie Médicale*, vol. 29, no. 4, pp. 352–355, 2019.

[7] S. M. Rudramurthy, S. A Shankarnarayan, S Dogra et al., "Mutation in the squalene epoxidase gene of Trichophyton interdigitale and Trichophyton rubrum associated with allylamine resistance," *Antimicrobial Agents and Chemotherapy*, vol. 62, no. 5, 2018.

35

Lymphocutaneous Sporotrichosis Refractory to First-Line Treatment

Walter Belda Jr.,[1,2] Luiz Felipe Domingues Passero,[3,4] and Ana Thereza Stradioto Casolato[1]

[1]*Dermatology Department, University of São Paulo, Medical School, Clinics Hospital, São Paulo, Brazil*
[2]*Laboratory of Pathology of Infectious Diseases, Medical School, University of São Paulo, São Paulo, Brazil*
[3]*São Paulo State University (UNESP), Institute of Biosciences, São Vicente, Presidente Prudente, Brazil*
[4]*São Paulo State University (UNESP), Institute for Advanced Studies of Ocean, São Vicente, Presidente Prudente, Brazil*

Correspondence should be addressed to Walter Belda Jr.; walterbelda@uol.com.br and Luiz Felipe Domingues Passero; felipepassero@yahoo.com.br

Academic Editor: Hristo Dobrev

Sporotrichosis is a fungal infection endemic in Latin America and has been attributed to the thermodimorphic fungus of the genus *Sporothrix*. Transmission to humans occurs during a traumatic injury with soil or organic material; additionally, lesions caused by infected cats play an important role in the epidemiology of the disease. The classic treatment of sporotrichosis is performed with itraconazole or potassium iodide; second-line medications, such as amphotericin B and terbinafine, can alternatively be used in cases of first-line drug failure. In the present study, a patient with lymphocutaneous sporotrichosis in the right upper limb exhibited intolerance to itraconazole and potassium iodide, additionally during the period of use; these drugs did not control skin lesions. In this patient, amphotericin B deoxycholate and its liposomal version were used in this patient; and complete recovery of the lesions was observed.

1. Introduction

Sporotrichosis is an infectious disease caused by the thermodimorphic fungus that belongs to the genus *Sporothrix*, and although cosmopolite, it is endemic in Latin America [1]. The main forms of transmission to humans are associated with traumatic injuries that occur with contaminated soil or organic material; infected cats are considered important vectors of this disease and are responsible for epidemic outbreaks in Latin America, such as Brazil [1, 2].

The clinical manifestations of sporotrichosis are classified as cutaneous and extracutaneous. Among the cutaneous forms, sporotrichosis can be further classified as lymphocutaneous, localized cutaneous, and cutaneous caused by multiple inoculations. In extracutaneous clinical form, different organs or systems can be affected. Furthermore, disseminated sporotrichosis can affect the skin, lungs, sinuses, liver, kidney, eyes, heart, and genitalia [3]. Classical sporotrichosis manifests between 2 and 4 weeks after injury and starts as a paponodular lesion at the site of inoculation and develops into ulcerated nodules that drain the seropurulent material. Frequently, this lesion spreads, and more nodules can be formed following the lymphatic vessels.

The gold standard for diagnosing sporotrichosis is to identify and isolate the etiologic agent, *Sporothrix* sp., from cutaneous lesions. Histopathological analysis can be suggestive, but it has low sensitivity due to a reduced number of fungal entities; however, it can increase after staining the tissue with PAS or Gomori; immunolabeling the etiologic agent in histological sections can also enhance the sensitivity of diagnosis [2].

Oral itraconazole, potassium iodide, and terbinafine as well as intravenous amphotericin B have been used in the treatment of sporotrichosis. In cutaneous and lymphocutaneous forms itraconazole is recommended as the first-choice drug for all patients [3, 4] at 200 mg per day until clinical cure. Patients receiving itraconazole therapy exhibit some tolerable side effects, such as headaches, nausea, vomiting, and epigastric pain. In cases of failure of treatment, 400 mg of itraconazole is used per day, divided into two doses. Additionally, itraconazole can be replaced by potassium iodide, initially with 3–5 drops three times a day, until 40–50 drops (4–6 g/day). This drug was chosen as the first-choice treatment for lymphocutaneous and localized clinical forms of sporotrichosis, but was replaced by itraconazole because the dose, counted in drops, is not as accurate as itraconazole. In addition, frequent side effects of potassium iodide include metallic taste in the mouth and gastrointestinal intolerance [3, 4]. Fluconazole has been considered the second-line treatment, but the efficacy of this drug is low compared to itraconazole and potassium iodide [5]. In severe forms of sporotrichosis, amphotericin B deoxycholate or the liposomal version has been used as the first-line drug in treatment, but after improvement of the lesions, it is replaced with itraconazole [6]; furthermore, patients with a compromised immune system also may be treated with amphotericin B when presenting with fixed cutaneous sporotrichosis [7]. In patients, amphotericin B can induce mild and severe side effects, such as fever, chills, headache, malaise, hypokalemia, hypomagnesemia, cardiotoxicity, and nephrotoxicity [8], which in fact is a huge drawback associated with the use of such a drug.

In the present case report, a patient with lymphocutaneous sporotrichosis, intolerant to first-line drugs, potassium iodide and itraconazole, was successfully treated with amphotericin B and presented a significant improvement of lesions.

2. Case Report

The case was a female patient, 61 years old, with lesions in the right upper limb that began 8 months before her appointment in the medical service of Hospital das Clínicas, Faculdade de Medicina da Universidade de São Paulo, Brazil. She was born in Barros Mendes (Bahia, Brazil), but residing in São Paulo city (São Paulo State, Brazil) for the last 45 years, working as a teacher. She has three healthy cats that regularly visit vets; according to her report, the cats did not scratch her before the onset of cutaneous lesions. One year before the appearance of skin lesions, she traveled to the countryside of São Paulo state (Registro town), and although she had contact with the Atlantic forest, skin injury was not observed. Additionally, between travel and appointment at the Hospital das Clínicas, she had no skin injuries or contact with plants and soil. One month after the appearance of the lesion, she was admitted to the Dermatology Service of the Hospital das Clinicas. The lesions were ulcerated, and the borders showed erythema and were infiltrated; the lesions were also covered with yellowish and hematic crusts. Furthermore, some ascendant subcutaneous nodular lesions were detected that suggest lymphangitis in the right upper limb (Figure 1(a)). Mobile and painless lymphadenopathy was detected in the right axillary area. The patient complained of pain in the lesions, and discrete hyaline exudation was verified, and no other local and systemic symptoms were observed. Skin fragments were collected to identify the etiologic agent of the lesions, as the morphology of the lesions suggested lymphocutaneous sporotrichosis, skin tuberculosis, or leishmaniasis. The histopathological study showed chronic granulomatous dermatitis with focal necrosis and neutrophil exudation of neutrophils (Figures 1(b) and 1(c)).

Fite-Faraco and Grocott staining did not evidence the presence of alcohol-acid-resistant bacilli or fungi, respectively. The immunohistochemistry reaction was not positive for BCG. Bacterioscopy and direct fungi research as well as culture of aerobic and anaerobic bacteria were negative. Skin samples cultured in agar-dextrose Sabouraud medium supplemented with chloramphenicol at 25°C allowed the growth of a whitish membranous culture, with a blackened peripheral halo (Figure 2(a)). Microscopically septate hyaline hyphae present in the apex conidiophores and bouquet-like structures were observed, suggesting a fungus belonging to the genus *Sporothrix* (Figures 2(b) and 2(c)). At 37°C, a white/yellowish colony with a smooth aspect was observed; additionally, yeasts were visualized at this temperature. Techniques of molecular biology were not used to identify species.

Based on these findings, lymphocutaneous sporotrichosis was diagnosed, and potassium iodide was prescribed at 1 g/mL; it was started with three drops per day and gradually increased as the patient tolerated the metallic taste. After one month of treatment, and using 25 drops of potassium iodide per day, the patient reported lack of appetite, nausea, and vomiting. Potassium iodide was replaced by itraconazole, which was administered orally for 12 days at 100 mg/day; as the patient became tolerant, the dose of this antifungal drug was increased to 200 mg/day. The patient reported constant nausea and emetic events after seven days of treatment; however, levels of alanine and aspartate transaminases, alkaline phosphatase, and gamma-glutamyl transferase were normal. Fifty days after the beginning of itraconazole therapy, the patient reported severe gastrointestinal alterations, and the intravenous antiemetic drug metoclopramide was administered to the patient; constant hydration was recommended. Ten days after this event, no improvement of skin lesions was observed. Due to the side effects of both first-line drugs and the resistance of the patient to take oral medicines, such as terbinafine or fluconazole, she was admitted to the Hospital das Clínicas to initiate a treatment with systemic amphotericin B. Additionally, it is important to observe that all these side effects were associated with the therapy with potassium iodide or itraconazole since the patient had no underlying diseases. Electrolytes, renal, and hepatic biochemical tests as well as electrocardiogram were performed, before beginning treatment. Amphotericin B deoxycholate at 50 mg/day (diluted in 500 mL of sodium chloride 0.9% and glucose 5% solution for 6 hours) was given during three days due to the inaccessibility of the liposomal formulation. At the beginning of treatment, episodes of nausea and vomiting were reported, but antiemetic medicines controlled these side effects. Biochemical tests were performed and revealed an increase of serum potassium and creatinine. Correction of electrolyte disturbance was carried out; and to compensate the biochemical alterations, the treatment was suspended for three days. A second set of treatment was performed with liposomal amphotericin B seven days after the infusion with amphotericin B deoxycholate, and it was administered at

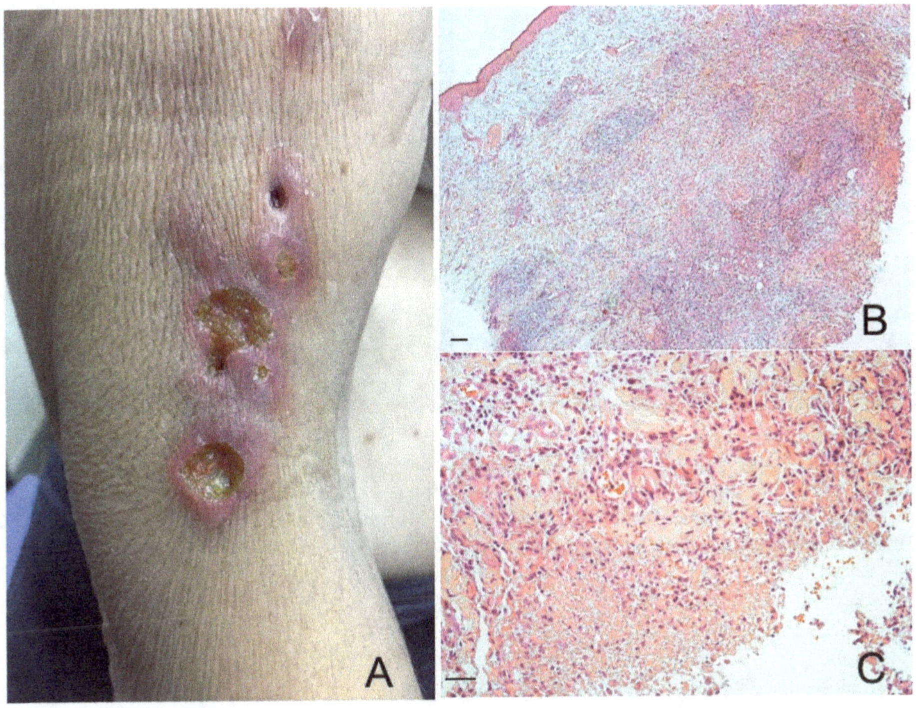

FIGURE 1: (a) Ulcerated lesions with borders showing erythema and infiltration. (b) Histological section showing the dense inflammatory infiltrate with the presence of granulomas; magnification 100x. (c) Focal necrosis and neutrophil exudation; magnification 200 ×. Histological sections were stained with hematoxylin and eosin. Bars = 5 μm.

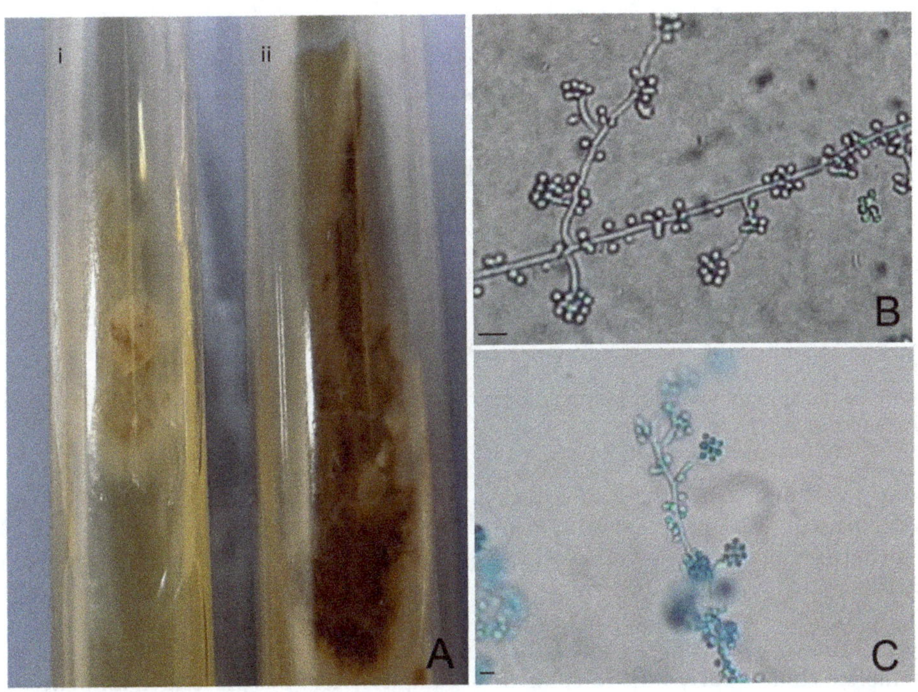

FIGURE 2: Skin samples were cultured in an agar-dextrose Sabouraud medium. (a) (i) In the sample cultured at 37°C, the fungi presented whitish/yellowish color with leveduriform aspect, and (ii) at 25°C, the fungi presented a brownish color that corresponded to the filamentous form of (b) fungi with conidiophore bouquet-like structures (c), magnification of 400x and 200x, respectively. Bars = 5 μm.

150 mg/day (diluted in 500 mL of sodium chloride 0.9% and glucose 5% solution for 6 hours) during 17 days. Clinical improvement of the lesions was observed during treatment (Figures 3(a) and 3(b)). A timeline containing the lesion appearance, diagnosis (Figure 4(a)), and treatment with iodide potassium, itraconazole (Figure 4(b)), or

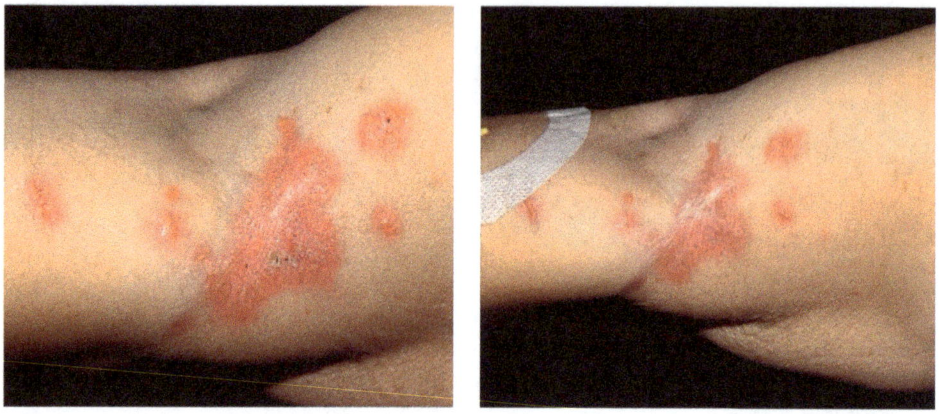

(a) (b)

Figure 3: (a) Morphological aspect of the lesions after infusion of 150 mg of amphotericin B deoxycholate and 2600 mg of liposomal amphotericin B presenting re-epithelization and absence of exudate. (b) Morphology of the lesion after infusion of 2600 mg of liposomal amphotericin B and 150 mg of amphotericin B deoxycholate, showing complete re-epithelization of ulcerated lesions and absence of exudation.

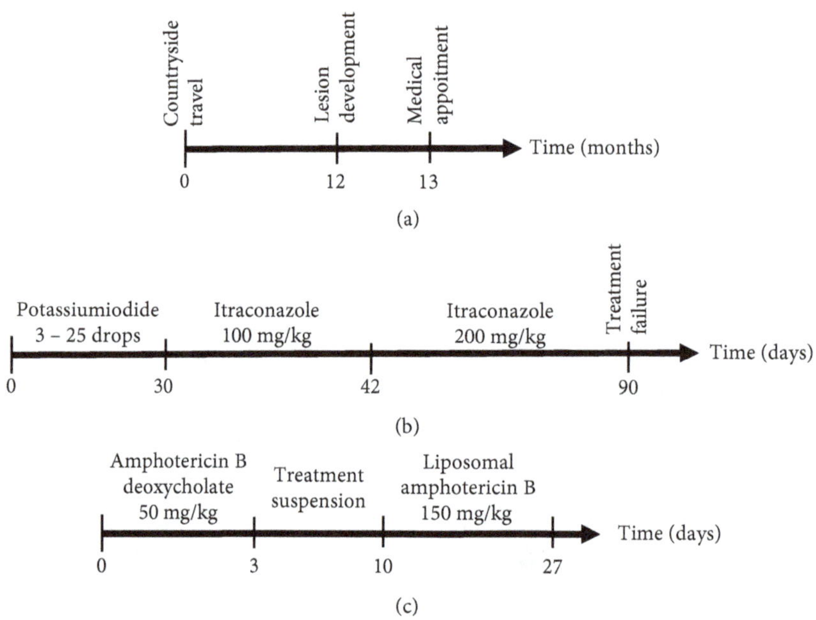

Figure 4: Timeline describing the appearance of the lesion (a); treatment with the first-line drugs potassium iodide and intraconazole (b); and treatment with amphotericin B (c).

amphotericin B (Figure 4(c)) summarizes the whole treatment performed in this patient. The treatment with liposomal amphotericin B did not change the levels of blood biochemical parameters.

The patient was infused with a total dose of 2600 mg of liposomal amphotericin B and 150 mg of amphotericin B deoxycholate until complete clinical cure, with re-epithelization of the ulcerated lesion and involution of lymphadenopathy. The follow-up has been performed monthly, and relapses were not recorded.

3. Discussion

Itraconazole has been used as first-line treatment in cutaneous and lymphocutaneous forms of sporotrichosis [9]. Similarly, potassium iodide, although an old drug, has been efficient at treating human cases [10]. Side effects of such drugs have been associated with gastrointestinal toxicity, as reported by the patient who was intolerant and presented lack of appetite, nausea, and vomiting without alteration of biochemical parameters [11]. Although highly toxic, amphotericin B is prescribed for patients with severe clinical forms, such as disseminated sporotrichosis [12–14]. Despite the toxicity of amphotericin B, this drug was used in lymphocutaneous clinical forms exclusively because the patient was intolerant to both first-line drug options. Although not the standard for the lymphocutaneous clinical form, intravenous treatment with amphotericin B was maintained, while improvement in clinical signals was observed. Amphotericin B topically applied was effective at healing fixed cutaneous sporotrichosis in an immunosuppressed patient that did not tolerate the first-line treatment [7]. In the present report, although the patient has no underlying diseases, the only tolerated treatment was amphotericin B. However, further studies need to be performed to understand the reasons of the refractoriness of the patient to the first-line drugs. Based on these findings, amphotericin B can be considered an interesting example of a successful nonconventional way to treat lymphocutaneous sporotrichosis in patients intolerant to first-line drugs.

Acknowledgments

The authors would like to thank HCFMUSP-LIM50.

References

[1] R. Orofino-Costa, P. M. de Macedo, A. M. Rodrigues, and A. R. Bernardes-Engemann, "Sporotrichosis: an update on epidemiology, etiopathogenesis, laboratory and clinical therapeutics," *Anais Brasileiros de Dermatologia*, vol. 92, no. 5, pp. 606–620, 2017.

[2] R. Arenas, C. Sánchez-Cardenas, L. Ramirez-Hobak, L. Ruíz Arriaga, and M. Vega Memije, "Sporotrichosis: from KOH to molecular biology," *Journal of Fungi*, vol. 4, no. 2, p. 62, 2018.

[3] V. K. Mahajan, "Sporotrichosis: an overview and therapeutic options," *Dermatology Research and Practice*, vol. 2014, Article ID 272376, 13 pages, 2014.

[4] R. O. Costa, P. M. de Macedo, A. Carvalhal, and A. R. Bernardes-Engemann, "Use of potassium iodide in dermatology: updates on an old drug," *Anais Brasileiros de Dermatologia*, vol. 88, no. 3, pp. 396–402, 2013.

[5] L. García Carnero, N. Lozoya Pérez, S. González Hernández, and J. Martínez Álvarez, "Immunity and treatment of sporotrichosis," *Journal of Fungi*, vol. 4, no. 3, p. 100, 2018.

[6] G. Verma, S. Verma, and R. Rattan, "Lymphocutaneous sporotrichosis of face with verrucous lesions: a case report," *Indian Dermatology Online Journal*, vol. 10, no. 3, p. 303, 2019.

[7] V. K. Mahajan, K. S. Mehta, P. S. Chauhan, M. Gupta, R. Sharma, and R. Rawat, "Fixed cutaneous sporotrichosis treated with topical amphotericin B in an immune suppressed patient," *Medical Mycology Case Reports*, vol. 7, pp. 23–25, 2015.

[8] R. Laniado-Laborín and M. N. Cabrales-Vargas, "Amphotericin B: side effects and toxicity," *Revista Iberoamericana de Micología*, vol. 26, no. 4, pp. 223–227, 2009.

[9] M. B. de Lima Barros, R. de Almeida Paes, and A. O. Schubach, "*Sporothrix schenckii* and sporotrichosis," *Clinical Microbiology Reviews*, vol. 24, no. 4, pp. 633–654, 2011.

[10] S. Xue, R. Gu, T. Wu, M. Zhang, and X. Wang, *Oral potassium iodide for the treatment of sporotrichosis*, vol. 2009, no. 4, Article ID CD006136, 2009.

[11] S. L. Xue and L. Li, "Oral potassium iodide for the treatment of sporotrichosis," *Mycopathologia*, vol. 167, no. 6, pp. 355-356, 2009.

[12] C. A. Kauffman, B. Bustamante, S. W. Chapman, and P. G. Pappas, "Clinical practice guidelines for the management of sporotrichosis: 2007 update by the infectious diseases society of America," *Clinical Infectious Diseases*, vol. 45, no. 10, pp. 1255–1265, 2007.

[13] P. E. Bunce, L. Yang, S. Chun, S. X. Zhang, M. A. Trinkaus, and L. M. Matukas, "Disseminated sporotrichosis in a patient with hairy cell leukemia treated with amphotericin B and posaconazole," *Medical Mycology*, vol. 50, no. 2, pp. 197–201, 2012.

[14] K. Ishida, R. A. Castro, J. J. Torrado et al., "Efficacy of a poly-aggregated formulation of amphotericin B in treating systemic sporotrichosis caused by *Sporothrix* brasiliensis," *Medical Mycology*, vol. 56, no. 3, pp. 288–296, 2018.

36

Mesenchymal Stem Cell Conditioned Media Ameliorate Psoriasis Vulgaris: A Case Study

Rajasekar Seetharaman,[1] Anjum Mahmood,[1] Prashant Kshatriya,[1] Divyang Patel,[1] and Anand Srivastava[1,2]

[1] *GIOSTAR Research Inc. Pvt. Ltd., Ahmedabad, Gujrat, India*
[2] *Global Institute of Stem Cell Therapy and Research, 4660 La Jolla Village Drive, San Diego, CA 92122, USA*

Correspondence should be addressed to Anand Srivastava; anand@giostar.com

Academic Editor: Jacek Cezary Szepietowski

Psoriasis, an autoimmune disease, affects a vast number of peoples around the world. In this report, we discuss our findings about a scalp psoriasis suffering patient with a Psoriasis Scalp Severity Index (PSSI) score of 28, who was treated with Mesenchymal stem cell conditioned media (MSC-CM). Remarkably, complete regression was recorded within a treatment period of one month only (PSSI score of 0). A number of bioactive factors like cytokines and growth factors secreted by MSCs in the conditioned medium are very likely to be the principle molecules which play a vital role in skin regeneration. Treatment using MSC-CM appears to be an effective tool for tackling the psoriatic problem and, thus, may offer a new avenue of therapy which could be considered as an alternative approach to overcome the limitations of the cell-based therapy.

1. Introduction

Psoriasis is a chronic disease thought to be of autoimmune origin which is characterized by patches on the skin and nails. It has been considered as a serious skin related problem affecting approximately 100 million individuals worldwide. About 2% of the world population and 0.44-2.8% of the Indian population were affected by psoriasis in 2016-2017 [1, 2]. Plaque, guttate, inverse, pustular, and erythrodermic are the five major types of psoriasis. Plaque psoriasis, also known as psoriasis vulgaris, is the most common form of the disease (about 90% of the cases) [3] which typically presents with red patches with white scales on top. Psoriasis vulgaris which commonly affects the areas includes scalp, knees, elbows, hands, nails, and feet [4].

Psoriasis, an autoimmune-inflammatory disease probably predisposed due to genetic makeup, is mediated by T-helper cells. Polymorphism, referred to as differences in DNA sequences of a gene, can be incurred by various external agents like chemicals, viruses, or radiation. Polymorphisms in genes of Th2 cytokine/regulatory T-cell (interleukin-10/IL10), Th1/Th17 cytokine (IL-12B and IL-23R), and tumour necrosis factor alpha (TNFAIP3; TNIP1) confer which increased other risks like cardiovascular diseases amongst psoriasis patients [5–7]. Single nucleotide alteration caused polymorphism in Th1 proinflammatory cytokine gene IL-2 [−330 (G/T)] which has been shown to be associated with greater disease severity in the Indian population [1]. On the other hand, another gene polymorphism occurring in Th-2 cytokine/regulatory T-cell (IL-4) has been shown to be protective against psoriasis [5]. Upregulation in the levels of inflammatory cytokines leads to psoriasis which also can be associated with an increased risk of psoriatic arthritis, lymphomas, cardiovascular risk, Crohn's disease, and depression [3]. There is no permanent cure for psoriasis, though steroid creams, vitamin D3 cream, ultraviolet light, and immune system suppressing medications (methotrexate) have been in wide use to help control the symptoms with some success [8, 9].

Mesenchymal stem cells (MSCs) are multipotent adult stem cells which have an excellent capacity to proliferate for an extended period of time while maintaining the undifferentiated cell status. The resulting daughter cells can differentiate into various types of cells of host tissues and thus help repair wear and tear incurred [10]. MSCs have a potential to serve as a powerful tool in cell-based therapy due to their tissue regenerative and host immune modulatory capabilities. The functions exhibited by MSCs have attracted a number of scientists and clinicians to investigate the mechanisms involved in their curative and tissue regeneration functions. A very few articles have reported the effectiveness of stromal vascular fraction (SVF)/MSC therapy in curing psoriasis by regulating the immune systems. Lee et al. [11] reported that human umbilical cord blood-derived mesenchymal stem cells (hUCB-MSCs) ameliorate psoriasis-like skin inflammation in mice and have regulatory effects on immune cells including $CD4^+$ T cells and dendritic cells. The first case study on intravenous infusion of SVF into psoriasis patient demonstrated a significant decrease in symptoms with a noticeable difference in skin appearance, psoriasis area, and severity index (PASI) score reduction (from 50.4 to 0.3) [12]. Chen *et al.* [13] reported that umbilical cord-derived MSC (UC-MSC) infusion effectively reduced psoriasis in human subjects. It was believed that MSCs' migration into the skin lesions and their immunomodulatory, autoimmune inhibitory, and paracrine effects were the principal factors behind the ameliorative effects. Other recent preclinical studies have shown that stem cell-derived conditioned media (CM) exhibit effective healing of psoriasis-like wounds and thus CM is an alternative for several cell-based therapies [14, 15]. The paracrine factors including growth factors, chemokines, and cytokines secreted from stem cells play a major role in wound healing [16] and these molecules are present in CM or spent medium harvested from cultured cells [17]. In short, CM can serve as a novel treatment approach in regenerative medicine which has been shown to have a successful outcome in preclinical studies. However, a very few reports are available on the clinical application of CM for treatment of any disease. Based on the principles and importance of CM, the present study was aimed at investigating the effect of MSC-CM on a patient suffering from psoriasis. This study is believed to be the first clinical report on the use of MSC-CM to treat psoriasis.

2. Case Report

2.1. Patient. A 38-year-old male patient, who was suffering from psoriasis vulgaris for 2 years, paid a visit to our centre. Preliminary examination of the patient showed that numerous erythematous plaques with numerous silvery scales present all over the scalp including the area behind the ears. The severity of the disease was assessed to be 28 on Psoriasis Scalp Severity Index (PSSI), calculated by the standard method which combines the severity (erythema, induration, and desquamation) and percentage of affected area.

2.2. Preparation of MSC-Conditioned Media. Adipose tissue was collected from a healthy volunteer by lipoaspiration by a plastic surgeon under the aseptic conditions in the O.T. About 100 ml of fat was aspirated out from the waist area and collected in a sterile container. The fat tissue contacting stem cells was processed in a biosafety laminar airflow chamber. MSCs were isolated from adipose tissue by standard enzymatic digestion method with 0.1% collagenase type I. Following the centrifugation, the resulting pellet was cultured in DMEM medium (Invitrogen, Paisley UK) supplemented with 10% foetal bovine serum (FBS) and 1% penicillin/streptomycin, at 37°C in humidified atmosphere containing 5% CO_2. The media were changed after every 3 days. About 5×10^6 MSCs of passage 2 were seeded in each T175 culture flask (n=10) containing 30 ml of DMEM medium supplemented with 10% FBS. MSCs were confirmed with spindle shaped morphology and free from any contamination (Figure 1) using a phase-contrast microscope. When cells attained 90% confluence at passage 2, the culture media were replaced with serum-free DMEM. After 72 h of incubation, resulting MSC-CM was collected, centrifuged at 2000 rpm for 5 min to remove the cell debris, filtered through 0.22-μm filter, and then concentrated (10 times) by ultrafiltration using centrifugal filtering units with a cut-off value of 3 kDa (Amicon Ultra-15; Millipore, MA), according to the manufacturer's instructions. The concentrated MSC-CM was aliquoted and stored at -20°C until use. MSC-CM was topically applied on the afflicted areas once a day over a period of one month. Clinical parameters like severity, changes, and clearance of psoriatic plaques were monitored at regular intervals.

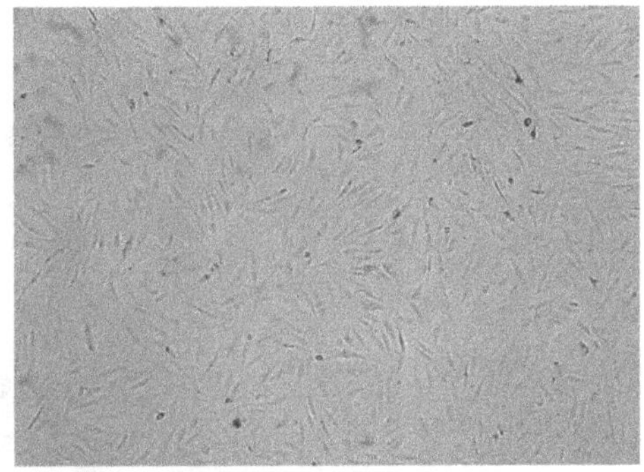

FIGURE 1: Phase-contrast microscopic image showing spindle shaped MSCs (× 100).

2.3. MSC-CM Ameliorates Psoriasis Vulgaris. Numerous psoriatic erythematous plaques with adhering silvery scales over the different regions of the scalp were observed before the treatment regimen started. In general, the number of the scales declined significantly within 2 weeks of topical application of MSC-CM. Interestingly, clearance of silvery scales and severity of psoriatic plaques were completely abolished within one month of the treatment (Figure 2). The PSSI score reduced to 0 from 28 and regression of the disease continued for 6 months of follow-up. The patient did not take any other medication during the follow-up period of six months and led an improved quality of life without any adverse side effects.

3. Discussion

Psoriasis is an autoimmune disease mediated by hyperactivity of T-helper cells. Increases in the levels of inflammatory cytokines triggered by T cells lead to psoriasis and

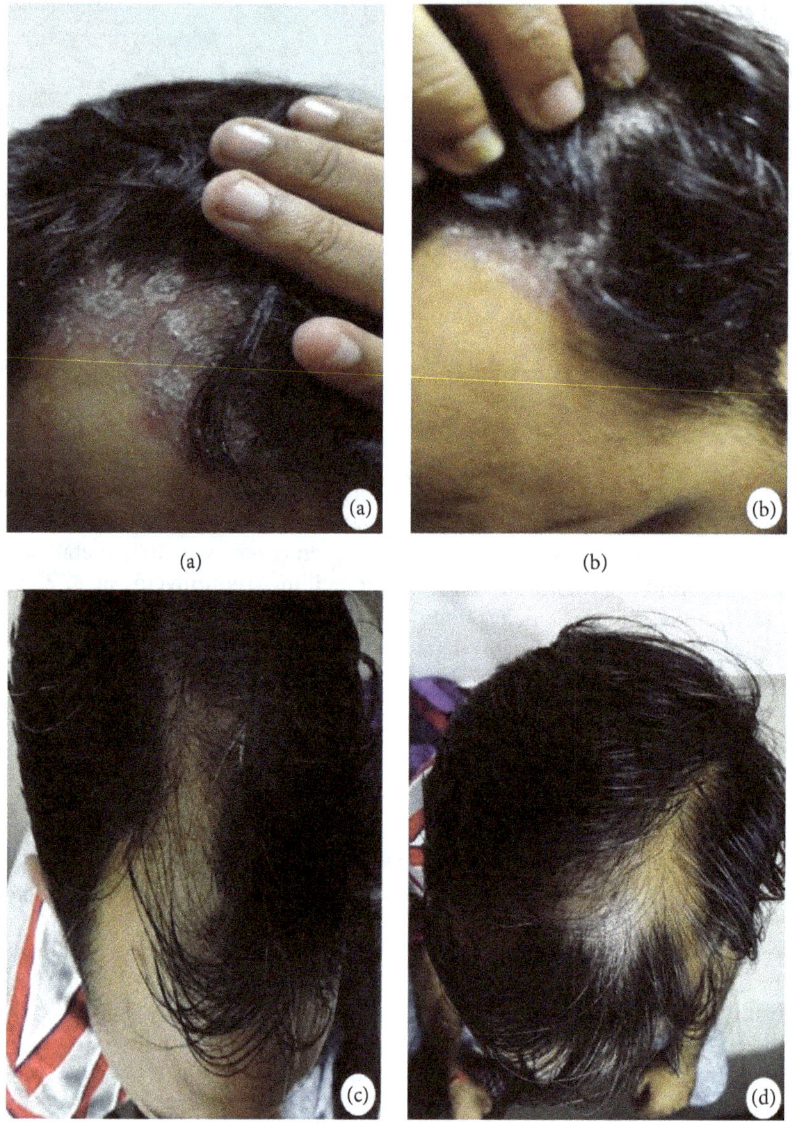

Figure 2: *Effect of MSC-CM on psoriasis vulgaris.* The scalp of patient showing numerous erythematous plaques with adherent silvery flakes before MSC-CM-treatment (a, b). Regression of psoriasis and a complete clearance of inflammatory erythematous plaques recorded after topical application of MSC-CM for a period of one month (c, d).

other associated diseases [3]. Therapies using multipotent MSCs have been shown to be effective in treating psoriasis and psoriasis-like other skin diseases. Clinical benefits may be attributed to MSCs engraftment or to their paracrine/immunomodulatory effects. However, transplanting MSCs come with few limitations like low survivability of cells in the host due to harsh microenvironment and cell loss because of poor or no cell adhesion [18]. Hence there is need of the hour to find an alternative for cell-based therapy.

Cell-free products of MSC origin are effective in wound healing and skin diseases. In this study, we demonstrated that MSC-CM can be used to treat patients with chronic psoriasis. Prior to MSC-CM treatment, the patient had received different medications but without any noticeable effective outcome. Remarkably, topical application of MSC-CM for a period of only one month completely abolished the erythematous plaques and resulted into a complete clearance of adherent silvery scales over the scalp. Further, the severity of psoriasis was completely reduced, from PSSI score of 28 to 0. This regeneration of tissue and improvement of qualitative appearance skin may be mediated by the growth factors, chemokines, and cytokines present in MSC-CM. Previous reports have shown that the paracrine factors secreted by MSC present in CM play a vital role in the healing of psoriasis-like wounds [16, 17]. Kim et al. [19] stated that adipose-derived stem cell (ADSC)-CM has regenerative effects on skin wounds. It stimulates both collagen synthesis, migration of dermal fibroblasts and promotes wound healing in animal models. ADSC-CM also upregulates the transcription of type I procollagen-alpha-1 chain gene of fibroblasts and induces Rho-associated kinase (RhoA-ROCK) signalling pathway, which leads to the proliferation of keratinocytes and dermal fibroblasts. In other studies [20, 21], MSC-CM promoted the recovery of skin burn wounds in rats, marked by an acceleration of wound closure, greater numbers of fibroblasts around and injured tissue and blood vessels, high epithelialization ratio, and high density of collagen fibres. It was suggested that basic fibroblast growth factor (bFGF) played an important role in the tissues regeneration of skin burn treated by MSC-CM.

In vitro and *in vivo* studies involving UC-MSC-CM demonstrated that its application caused an increase in the proliferation and migration of dermal fibroblasts, decrease in the ratio of transforming growth factor-$\beta 1/\beta 3$, and an increase in the ratio of matrix metalloproteinase over counter agent tissue inhibitor of metalloproteinases [22]. Similarly, human embryonic stem cell (hESC)-derived endothelial precursor cells CM is a rich source of a number of growth factors like epidermal growth factor (EGF), bFGF, fractalkine, granulocyte-macrophage colony-stimulating factor (GM-CSF), and interleukin (IL)-6. It was successfully used in the treatment of excisional wound healing in rats [23]. A comparative study revealed that wound healing by bone-marrow derived mesenchymal stem cell (BMMSC)-CM was significantly higher than that by fibroblast-CM [16]. The fact that BMMSC-CM had higher levels of paracrine factors than those in fibroblast-CM indicated the importance of origin of cells played a significant role in the production of paracrine factors. Other growth factors like Vascular endothelial growth factor (VEGF), insulin like growth factor (IGF), EGF, keratinocyte growth factor (KGF), angioprotein-1 (Ang-1), stromal derived factor-1, and erythropoietin (EPO) were also present in BMMSC-CM. With the supporting evidence of previous reports, the ameliorative effect of MSC-CM exhibited in this present study could be attributed to the presence of numerous growth factors secreted by MSCs in the media.

4. Conclusions

This is the first case report which demonstrates the ameliorative effect of MSC-CM on psoriasis vulgaris. MSC-CM is likely to have a wide range of cytokines and growth factors which can directly act on resident skin cells and thus can help in the skin regeneration. The active bioactive ingredients and their needed combination are yet to be determined. Use of MSC-CM instead of direct implantation of MSCs to tackle the issue offers an alternative approach which overcomes a number of limitations of cell-based therapy. In conclusion, treatment using MSC-CM appears to be highly effective for the treatment of psoriasis and may represent a new avenue of therapy. Further investigations for addressing a number of question provoked by the findings reported here, such as long-term effects (over a period of years), induced changes at cellular and histological levels, and identification of involved bioactive molecules, demand more studies.

Consent

The patient and the volunteer, participating in the study, were informed about the procedures and their consent was obtained in advance.

References

[1] D. M. Thappa and M. Munisamy, "Research on psoriasis in India: Where do we stand?" *Indian Journal of Medical Research*, vol. 146, no. 2, pp. 147–149, 2017.

[2] WHO, *Global Report on Psoriasis*, 2016.

[3] W. H. Boehncke and M. P. Schon, "Psoriasos," *Lancet*, vol. 386, pp. 983–994, 2015.

[4] C. G. Helmick, H. Lee-Han, S. C. Hirsch, T. L. Baird, and C. L. Bartlett, "Prevalence of psoriasis among adults in the U.S.: 2003-2006 and 2009-2010 national health and nutrition examination surveys," *American Journal of Preventive Medicine*, vol. 47, no. 1, pp. 37–45, 2014.

[5] S. Indhumathi, M. Rajappa, L. Chandrashekar, P. H. Ananthanarayanan, D. M. Thappa, and V. S. Negi, "TNFAIP3 and TNIP1 polymorphisms confer psoriasis risk in South Indian Tamils," *British Journal of Biomedical Science*, vol. 72, no. 4, pp. 168–173, 2015.

[6] S. Indhumathi, M. Rajappa, L. Chandrashekar, P. H. Ananthanarayanan, D. M. Thappa, and V. S. Negi, "Investigation of association of the IL-12B and IL-23R genetic variations with psoriatic risk in a South Indian Tamil cohort," *Human Immunology*, vol. 77, no. 1, pp. 54–62, 2016.

[7] S. Indhumathi, M. Rajappa, L. Chandrashekar, P. H. Ananthanarayanan, D. M. Thappa, and V. S. Negi, "T helper-2 cytokine/regulatory T-cell gene polymorphisms and their relation with risk of psoriasis in a South Indian Tamil cohort," *Human Immunology*, vol. 78, no. 2, pp. 209–215, 2017.

[8] A. Menter and C. E. Griffiths, "Current and future management of psoriasis," *The Lancet*, vol. 370, no. 9583, pp. 272–284, 2007.

[9] A. Menter, A. Gottlieb, S. R. Feldman et al., "Guidelines of care for the management of psoriasis and psoriatic arthritis. Section 1. Overview of psoriasis and guidelines of care for the treatment of psoriasis with biologics," *Journal of the American Academy of Dermatology*, vol. 58, no. 5, pp. 826–850, 2008.

[10] R. S. Mahla, "Stem cells applications in regenerative medicine and disease therapeutics," *International Journal of Cell Biology*, vol. 2016, Article ID 6940283, 24 pages, 2016.

[11] Y. S. Lee, S. K. Sah, J. H. Lee, K.-W. Seo, K.-S. Kang, and T.-Y. Kim, "Human umbilical cord blood-derived mesenchymal stem cells ameliorate psoriasis-like skin inflammation in mice," *Biochemistry and Biophysics Reports*, vol. 9, pp. 281–288, 2017.

[12] K. Comella, M. Parlo, R. Daly, and K. Dominessy, "First-in-man intravenous implantation of stromal vascular fraction in psoriasis: A case study," *International Medical Case Reports Journal*, vol. 11, pp. 59–64, 2018.

[13] H. Chen, J. Niu, H. Ning et al., "Treatment of psoriasis with mesenchymal stem cells," *American Journal of Medicine*, vol. 129, no. 3, pp. e13–e14, 2016.

[14] J. A. Pawitan, "Prospect of stem cell conditioned medium in regenerative medicine," *BioMed Research International*, vol. 2014, Article ID 965849, 14 pages, 2014.

[15] M. N. M. Walter, K. T. Wright, H. R. Fuller, S. MacNeil, and W. E. B. Johnson, "Mesenchymal stem cell-conditioned medium accelerates skin wound healing: an in vitro study of fibroblast and keratinocyte scratch assays," *Experimental Cell Research*, vol. 316, no. 7, pp. 1271–1281, 2010.

[16] L. Chen, E. E. Tredget, P. Y. G. Wu, Y. Wu, and Y. Wu, "Paracrine factors of mesenchymal stem cells recruit macrophages and endothelial lineage cells and enhance wound healing," *Plos One*, vol. 3, no. 4, Article ID e1886, 2008.

[17] R. Shohara, A. Yamamoto, and S. Takikawa, "Mesenchymal stromal cells of human umbilical cord Wharton's jelly accelerate wound healing by paracrine mechanisms," *Cytotherapy*, vol. 14, no. 10, pp. 1171–1181, 2012.

[18] S. Lee, E. Choi, M. J. Cha, and K. C. Hwang, "Cell adhesion and long-term survival of transplanted mesenchymal stem cells: a prerequisite for cell therapy," *Oxidative Medicine and Cellular Longevity*, vol. 2015, Article ID 632902, 9 pages, 2015.

[19] W.-S. Kim, B.-S. Park, and J.-H. Sung, "Protective role of adipose-derived stem cells and their soluble factors in photoaging," *Archives of Dermatological Research*, vol. 301, no. 5, pp. 329–336, 2009.

[20] I. Padeta, W. S. Nugroho, D. L. Kusindarta, Y. H. Fibrianto, and T. Budipitojo, "Mesenchymal stem cell-conditioned medium promote therecovery of skin burn wound," *Asian Journal of Animal and Veterinary Advances*, vol. 12, no. 3, pp. 132–141, 2017.

[21] T. Tarcisia, L. Damayanti, R. D. Antarianto, Y. Moenadjat, and J. A. Pawitan, "Adipose derived stem cell conditioned medium effect on proliferation phase of wound healing in sprague dawley rat," *Medical Journal of Indonesia*, vol. 26, no. 4, pp. 239–245, 2017.

[22] M. Li, F. Luan, Y. Zhao et al., "Mesenchymal stem cell-conditioned medium accelerates wound healing with fewer scars," *International Wound Journal*, vol. 14, no. 1, pp. 64–73, 2017.

[23] M. J. Lee, J. Kim, K. I. Lee, J. M. Shin, J. I. Chae, and H. M. Chung, "Enhancement of wound healing by secretory factors of endothelial precursor cells derived from human embryonic stem cells," *Cytotherapy*, vol. 13, no. 2, pp. 165–178, 2011.

Oral White Sponge Nevus: An Exceptional Differential Diagnosis in Childhood

Fatima zahra Elfatoiki, Sophia Capatas, Hayat Dahbi Skali, Fouzia Hali, Hicham Attar, and Soumia Chiheb

Department of Dermatology, Ibn Rochd UHC, 1 Quartier des Hopitaux 20000, Casablanca, Morocco

Correspondence should be addressed to Fatima zahra Elfatoiki; fatiza59@hotmail.fr

Academic Editor: Tak-Wah Wong

White sponge nevus is an autosomal dominant skin disorder characterized by white, irregular, diffuse plaques mainly affecting the oral mucosa. Histological findings of white sponge nevus are characteristic but not pathognomonic. We report a case of an oral white sponge nevus in a 6-year-old girl, which poses a problem in differential diagnosis with oral candidiasis. No treatment was performed because of the benign and asymptomatic nature of the lesions.

1. Background

White sponge nevus is a rare hereditary mucosal disorder characterized by asymptomatic spongy white plaques that affect oral mucosa and less frequently nasal, esophageal, rectal, and genial mucosa. Oral white sponge nevus appears as white or gray diffuse plaques thickened with multiple furrows and spongy texture located onbuccal, labial, gingival mucosa and floor of the mouth [1].

2. Case Report

A 6-year-old girl without any parental consanguinity, presented to our Department of Dermatology with chronic white lesions of oral mucosa that appear at the age of 2 years according to her mother. She was treated as mucosal candidiasis for more than 3 years without any result. There were no other family members affected by similar lesions. The lesions were asymptomatic except of some episodic burning sensations when eating acid or spicy food.

Cutaneous examination showed white irregular plaques with well-defined borders and symmetric distribution on the buccal mucosa (Figure 1). There was no associated erythema, and the plaques did not scrape off when using a tongue blade. There were no similar lesions elsewhere on the other mucosae. Histopathological examination showed superficial parakeratosis, acanthosis, and spongiosis with perinuclear eosinophilic condensation of epithelial cells. A minimal lymphocytic infiltration was present in the stroma. PAS coloration was negative. These features were characteristic of oral white sponge nevus. The genetic study was not performed.

Because of the benign and asymptomatic nature of the lesions, no medication was performed and the fungal treatment was stopped.

3. Discussion

White sponge nevus is an autosomal dominant genodermatosis that is often manifested in early childhood and showed no gender preference [2]. In our case, the lesions appear at the age of 2 years and were treated as oral candidiasis for many years.

The autosomal dominant characteristic of white sponge nevus shows irregular penetrance and variable expressivity in the same family. In our case, no similar lesions were found in parents or in siblings. The mutations concern the Keratin 4 or Keratin 13 genes, encoding mucosa-specific keratin intermediate filament proteins Keratin 4 and Keratin 13, "respectively," that are important for the assembly of keratin

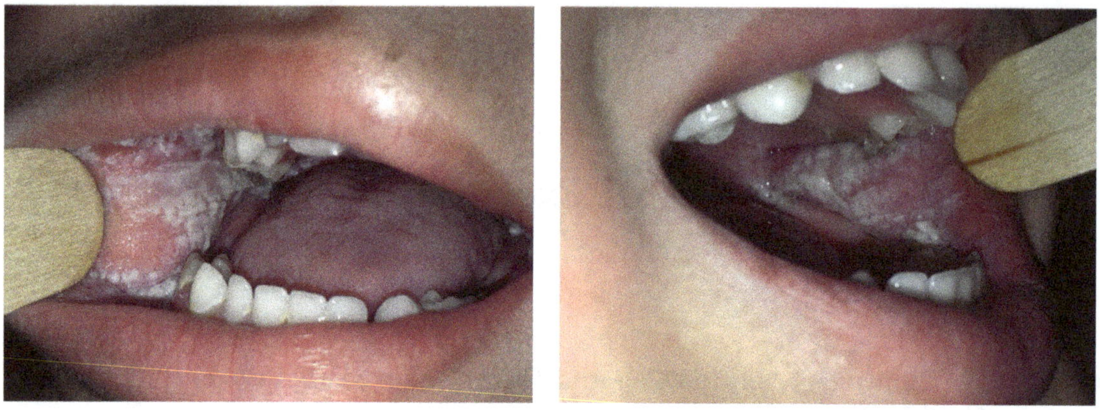

(a) (b)

Figure 1: White irregular plaques with well-defined borders and symmetric distribution on the buccal mucosa.

filaments [3, 4]. Liu et al. have recently compared sporadic and familial cases of white sponge nevus and concluded that only one of the five sporadic cases had keratin mutation [5]. The present case is probably sporadic without any similar familial cases especially in parents and siblings.

The lesions are seen usually in oral mucosa bilaterally as symmetrical, thickened, white, velvety, diffuse plaques that affect the buccal mucosa as observed in our case. The affected mucosa appears folded with a soft or spongy texture [6]. The less common intraoral location of white sponge nevus includes the tongue, labial mucosa, soft palate, alveolar mucosa, and floor of the mouth [7].

The differential diagnosis of oral white sponge nevus in childhood is made with other conditions presenting as white lesions on the oral mucosa [8]. These include other congenital disorders such as leukoedema, follicular keratosis, dyskeratosis congenita, hereditary benign intraepithelial dyskeratosis, and oral lesions of pachyonychia congenita and Darier disease. The acquired conditions include focal epithelial hyperplasia and oral florid papillomatosis associated with human papillomavirus. Oral candidiasis is difficult to differentiate from an oral white sponge nevus. This diagnosis is excluded by fungal examination and responsiveness to antifungal agents. Oral lichen planus may also be confused with an oral white sponge nevus, but this disorder is less common in young people [8].

The histological findings are characteristic of white sponge nevus. The histological features include acanthosis, hyperparakeratosis, and vacuolization of keratinocytes with a characteristic perinuclear eosinophilic condensation which is not necessarily pathognomonic [9].

Malignant transformation of a white sponge nevus is exceptional. Downham and Plezia reported the occurrence of an oral squamous-cell carcinoma within a white sponge nevus. This malignant transformation might be induced by chronic prednisone use, and no other similar cases were reported [10].

There is no treatment required in case of asymptomatic oral white sponge nevus. Various molecules were tested to reduce the clinical presentation of the white sponge nevus. These include beta-carotene, antibiotics (penicillin, azithromycin, etc.), antihistamines, local applications of retinoic acid, tetracycline mouth rinses, surgical resection, and laser ablation, but without any success [9].

In conclusion, our case illustrates the rarity of the oral white sponge nevus and its resemblance with other diagnoses more common in the oral cavity. The diagnosis of oral white sponge nevus should be established earlier by physicians to avoid unnecessary treatment.

References

[1] J. A. Regezi, J. J. Scuibba, and R. C. Jordan, *Oral Pathology Clinical Pathologic Correlations*pp. 80-81, Saunders Elsevier, Philadelphia, PA, USA, 6th edition, 2012.

[2] C. Quintella, G. Janson, L. R. Azevedo, and J. H. Damante, "Orthodontic therapy in a patient with white sponge nevus," *American Journal of Orthodontics and Dentofacial Orthopedics*, vol. 125, no. 4, pp. 497–499, 2004.

[3] Y. Shibuya, J. Zhang, S. Yokoo, M. Umeda, and T. Komori, "Constitutional mutation of keratin 13 gene in familial white sponge nevus," *Oral Surgery, Oral Medicine, Oral Pathology, Oral Radiology, and Endodontology*, vol. 96, no. 5, pp. 561–565, 2003.

[4] A. Terrinoni, E. Candi, S. Oddi et al., "A glutamine insertion in the 1A alpha helical domain of the keratin 4 gene in a familial case of white sponge nevus," *Journal of Investigative Dermatology*, vol. 114, no. 2, pp. 388–391, 2000.

[5] X. Liu, Q. Li, Y. Gao, S. Song, and H. Hua, "Mutational analysis in familial and sporadic patients with white sponge naevus," *British Journal of Dermatology*, vol. 165, no. 2, pp. 448–451, 2011.

[6] R. Rajendran, "Diseases of the skin," in *Shafer's Textbook of Oral Pathology*, R. Rajendran and B. Sivapathasundharam, Eds., pp. 821-822, Elsevier, New Delhi, India, 7th edition, 2012.

[7] B. W. Neville, D. D. Damn, C. M. Allen et al., *Oral and Maxillofacial Pathology*, Elsevier, Philadelphia, PA, USA, 2nd edition, 2002.

[8] M. Sobhan, P. Alirezaei, M. Farshchian, G Eshghi, H. R Ghasemi Basir, and L Khezrian, "White sponge nevus:

report of a case and review of the literature," *Acta Medica Iranica*, vol. 55, no. 8, pp. 533–535, 2017.

[9] N. Sanjeeta, D. Nandini, T. Premlata, and S. Banerjee, "White sponge nevus: report of three cases in a single family," *Journal of Oral and Maxillofacial Pathology*, vol. 20, no. 2, pp. 300–303, 2016.

[10] T. F. Downham Jr. and R. A. Plezia, "Oral squamous-cell carcinoma within a white-sponge nevus," *The Journal of Dermatologic Surgery and Oncology*, vol. 4, no. 6, pp. 470–472, 1978.

38

Brooke–Spiegler Syndrome: Familial Cylindromatosis, a Rare Variant of a Rare Familial Syndrome

Harsh Patel,[1] William Naber,[1] Austin Cusick,[2] and Craig Oser[3]

[1]*Ohio University, Heritage College of Osteopathic Medicine, 191 W Union St, Athens, OH 45701, USA*
[2]*Riverside Methodist Hospital, 3535 Olentangy River Rd., Columbus, OH 43214, USA*
[3]*Oser Plastic Surgery and Med Spa, 1 Robinson Plaza Suite 230, Pittsburgh, PA 15205, USA*

Correspondence should be addressed to Austin Cusick; ac830312@ohio.edu

Academic Editor: Alireza Firooz

Brooke–Spiegler Syndrome (BSS) is a rare autosomal dominant familial disorder resulting in dermatologic neoplasms of copious nodular appendages. Here, we report a case of Familial Cylindromatosis (FC), a subtype of BSS, in a patient with the largest cylindroma of $7.4 \times 5.6 \times 3.8$ cm on the scalp. The patient had undiagnosed cylindromas growing for 36 years at presentation; however, he did not seek out healthcare evaluation. Excision and pathologic investigation of three large masses from different body sites determined a shared phenotype of cylindromas. Subsequent evaluation of the patient's son separately, after primary patient excision, confirmed cylindroma development as well. The pathologic evidence of cylindromas in the patient with a new history of family incidence confirmed the diagnosis of the FC variant of BSS.

1. Introduction

Brooke–Spiegler Syndrome (BSS), aptly named after its first descriptors in the late 1800s, is a rare autosomal dominant familial disorder with an unknown incidence and prevalence, resulting in dermatologic neoplasms of copious nodular appendages [1]. This condition first presents as 0.5 to 3.0 cm head nodules in adolescence with a 6–9.6 : 1 female to male ratio and has three common adnexal neoplasms: spiradenoma, cylindroma, and trichoepithelioma [1]. The Multiple Familial Trichoepitheliomas (MFT), formally Brooke–Foredyce Trichoepitheliomas, and Familial Cylindromatosis (FC), formally Ancell–Spiegler Cylindromas, are considered two distinct variants consisting only of their predominate histological subtype [2].

The FC and MFT subtypes are associated with CYLD gene mutations on chromosome 16q12-913 [2]. This tumor suppressor gene impedes the Tumor Necrosis Factor-alpha pathway by reducing the expression of nuclear factor kappa B (NF-kB), a transcription factor with a key role in the antiapoptotic process [2, 3]. BSS, FC, and MFT variants have simultaneously presented in patients, suggesting these seemingly distinct subtypes are actually the end result of phenotypic variability within the same disease.

Creating an effective treatment plan with careful follow-up is imperative as malignant transformation occurs in 5–10% of patients with BSS [1]. Considering the malignancy risk with inadequate treatment, we present a case of FC found in a father and son of a rural medically underserved community with poor medical accessibility. The patients cited their poor healthcare access delayed the evaluation of their conditions substantially. From this novel case, we demonstrate a successful treatment modality for substantial BSS masses and highlight the importance of proper medical care in underserved areas.

2. Case Presentation

A 54-year-old male presented to the office with several subcutaneous nodular masses ranging in size on the scalp, groin, and back. The patient reports he had these nodules at age 18, but they have slowly grown over the years. The largest nodules were selected for surgical excision from each region. The nodules removed included a scalp lesion ($7.4 \times 5.6 \times 3.8$ cm)

(Figure 1), right groin (4.7 × 2.7 × 1.9 cm), and upper back (4.4 × 3.5 × 3.2 cm). After excision, the three nodules had a similar gross appearance, gray-tan, firm, nodular mass. Scalp and back lesions were sent for frozen sectioning during the procedure but were inconclusive on the specific pathology. Frozen sectioning did raise concern for possible malignancy. Permanent sectioning revealed an irregular globular jigsaw of basaloid cell morphology of the dermis in all specimens. Hyaline droplets and focal ductal differentiation were also present in all specimens. No nuclear pleomorphism or mitotic elements were present. The tumor cells were positive for cytokeratin 7 (CK7), periodic acid-Schiff (PAS), and epithelial membrane antigen (EMA). These histologic findings were consistent with multiple cylindromas. The presence of multiple cylindromas raised concern for potential familial diseases such as Brooke–Spiegler syndrome. On follow-up, the patient discussed that his son had similar appearing nodules. On follow-up, the patient reported his son also had subsequent surgical resection. His lesions were determined to be cylindromas as well, solidifying a familial component.

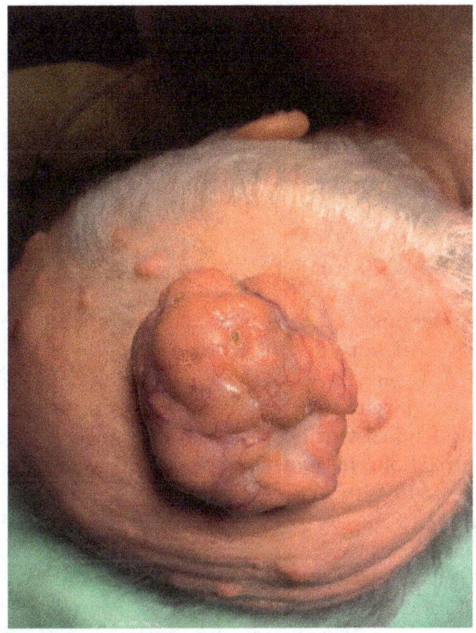

Figure 1: Cylindroma presentation on the patient's head, before surgical excision.

3. Discussion

Brooke–Spiegler Syndrome is associated with a mutation of CYLD, a tumor suppressor gene. The gene codes for a deubiquitinating enzyme by removing the lysine 63-linked polyubiquitin chain from substrates. Subsequently, it impedes the NF-kB and c-Jun N-terminal kinase pathways [4]. The majority of the mutations are frameshift, nonsense, and missense, which lead to truncated proteins. Genetic evaluation of patients presenting with the classic BSS phenotype demonstrates germline CYLD mutation in 80–85% of cases, while the MFT phenotype demonstrates a germline mutation in 40–45% cases [4]. Interestingly, the clinical severity of the disease does not correlate with the genotype, and the phenotypic expression is variable between subsequent generations with the same germline mutations [4].

Cylindromas are usually benign slow-growing tumors presenting as red or pink dermal nodules with arborizing telangiectasias [5]. Histologically, cylindromas and spiradenomas are categorized as follicular tumors specifically derived from hair follicle bulge [6]. Cylindroma is comprised of tumor isles that are surrounded by a hyaline eosinophilic sheath. Within each island, there is an outer layer of poorly differentiated epithelial tumor cells with small dark nuclei along with well-differentiated inner cells with big pale nuclei [7]. Historically, both cylindromas and spiradenomas have been considered driven from an eccrine origin, but this has been recently questioned with new histochemistry techniques. Recent research shows that both tumors are found to be CD200 positive, an immunoprotective membranous molecule. CD200 is highly specific for the hair follicle bulges, and it further supports the common locations of these tumors on the scalp and face [6].

Evaluation and successful diagnosis is important as to rule out other syndromic pathologies and possible malignant potential. Syndromic considerations for a differential diagnosis included neurofibromatosis, basal cell nevus syndrome, toxic-exposure-related incidence, and tuberous sclerosis. The differential diagnosis of a particular lesion should include benign lesions such as those shared in the abovementioned syndromic disease presentation; however, due to size and uniqueness in the removed lesions, malignant cylindromas were to be considered.

Due to this condition's rarity, treatment modalities vary. Usually, surgical interventions, such as electro cryosurgery, laser surgery, and radiosurgery, have all been utilized [1]. Besides the surgical approach to treatment, medications including aspirin, adalimumab, topical imiquimod, and vismodegib have been trialed with varying success [1]. In 2016, Mulder et al. reported the use of intralesional triamcinolone acetonide injection as a treatment modality for cylindromas. They hypothesized that corticosteroids would lead to regression of the tumor since it suppresses the NF-kB pathway. Clinically, this treatment resulted in initial regression of the tumors, but the neoplasms began to regrow after a couple of months [8]. Further investigation of medical management could provide alternative treatments for patients with economic challenges.

We report this case to add to the incidence report of this rare variant of the rare syndrome. Moreover, we also want to highlight that our patient had cylindromas beyond his head and neck area including significantly large cylindromas in the upper back and groin. The largest cylindroma on the head measured at 7.4 × 5.6 × 3.8 cm over the period of 36 years. The unique presentation of multiple large nodules on the head and extending to other areas of the body may be secondary to socioeconomic challenges. Being in a rural area of the United States, the patient elected to delay healthcare evaluation. The concern with regards to this delay in evaluation could have allowed for lesions to grow further and possible malignant transformation, adding to the uniqueness of this case.

Acknowledgments

The authors thank Joseph J Sreenan, MD FCAP, FASCP, for his work in proofing the manuscript and guidance and Ohio University Heritage College of Osteopathic Medicine Office of Research and Grants for funding the publishing cost (10-100000-250410-0000-20).

References

[1] W. Mohiuddin, J. Laun, and W. Cruse, "Brooke-spiegler syndrome," *Eplasty*, vol. 18, 2018.

[2] S. Bowen, M. Gill, D. A. Lee et al., "Mutations in the CYLD gene in brooke-spiegler syndrome, familial cylindromatosis, and multiple familial trichoepithelioma: lack of genotype-phenotype correlation," *Journal of Investigative Dermatology*, vol. 124, no. 5, pp. 919-920, 2005.

[3] S. Lucas-Truyols, C. Lloret-Ruiz, F. Millán-Parrilla, and E. Gimeno-Carpio, "Método simple y efectivo para el tratamiento de los cilindromas en el síndrome de Brooke-Spiegler," *Actas Dermo-Sifiliográficas*, vol. 108, no. 7, pp. 692–694, 2017.

[4] D. V. Kazakov, "Brooke-spiegler syndrome and phenotypic variants: an update," *Head and Neck Pathology*, vol. 10, no. 2, pp. 125–130, 2016.

[5] P. Zaballos, I. Gómez-Martín, J. M. Martin, and J. Bañuls, "Dermoscopy of adnexal tumors," *Dermatologic Clinics*, vol. 36, no. 4, pp. 397–412, 2018.

[6] K. Sellheyer, "Spiradenoma and cylindroma originate from the hair follicle bulge and not from the eccrine sweat gland: an immunohistochemical study with CD200 and other stem cell markers," *Journal of Cutaneous Pathology*, vol. 42, no. 2, pp. 90–101, 2015.

[7] C. Jordão, T. C. de Magalhães, T. Cuzzi, and M. Ramos-e-Silva, "Cylindroma: an update," *International Journal of Dermatology*, vol. 54, no. 3, pp. 275–278, 2015.

[8] K. M. Mulder, M. B. Crijns, and R. van Doorn, "Efficacy of intralesional corticosteroids in the treatment of cylindromas," *Clinical and Experimental Dermatology*, vol. 41, no. 5, pp. 578–580, 2016.

39

Deep Venous Thrombosis in Patients with Erythema Nodosum Leprosum in the use of Thalidomide and Systemic Corticosteroid in Reference Service in Belo Horizonte, Minas Gerais

Luiz Alberto Bomjardim Pôrto[1] **Maria Aparecida de Faria Grossi,**[2] **Edilamar Silva de Alecrim,**[1] **Marcus Henrique de Souza Brito Xavier,**[3] **Frederico Paiva e Silva,**[1] **Amalia Sathler Pires,**[1] **Fabianny Sanglard da Silva,**[1] **and Sandra Lyon**[1]

[1]*Dermatology Service Eduardo de Menezes Hospital, FHEMIG, Belo Horizonte, Minas Gerais, Brazil*
[2]*Secretary of State for Health, Belo Horizonte, Minas Gerais, Brazil*
[3]*Dermatology Service Alberto Cavalcante Hospital, Belo Horizonte, Minas Gerais, Brazil*

Correspondence should be addressed to Luiz Alberto Bomjardim Pôrto; luizalbertobp@yahoo.com.br

Academic Editor: Alireza Firooz

Introduction. Erythema nodosum leprosum (ENL) is a type of lepra reaction treated with corticosteroids and thalidomide, but this association increases the risk of deep venous thrombosis (DVT). *Objective.* To report cases of ENL with DVT in the use of thalidomide/corticosteroid associated. *Methodology.* The study was conducted between December 2015 and December 2016 at the Eduardo de Menezes Hospital (HEM-FHEMIG). *Results.* A clinical case series of 16 patients, eight from HEM-FHEMIG and eight from the literature. DVT occurred on 4 continents, mainly in adults and men. All patients were multibacillary; four people had pulmonary embolism (PE); there were 11 unilateral and five bilateral DVT cases; 12 cases were proximal, two distal, and two unspecified. Pharmacological thromboprophylaxis was used on two individuals. Outcome after DVT, 14 patients improved, one had sequelae, and one died. *Discussion.* DVT increased in association with thalidomide/corticosteroid in multiple myeloma, but this complication is poorly described in ENL. In proximal DVT, there was a greater risk of PE and sequelae venous insufficiency. After DVT, start anticoagulation. ASA 100mg/day as prophylaxis for DVT in case of this drug association in ENL is recommended. *Conclusion.* The article illustrates the incidence increase of DVT because of the thalidomide/corticosteroid combination in ENL. When this association is necessary, use ASA 100mg/day as prophylaxis.

1. Introduction

According to the World Health Organization (WHO), there were 210671 new cases of leprosy, in 2017 which represents a detection rate of 2.77 cases per 100 thousand inhabitants. Brazil has high burden for an illness, being the second with the highest number of new cases registered in the world [1].

Leprosy is a chronic infection caused by Mycobacterium leprae that primarily attacks the skin and peripheral nerves. The clinical presentation depends on the genetically determined cellular immunity of the patient. Accordingly, the disease is often categorized as multibacillary or paucibacillary (lepromatous or tuberculoid) which determines the type of therapeutic scheme [2].

Leprosy reactions are acute inflammatory episodes that may occur multiple times during the course of the disease or after treatment, manifesting as type 1 reaction or type 2 reaction known as erythema nodosum leprosum (ENL), whose treatment of choice is thalidomide [3–5]. The use of thalidomide associated with corticosteroids, cyclophosphamide, and doxorubicin may increase thromboembolic risk [6]. There are studies associating a 10%

Table 1: Reports of ENL complicated by thrombosis during thalidomide/corticosteroids therapy.

N	COUNTRY	AGE (YEARS)	GENDER	TYPE OF LEPROSY	MDT	COMORBITIES	REFERENCE
1	BRAZIL	43	M	LL	No	No	CASE 1
2	BRAZIL	39	M	BL	Yes	Cutaneous leishmaniasis	CASE 2
3	BRAZIL	57	F	LL	MOC	No	CASE 3
4	BRAZIL	40	M	LL	No	HIV+	CASE 4
5	BRAZIL	54	M	LL	Yes	No	CASE 5
6	BRAZIL	34	F	LL	No	Diabetes, ex-alcoholic, asthma and mood disorder	CASE 6
7	BRAZIL	55	M	LL	No	No	CASE 7
8	BRAZIL	71	F	LL	No	HIV+ e diabetes	CASE 8
9	SPAIN	43	M	B	No	No	Petiti-Martin et al. 2013
10	ÍNDIA	35	M	LL	Yes	No	LLetricheLLLLel et al. 2008
11	USA	39	M	B	Yes	No	Fabi et al. 2009
12	ÍNDIA	37	F	MB	Yes	No	Sharma et al. 2004
13	PORTUGAL	33	M	B	Yes	HIV+	Medeiros et al. 2009
14	JAPAN	58	M	B	Yes	HL; HTN	Sayaka et al 201
15	BRAZIL	75	M	BL	No	No	Brito et al. 2010
16	SRI LANKA	60	M	LL	Yes	No	Ahamed et al 2011 9:2.

B, borderline leprosy; BL, borderline lepromatous leprosy; ENL, erythema nodosum leprosum; F, female; HL hyperlipidemia; HTN, hypertension; LL, lepromatous leprosy; M, male; MB, multibacillary; MDT, multi-drug therapy.

increase in the risk of deep venous thrombosis (DVT) with thalidomide in combination with systemic corticosteroids [5, 7].

Thrombosis is linked to an imbalance of the fibrinolytic system and has as risk factors previous diseases, use of medication and alteration, of pro- or anticoagulant factors [8].

In the literature review, eight patients with leprosy erythema nodosum treated with thalidomide associated with systemic corticosteroids presented thrombotic events [5–12].

In this series, we present eight cases of DVT in individuals with leprosy and type 2 reaction.

2. Objective

The present study aims to report clinical cases of patients with ENL with the outcome of DVT during the use of thalidomide and systemic corticosteroids.

3. Methodology

The study was conducted between December 2015 and December 2016, at the Hospital Eduardo de Menezes of the Hospital Foundation of the State of Minas Gerais (HEM-FHEMIG). HEM-FHEMIG is a Regional Reference Center for Health Dermatology and Infectious Diseases [13].

The preparation of this series of cases took into account anamnesis, clinical examination, and propaedeutic exams. A review of the literature on "deep vein thrombosis" related to the use of systemic corticosteroid therapy and thalidomide was performed. The research was done in publications made after 2004, in English and Portuguese, using the following health sciences descriptors: Pubmed, google academic, LILLACS, and Epistemonikos. There were few manuscripts on this subject, most of which were case reports.

Patient images were stored with appropriate descriptions in the DermatologiaWeb Software and later selected for the article. The DermatologiaWeb system is used for photographic documentation of patients in a digital virtual way. It includes photo storage functionality and the comparison function of the most recent images with the oldest images of the same lesion or of the same part of the body [14, 15].

4. Clinical Case Series

Table 1 presents a series of 16 clinical cases of DVT in ENL patients in the period of thalidomide and corticosteroid use, of which eight were followed in the HEM-FHEMIG and the other cases coming from reports of cases found in the English and Portuguese language literature. Thus, it is observed that such complication was described in in North America (1), South America (9), Europe (2), and Asia (4).

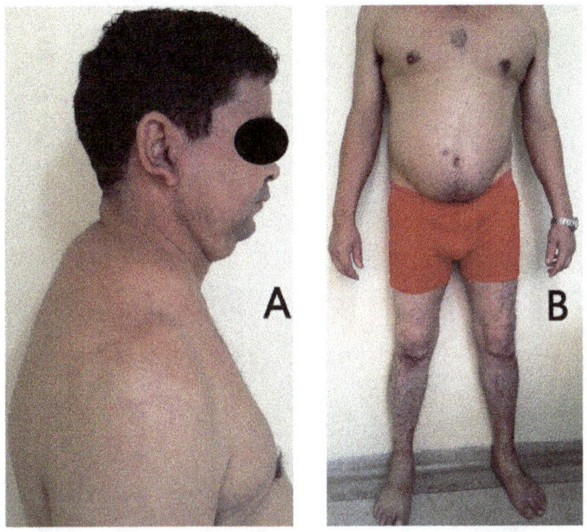

(a) (b)

FIGURE 1: (a) Case 1: patient with Cushing's syndrome secondary to systemic corticosteroid; (b) Case 1: patient without edema after recovered DVT in right leg.

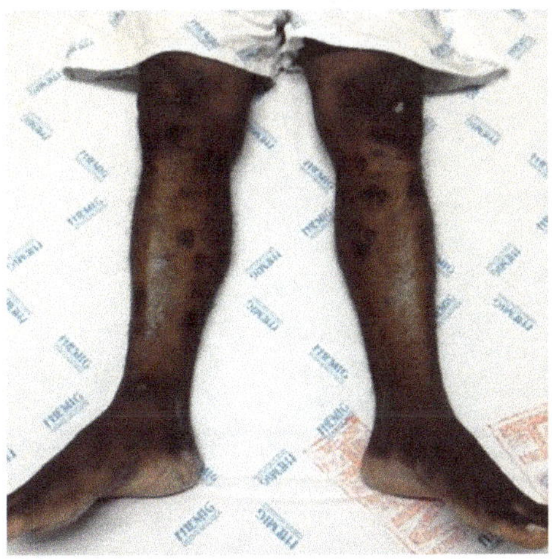

FIGURE 2: Case 2: patient without edema after recovered DVT in both legs.

The patients' age range was 33 to 75 years (mean of 48.3 years). There was a predominance of males in the proportion of 12:4. All 16 patients were multibacillary in the lepromatous leprosy (9), borderline (3), and borderline lepromatous (3) forms and were not subclassified (1). Three patients had HIV-AIDS, one had cutaneous leishmaniasis, one had hypertension and dyslipidemia, one had diabetes, and one had diabetes, asthma, alcoholism, and a mood disorder.

Table 2 presents the characteristics of the DVT and pulmonary embolism (PE) in these 16 clinical cases. Among the 16 patients described with DVT, four also presented PE. Most patients had unilateral DVT (68,8%) and the proximal veins were more affected (75%). Drug thromboprophylaxis was performed in two patients: in case number 2, prophylactic enoxaparin was used; in case 6, acetylsalicylic acid (ASA) was used. In three patients, there were changes in the coagulation system, even without the use of medication thromboprophylaxis at the time of diagnosis of the thrombotic event.

Three patients presented risk factors commonly associated with thrombosis: case 2 was hospitalized for bacterial sepsis prior to the diagnosis of DVT; case 6 was a smoker and an injectable contraceptive user; and case 12 used cyclophosphamide to treat ENL.

Regarding the outcome of the cases, the majority (87.5%) did not present any complications. However, one patient remained with chronic lymphedema in one lower limb and another patient died whose cause was not identified.

Soon after the diagnosis of thrombosis, all were anticoagulated with enoxaparin and subsequently warfarin, except for the third clinical case described in this article for refusal of treatment.

There are five figures of the patients to illustrate the cases from HEM-FHEMIG. Figure 1(a) is about case 1 with Cushing's syndrome secondary to systemic corticosteroid. Figures 1(b), 2, and 5 are about cases 1, 2, and 6 without edema of the legs after recovered DVT. Figure 3 is about case 4 with edema during acute DVT in right leg. Figure 4 is about case 5 with edema after recovered DVT in left leg.

Table 2: Reports of DVT and PE.

N	DVT	PE	COAGULATION DISTURB	PHARMARCOLOGICAL PROPHLAXIS	RISK FACTOR TO DVT	OUTCOME AFTER DVT	REFERENCE
1	Unilateral proximal	No	No	No	No	Recovered	CASE 1
2	Bilateral proximal	No	No	Enoxaparina	Bacterial sepsis	Recovered	CASE 2
3	Bilateral proximal	No	No	No	No	Recovered	CASE 3
4	Unilateral proximal	No	No	No	No	Edema unilateral and death	CASE 4
5	Unilateral proximal	No	No	No	No	Edema unilateral	CASE 5
6	Unilateral distal	No	No	ASA	Smoking and medroxyprogesterone	Recovered	CASE 6
7	Unilateral distal	No	No	No	No	Recovered	CASE 7
8	Unilateral	No	No	No	No	Recovered	CASE 8
9	Unilateral proximal	No	Thrombophilia	No	No	Recovered	Petiti-Martin et al., 2013
10	Bilateral proximal	No	No	No	No	Recovered	LLetricheLLLLel et al., 2008
11	Unilateral proximal	Yes Bilateral	No	No	No	Recovered	Fabi et al., 2009
12	Unilateral proximal	No	No	No	Cyclophosphamide	Recovered	Sharma et al., 2004
13	Bilateral proximal	Yes	No	No	No	Recovered	Medeiros et al.,2009
14	Bilateral	Yes Bilateral	No	No	No	Recovered	Sayaka et al., 201
15	Unilateral proximal	No	Coagulogram disturb	No	No	Recovered	Brito et al., 2010
16	Unilateral proximal	Yes Bilateral	Thrombocytopenia 90.000	No	No	Recovered	Ahamed et al., 2011 9:2.

DVT, deep vein thrombosis; PE, pulmonary embolism; ASA, acetyl salicylic acid.

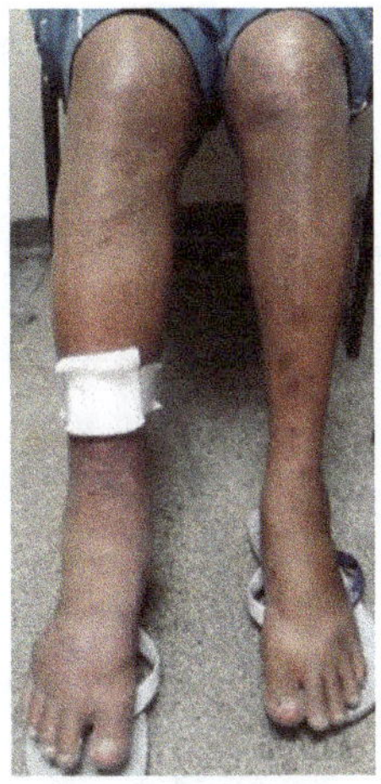

FIGURE 3: Case 4: patient with edema during acute DVT in right leg.

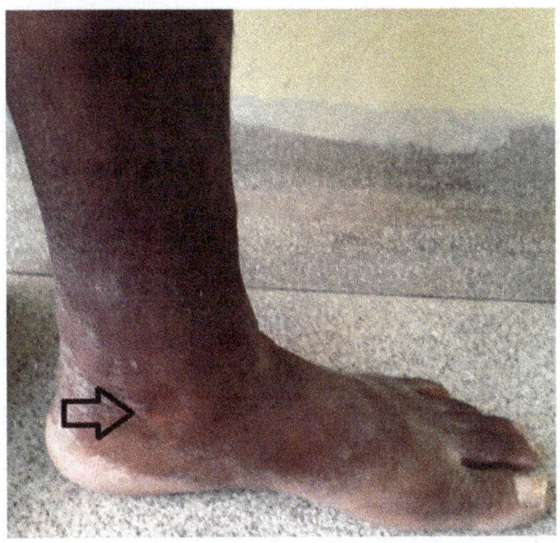

FIGURE 4: Case 5: patient with edema after recovered DVT in left leg.

Between 2014 and 2015, we followed 120 patients in the HEM-FHEMIG dermatology service using Thalidomide and oral corticosteroid for the treatment of ENL. In this period, we observed eight cases of DVT, which means an incidence of 6.66% of cases of thromboembolic events among those individuals.

5. Discussion

The drugs used in the treatment of ENL are thalidomide, oral corticosteroids, clofazimine, azathioprine, mycophenolate mofetila, methotrexate, and immunoglobulin G. Thalidomide is used in the treatment of ENL because of its anti-inflammatory property which is attributed to the inhibition of cytokines, TNF-alpha, endothelial growth factor, and fibroblast growth factor. The association of thalidomide with corticosteroid generates alterations in endothelial cell function, modifies the Th-1 cellular response, and increases the secretion of interferon-gamma and interleukin-2. The drug is also used in the treatment of multiple myeloma and renal carcinoma [8].

Thromboembolic events have been described in the association of thalidomide and corticosteroid in the treatment of multiple myeloma, but there are few reports when these drugs are used in the treatment of ENL. In addition, despite the existence of reports of prophylactic anticoagulation in individuals with multiple myeloma using the combination of thalidomide and corticosteroid, we did not find in the literature this prophylaxis for ENL [10].

Clinical suspicion of DVT should be confirmed by a complementary propaedeutic, in order to identify the involved vessel and the extent of thrombosis, since the risk of PE due to proximal DVT is greater, as well as the severity of chronic venous insufficiency [11, 16].

In studies with multiple myeloma patients, the incidence of DVT at the time of use of thalidomide alone is in the range of 2-3% and increases to 12-26% in the case of combination of thalidomide and dexamethasone without prophylactic anticoagulation, but the anticoagulation reduces the chances of DVT [17, 18].

In the results of this article, HEM-FHEMIG presented a 6.66% incidence of thrombosis in patients using Thalidomide for the treatment of ENL, which is more than twice as described in patients with multiple myeloma in use of thalidomide. We believe that this difference is due to the

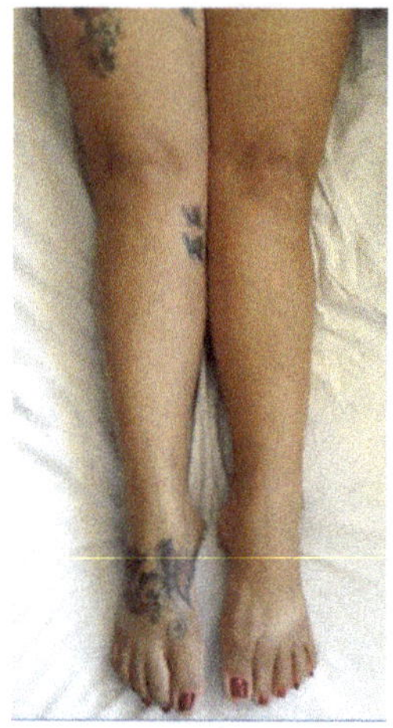

FIGURE 5: Case 6: patient without edema after recovered DVT in right leg.

frequent association of corticosteroid and thalidomide in our patients.

In Brazil, the Ministry of Health recommends ASA 100mg/day as prophylaxis for DVT in case of combination of thalidomide and corticosteroid for the treatment of ENL [4, 19].

A study of adverse effects of thalidomide was performed in HEM-FHEMIG and DVT were recorded in the use of the association thalidomide and systemic corticosteroid in patients with ENL [20]. HEM-FHEMIG is a Reference Center of leprosy and is aware in order to ensure timely diagnosis, treatment and prevention of complications [21, 22].

The risk factors commonly associated with DVT are smoking, drug use, immobility, cancer, heart disease, inflammatory bowel disease, and previous history of thrombotic events [9].

The risk of DVT is related to genetic factors and is higher in blacks, intermediate in Caucasians, and lower in Asians. The incidence and prevalence of DVT are also strongly related to age, increasing almost 90-fold from 15 to 80 years of age. There is no definitive data on frequency between genders. Contraceptive use and HIV infection increase the incidence of DVT [23].

The increase in thromboembolic events in patients with ENL in treatment with thalidomide and corticosteroid is not related to genetic events of thrombophilia, but rather the association of the two medications [24].

6. Conclusion

The increased risk of thromboembolic events in ENL patients is not related to genetic events of thrombophilia and should be considered when prescribing the combination thalidomide and corticosteroids.

When this association is necessary, the use of ASA 100mg/day prophylaxis for DVT should be evaluated and the occurrence of DVT should be monitored to avoid complications.

Consent

Informed consent was taken from all the patients, including the patients who allowed photographic registration.

References

[1] World Health Organization, *Weekly Epidemiological Record*, vol. 93, no. 35, Genebra, Switzerland, 2015.

[2] World Health Organization, *Leprosy Elimination*, World Health Organization, Geneva, Switzerland, 2017.

[3] Organização Mundial da Saúde, *Estratégia Global Aprimorada Para Redução Adicional Da Carga Da Hanseníase: 2011-2015: Diretrizes Operacionais (Atualizadas)*, vol. 70, Organização Mundial da Saúde. Brasília: Organização Pan-Americana da Saúde, 2010.

[4] *Guia Prático Sobre A Hanseníase*, Ministério da Saúde, Secretaria de Vigilância em Saúde, Departamento de Vigilância das Doenças Transmissíveis, 2017.

[5] G. H. Petiti-Martin, M. Villar-Buill, I. Hera et al., "Deep vein thrombosis in a patient with lepromatous leprosy receiving thalidomide to treat leprosy reaction," *Actas Dermo-Sifiliográficas*, vol. 104, no. 1, pp. 67–70, 2013.

[6] T. P. Vetrichevvel, G. A. Pise, and D. M. Thappa, "A case report of venous thrombosis in a leprosy patient treated with corticosteroid and thalidomide," *Leprosy Review*, vol. 79, no. 2, pp. 193–195, 2008.

[7] S. G. Fabi, C. Hill, J. N. Witherspoon, S. L. Boone, and D. P. West, "Frequency of thromboembolic events associated with thalidomide in the non-cancer setting: a case report and review of the literature," *Journal of Drugs in Dermatology (JDD)*, vol. 8, no. 8, pp. 765–769, 2009.

[8] N. L. Sharma, V. Sharma, V. Shanker, V. K. Mahajan, and S. Sarin, "Deep vein thrombosis: a rare complication of thalidomide therapy in recurrent erythema nodosum leprosum," *International Journal of Leprosy and Other Mycobacterial Diseases*, vol. 72, no. 4, pp. 483–485, 2004.

[9] S. Medeiros, C. Fernandes, N. Martins et al., "Hansen's disease in an HIV patient complicated by deep vein thrombosis: a

rare complication of thalidomide therapy," *European Journal of Dermatology*, vol. 19, no. 3, pp. 272-273, 2009.

[10] Y. Yamamoto, A. Hosokawa, K. Hagiwara, H. Uezato, and K. Takahashi, "Deep venous thrombosis and pulmonary embolism secondary to co-administration of thalidomide and oral corticosteroid in a patient with leprosy," *The Journal of Dermatology*, vol. 39, no. 8, pp. 711–714, 2012.

[11] E. O. X. Brito, S. M. F. Queen, C. A. A. Pires, and E. L. R. Daxbacher, "Trombose venosa profunda em um paciente com reação hansênica em uso de Talidomida e corticóide: um raro efeito adverso?" *Hansenologia Internationalis*, vol. 35, no. 1, pp. 53–56, 2010.

[12] R. Ahamed, W. Bandula, and R. Chamara, "An unexpected case of venous and pulmonary thrombo-embolism in a patient treated with thalidomide for refractory erythema nodosum leprosum: a case report," *Thrombosis Journal*, vol. 9, no. 2, 2011.

[13] E. S. Alecrim, *Avaliação de fatores associados à soropositividade do teste ML Flow e à reatividade ao Teste de Mitsuda em contatos de casos-índice de hanseníase em um centro de referência em Minas Gerais (MS thesis)*, Brasil. Dissertação, 2017.

[14] L. A. B. Porto, *Prontuário eletrônico de Imagens Na Dermatologia, Medicina E Cirurgia Estética: Relato De Caso. 37f. 2016. Monografia (Pós-Graduação Lato Sensu em Medicina e Cirurgia Estética). Orientadora: Dra. Sandra Lyon*, Instituto de Dermatologia Medicina e Cirurgia Estética, Belo Horizonte, Brazil, 2016.

[15] L. A. B. PORTO, *DermatologiaWEB - Um software para os Dermatologistas*, 2018, http://drluizporto.com.br/dermascopiaweb-um-softwares-para-os-dermatologista.

[16] M. Giannini, H. A. Rollo, and F. H. Maffei, "O papel do mapeamento dúplex no diagnóstico da trombose venosa profunda assintomática dos membros inferiores," *Jornal Vascular Brasileiro*, vol. 4, no. 3, pp. 290–296, 2005.

[17] S. V. Rajkumar, "Thalidomide therapy and deep venous thrombosis in multiple myeloma," *Mayo Clinic Proceedings*, vol. 80, no. 12, pp. 1549–1551, 2005.

[18] R. N. El Accaoui, W. A. Shamseddeen, and A. T. Taher, "Thalidomide and thrombosis - a meta-analysis," *Thrombosis and Haemostasis*, vol. 97, no. 6, pp. 1031–1036, 2007.

[19] Ministério da Saúde, *Diretrizes Para Vigilância, Atenção E Eliminação Da Hanseníase Como Problema De Saúde Públic*, 2016, Manual Técnico-Operacional.

[20] P. L. Drummond, R. M. Santos, G. O. Carvalho, and C. A. Pádua, "Adverse events in patients with leprosy on treatment with thalidomide," *Journal of the Brazilian Society of Tropical Medicine*, vol. 52, Article ID e20180385, 2019.

[21] E. S. Alecrim, E. S. C. Menezes, E. C. Gomes et al., "Diagnóstico tardio de hanseníase em criança: relato de caso," *Revista Amrigs*, vol. 62, p. 72, 2018.

[22] E. S. Alecrim, A. T. Chaves, L. A. Pôrto, M. A. Grossi, S. Lyon, and M. O. Rocha, "Reading of the Mitsuda test: comparison between diameter and total area by means of a computerized method," *Revista do Instituto de Medicina Tropical de São Paulo*, vol. 61, pp. 1–5, 2019.

[23] M. Montagnana, E. J. Favaloro, M. Franchini, G. C. Guidi, and G. Lippi, "The role of ethnicity, age and gender in venous thromboembolism," *Journal of Thrombosis and Thrombolysis*, vol. 29, no. 4, pp. 489–496, 2010.

[24] A. M. F. Roselino, P. Louzada Júnior, M. J. F. Brochado et al., "Trombose e pacientes com hanseníase em tratamento com talidomida e corticóide para reação tipo 2 não está relacionado fatores genéticos de trombofilia," *Hansenologia Internationalis*, vol. 30, no. 1, pp. 128-129, 2005.

40

Calcinosis Cutis Associated with Chronic Sclerodermoid Graft versus Host Disease: A Case and Review of the Literature

Jacqueline Deen, Lisa Byrom, and Ivan Robertson

Department of Dermatology, Royal Brisbane and Women's Hospital, Brisbane, Queensland, Australia

Correspondence should be addressed to Jacqueline Deen; jacqui.deen@gmail.com

Academic Editor: Alireza Firooz

We present a rare case of calcinosis cutis associated with chronic sclerodermoid graft versus host disease in a 59-year-old male, 13 years following allogenic bone marrow transplantation. The etiology of calcification was thought to be dystrophic. Further research is needed to understand the link between calcinosis cutis and chronic sclerodermoid graft versus host disease to assist with selecting appropriate management for these patients.

1. Introduction

Calcinosis cutis is a descriptive term for the deposition of insoluble calcium salts in the dermis and subcutaneous tissue and is associated with a number of underlying disorders. The underlying cause of this condition remains unknown. Serum calcium, phosphate, and parathyroid hormone are typically normal, although there may be reduced excretion of calcium and phosphate. There are five different types based upon etiology of calcium deposition: dystrophic, metastatic, iatrogenic, idiopathic, and calciphylaxis [1]. The most common form is the dystrophic type, which results from local tissue trauma, in the setting of normal calcium homeostasis. The clinical presentation varies in severity from asymptomatic (incidental finding on radiologic imaging) to subcutaneous nodules and plaques, which may cause associated pain or functional impairment. Dystrophic calcinosis cutis is most frequently associated with autoimmune connective tissue diseases such as dermatomyositis, systemic lupus erythematosus, and systemic sclerosis. It may also occur in patients with cutaneous neoplasms, panniculitis, porphyria cutaneous tarda, genodermatoses, localized trauma, or infection [1, 2].

Metastatic calcification occurs from abnormal calcium and phosphate metabolism, and the most common underlying cause is chronic renal failure. Iatrogenic calcinosis occurs from the deposition of calcium salts in the skin secondary to medical interventions, typically intravenous calcium gluconate and calcium chloride. Idiopathic calcification occurs in the absence of an underlying tissue injury or metabolic disorder. The final subtype, calciphylaxis, is a calcific vasculopathy of small and medium-sized blood vessels in the dermis and subcutaneous tissue, usually associated with end-stage renal failure [1, 3].

We present a rare case of calcinosis cutis associated with chronic sclerodermoid graft versus host disease. To our knowledge, this is the third reported case in the literature.

2. Case Report

A 59-year-old male presented for routine dermatology follow-up, 13 years following allogenic bone marrow transplantation (BMT) for grade 3 follicular non-Hodgkin lymphoma. The patient had a background history of sclerodermoid graft versus host disease (GVHD), which developed 12 months after BMT and was confirmed by cutaneous biopsy (Figure 1). He had multiorgan involvement, including the skin, eyes, oral cavity, joints, and lungs (restrictive lung disease). His GVHD was refractory to multiple systemic treatments including prednisolone, intravenous immunoglobulin (IVIG), cyclosporine, methotrexate, mycophenolate mofetil, tacrolimus, thalidomide,

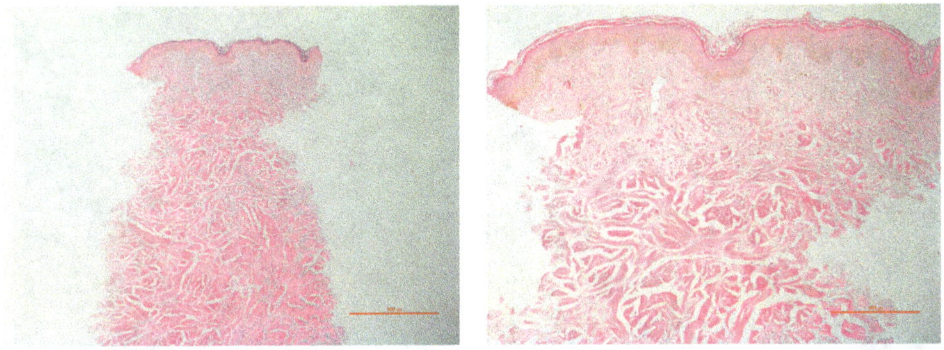

(a) (b)

Figure 1: Histopathology demonstrating sclerodermoid graft versus host disease. (a), (b) A normal *epidermis* with no lichenoid reaction pattern. Within the deep reticular dermis, there are broad bundles of collagen running parallel to the skin surface. Figure 1(b) shows mild pigment incontinence in the superficial dermis. A mild perivascular lymphocytic infiltrate is present within the deep dermis. There is no malignant infiltrate and no viral cytopathic changes or fungal organisms identified (hematoxylin and eosin staining, 1(a) original magnification × 40, 1(b) original magnification × 100).

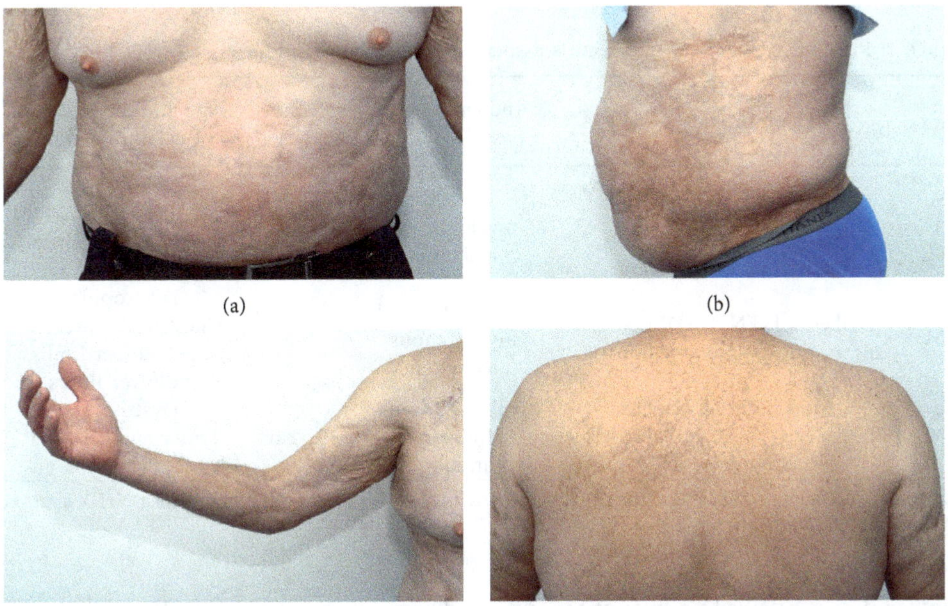

(a) (b) (c) (d)

Figure 2: Clinical photographs showing hyperpigmented, indurated plaques of the abdomen. (a), (b) The right forearm and (c), (d) upper back.

psoralen and ultraviolet A (PUVA), and ultraviolet A1 (UVA1).

The patient's non-Hodgkin lymphoma was diagnosed 15 years prior, and after failing chemotherapy and autologous stem cell transplantation, he underwent a BMT from an unrelated female donor with ABO compatibility. His other past medical history was significant for steroid-induced diabetes mellitus and a previous left leg deep vein thrombosis. His medications included warfarin, allopurinol, intravenous immunoglobulin, celecoxib, lubricant eye drops, prophylactic trimethoprim/sulfamethoxazole, and valaciclovir. There were no known drug allergies; the patient was a nonsmoker and worked as a pastor.

On examination, there were indurated, woody, thickened plaques on the upper arms, forearms, and trunk, clinically consistent with sclerodermoid changes (Figure 2). There were fixed flexion deformities of the bilateral elbows and perioral skin tightening with a decreased oral aperture. As an incidental finding, there were multiple, small, nontender, stone-hard nodules palpable over the trunk and bilateral upper limbs. There was no evidence clinically of autoimmune connective tissue disease including no nail fold telangiectasia, Raynaud's disease, sclerodactyly, or a photodistributed rash. Muscle power was graded 5/5 for the upper and lower limbs.

Baseline bloods including a complete blood count, urea and electrolytes, and liver function were unremarkable, and the patient's renal function was stable (creatinine 123 μmol/L, eGFR 55 mL/min). Corrected calcium, phosphate, and parathyroid hormone were within normal limits. ANA was negative.

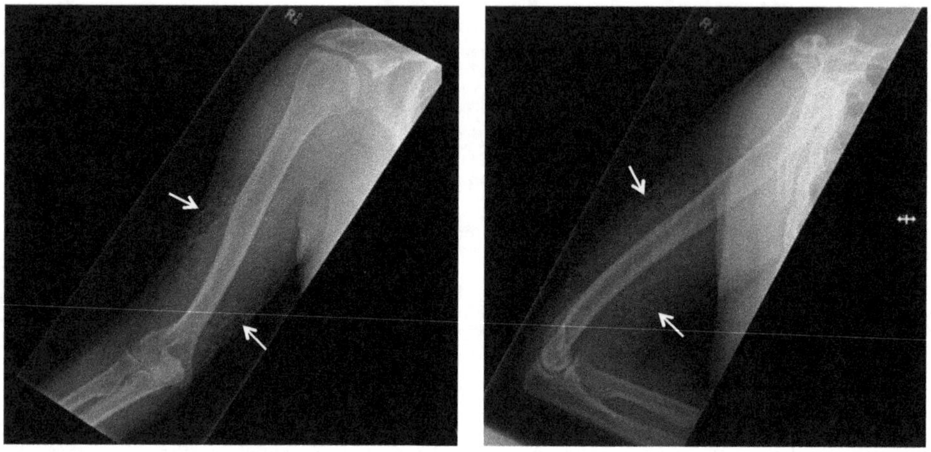

(a) (b)

Figure 3: Radiographs of the anterior (a) and posterior (b) right arm and forearm show extensive linear and irregular calcifications (arrows) in the field of view. The distribution of the calcified foci includes the subcutaneous fat.

Table 1: Previous cases of calcinosis cutis associated with sclerodermoid graft versus host disease.

Case	Age[†]	Sex	Comorbidities	Indication for BMT	Time interval*	Type and distribution of calcinosis cutis	Biochemistry (calcium and phosphate)
Lipshutz et al. [9]	54	F	T2DM, peripheral neuropathy, diabetic nephropathy, hyperlipidemia, pericarditis, anxiety, and depression	Acute myelogenous leukemia	11 years	Dystrophic Left iliac spines, proximal, and distal lower legs	Calcium (N) Phosphate (low)
Man et al. [10]	60	M	Diabetes, HTN, CAD, gastric ulcers, and pulmonary fibrosis	Acute myelogenous leukemia	N.S	Dystrophic Chest wall, anterior thighs, upper limbs, andlower limbs	Serum calcium (N) Phosphate (N.S)
Current case	59	M	Steroid induced diabetes, pulmonary GVHD, and restrictive lung disease	Follicular non-Hodgkin's lymphoma	12 years	Dystrophic Trunk and bilateral upper limbs	Serum calcium (N) Phosphate (N)

[†]Age in years, F: female, M: male, T2DM: type 2 diabetes mellitus, HTN: hypertension, CAD: coronary artery disease, GVHD: graft versus host disease, *time interval between GVHD and calcinosis cutis, N.S: not stated, N: normal.

Radiographs showed diffuse calcified nodules of the soft tissue overlaying the right humerus and proximal radius and ulnar (Figure 3), indicative of calcinosis cutis. Treatment was not initiated, as the patient was asymptomatic, and there was no evidence of lesion extrusion.

3. Discussion

Graft versus host disease has numerous cutaneous manifestations that are traditionally divided into acute and chronic forms based on the time of onset. Acute GVHD occurs within 100 days of transplantation, while chronic forms present after 100 days [4]. However, since signs of acute and chronic GVHD can present outside of these time periods, there has been increased use of clinical findings, rather than a designated time period to differentiate between acute and chronic GVHD [5].

Chronic GVHD has an incidence of approximately 40% in BMT recipients, although this is variable (between 6 and 80%) depending upon the presence of risk factors and diagnostic criteria used. The risk factors associated with chronic GVHD are well described, including an unrelated donor, donor-recipient sex mismatch, and older age (>40 years) of the recipient at the time of the BMT [6, 7]. In a multivariate analysis by Skert et al., significant predictors for the development of skin sclerosis in chronic GVHD were defined as disorders of pigmentation, eosinophilia, and autoimmunity [8]. Our patient had many risk factors for development of GVHD and, however, did not have any risk factors for development of sclerodermoid subtype.

Calcinosis cutis associated with sclerodermoid GVHD remains an interesting yet rarely discussed topic in the literature (Table 1) [9, 10]. In the two previously published cases and in our patient, the patient age was greater than 50 years, serum calcium was normal, the time interval between the initial diagnosis of sclerodermoid GVHD and the development of calcinosis cutis was greater than 10 years (average 11.5 years), and the aetiology of calcification was thought to be dystrophic, related to chronic sclerodermoid change. Furthermore, the distribution of calcinosis cutis involved tissues affected by sclerodermatous changes; thus, it is likely that the calcification is secondary to tissue injury related to chronic GVHD.

Treatment of calcinosis cutis is difficult as data on efficacy is limited and conflicting. The literature is mainly based on treatments for dystrophic calcinosis in patients with autoimmune conditions such as dermatomyositis and systemic sclerosis. Previous reported treatments include diltiazem, bisphosphonates, sodium thiosulfate, and surgical excision (mainstay of treatment) [11, 12].

Further research is needed to understand the link between calcinosis cutis and chronic sclerodermoid GVHD. The recently published prediction model for development of sclerodermoid GVHD suggests an immunological explanation and guides early identification and treatment [8]. This case adds an additional unique cutaneous manifestation of GVHD to the current literature.

References

[1] N. Reiter, L. El-Shabrawi, B. Leinweber, A. Berghold, and E. Aberer, "Calcinosis cutis," *Journal of the American Academy of Dermatology*, vol. 65, no. 1, pp. 1–12, 2011.

[2] N. Boulman, G. Slobodin, M. Rozenbaum, and I. Rosner, "Calcinosis in rheumatic diseases," *Seminars in Arthritis and Rheumatism*, vol. 34, no. 6, pp. 805–812, 2005.

[3] J. S. Walsh and J. A. Fairley, "Calcifying disorders of the skin," *Journal of the American Academy of Dermatology*, vol. 33, no. 5, pp. 693–706, 1995.

[4] P. Häusermann, R. B. Walter, J. Halter et al., "Cutaneous graft-versus-host disease: a guide for the dermatologist," *Dermatology*, vol. 216, no. 4, pp. 287–304, 2008.

[5] A. H. Filipovich, D. Weisdorf, S. Pavletic et al., "National Institutes of Health consensus development project on criteria for clinical trials in chronic graft-versus-host disease: I. Diagnosis and staging working group report," *Biology of Blood and Marrow Transplantation*, vol. 11, no. 12, pp. 945–956, 2005.

[6] M. E. D. Flowers, Y. Inamoto, P. A. Carpenter et al., "Comparative analysis of risk factors for acute graft-versus-host disease and for chronic graft-versus-host disease according to National Institutes of Health consensus criteria," *Blood*, vol. 117, no. 11, pp. 3214–3219, 2011.

[7] E. W. Cowen, "Graft-versus-host disease," in *Dermatology*, J. L. Bolognia, J. L. Jorizzo, and J. V. Schaffer, Eds., vol. 3, 3rd edition, 2012.

[8] C. Skert, F. Patriarca, A. Sperotto et al., "Sclerodermatous chronic graft-versus-host disease after aloogenic hematopoietic stem cell transplantation: incidence, predictors and outcomes," *Haematologica*, vol. 91, no. 2, pp. 258–261, 2006.

[9] G. H. Lipshutz and F. S. Chew, "Calcinosis cutis related to sclerodermatous chronic graft versus host disease," *Radiology Case Reports*, vol. 3, no. 4, p. 242, 2008.

[10] J. Man, M. Kalisiak, I. W. J. Birchall, and T. G. Salopek, "Chronic cutaneous graft-versus-host disease manifesting as calcinosis cutis universalis on a background of widespread sclerodermatoid changes," *Journal of Cutaneous Medicine and Surgery*, vol. 14, no. 5, pp. 249–253, 2010.

[11] A. Valenzuela, P. Song, and L. Chung, "Calcinosis in scleroderma," *Current Opinion in Rheumatology*, vol. 30, no. 6, pp. 554–561, 2018.

[12] H. Traineau, R. Aggarwal, J.-B. Monfort et al., "Treatment of calcinosis cutis in systemic sclerosis and dermatomyositis: a review of the literature," *Journal of the American Academy of Dermatology*, vol. 82, no. 2, pp. 317–325, 2020.

41

Vitiligo Associated with Melanoma in a Malagasy Woman

I. M. Ranaivo[1] **F. A. Sendrasoa**[2] **M. Andrianarison,**[2] **M. Razakanaivo,**[3] **L. S. Ramarozatovo,**[2] **F. Rafaramino,**[3] **and F. Rapelanoro Rabenja**[2]

[1]*Department of Dermatology, University Hospital Morafeno, Toamasina, Madagascar*
[2]*Department of Dermatology, University Hospital Joseph Raseta Befelatanana, Antananarivo, Madagascar*
[3]*Department of Oncology, University Hospital Joseph Ravoahangy Andrianavalona, Antananarivo, Madagascar*

Correspondence should be addressed to I. M. Ranaivo; irinamami@yahoo.fr

Academic Editor: Ravi Krishnan

Malignant melanoma is the first fatal skin cancer. Vitiligo is a leukoderma or a multifactorial depigmentation acquired but especially of autoimmune origin. We report the first Malagasy case affected by both melanoma and Vitiligo. The appearance of Vitiligo during a melanoma could testify to an immunological response against melanocytes. Despite the association of melanoma and Vitiligo, the prognosis of melanoma is still fatal.

1. Introduction

Malignant melanoma is the most aggressive malignant tumor of skin cancer. Vitiligo is a multifactorial acquired leukoderma. The association of a malignant melanoma with various clinical forms of skin depigmentation is known in particular the association with a Vitiligo [1]. We report the first Malagasy case of melanoma associated with and Vitiligo.

2. Case Presentation

A 44-year-old woman, farmer, presented asymptomatic skin depigmentations associated with a non-painful right inguinal swelling evolving for 6 months. Two years ago, she had an excision of a tumor lesion pigmented in the pressure zone of right heel, but no histology screen was performed. The pigmented lesion of the heel recurred one year later, motivating a second surgical resection of which histology analysis shown specific signs of lentiginous melanoma, Breslow >4 mm, Clark IV, with ulceration and positive margin. She had no family history of melanoma or Vitiligo. Physical examination show that the patient was in good general condition. She had multiple achromic patches varying in size from a few millimeters to 20 cm in diameter, in the face (Figure 1), chest, arms, thighs, right inguinal swelling, and backs of the feet. She had also a hard right inguinal lymphadenopathy 15 cm in diameter adhering to the deep plane (Figure 2). On the right heel, she had a pigmented ulcero-crusty lesion of 4 cm in diameter (Figure 3).

The rest of the physical examination was normal. The extension assessment found liver metastases and necrotic lymphadenopathy on the right iliac chain. Then, a diagnosis of acral lentiginous melanoma, Stage IV according to American Joint Committee on Cancer 2009 (AJCC) associated with recent generalized Vitiligo was made. She received palliative treatment. Unfortunately she died 2 months later.

3. Discussion

In Madagascar skin cancers account for 9% of cancers and melanomas account for 23% of malignant skin tumors [2]. Vitiligo is an acquired leukoderma due to destruction or loss of melanocytes. It is probably a multifactorial disease: genetic and environmental factors as well as autoimmune and auto-inflammatory mechanisms have been advanced [3–5]. Various pathogenetic mechanisms have been suggested, most evidence supports an autoimmune basis for the Vitiligo. Different genome-wide association studies of generalized Vitiligo have been reported, identifying a total of 17 confirmed generalized Vitiligo susceptibility loci. Almost all of these genes encode

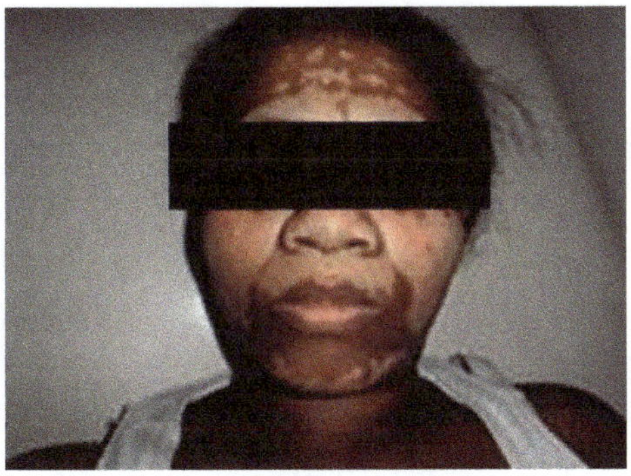

Figure 1: Facial achromic lesions (archive of the Department of Dermatology, Joseph Raseta Befelatanana University Hospital, Antananarivo, Madagascar).

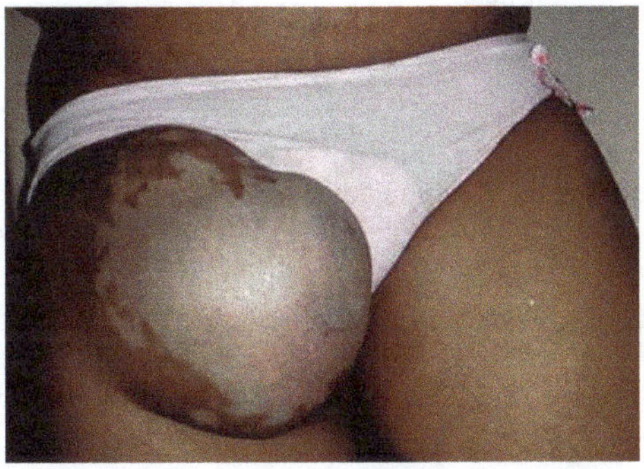

Figure 2: Achromic lesion with right inguinal swelling (archive of the Department of Dermatology, Joseph Raseta Befelatanana University Hospital, Antananarivo, Madagascar).

immunoregulatory proteins. In melanocytes HLA-A∗02:01 presents the major Vitiligo autoimmune antigen, TYR (encoding tyrosinase), which in turn, activates and recruits anti-melanocytes auto-reactive cytotoxic T lymphocytes to the skin within the target and destroy melanocytes. Moreover, the biological interaction between these generalized Vitiligo susceptibility genes, HLA-A and TYR, points to show inverse relationship between susceptibility to generalized Vitiligo versus malignant melanoma, suggesting that generalized Vitiligo may result, in part, from dysregulation of normal processes of immune surveillance against melanoma. Unfortunately, we could not do genetic study for our patient to confirm this hypothesis [6, 7].

Vitiligo-like lesions may appear during primary or metastatic melanoma [8]. It affects 3% to 6% of melanoma cases. Leukoderma can precede, from a few months to several years, the appearance of melanoma [1, 9]. Or it can appear on primary or metastatic melanoma spontaneously or during melanoma treatment. The development of Vitiligo during melanoma maybe the result of an immunological response against melanocytes. Humoral and cellular immunity is involved [9]. In particular, the antityrosinase antibodies and the CD8 + oligoclonal in vitro T lymphocytes were involved in the destruction of normal melanocytes during the immune response to melanoma antigens [10, 11]. During immunotherapy by pembrolizumab in patients with metastatic melanoma, the appearance of Vitiligo demonstrates a good therapeutic response [12]. In common Vitiligo, there is a greater history of autoimmune disease and family history of Vitiligo compared to patients with Vitiligo-like lesions during melanoma. Achromic lesions can localize around cutaneous and distant metastases. They are often generalized bilateral, symmetrical and without Koebner phenomenon in case of Vitiligo associated with melanoma [10, 13]. For our patient she had a generalized Vitiligo with achromic lesion next to lymph node metastasis. Although the presence of Vitiligo indicates a strong immune response against melanoma, our patient died quickly. In Madagascar the management of melanoma especially in the metastatic stage is disappointing. The treatment is expensive, we do not have molecular biology yet. Immunotherapy and targeted therapy are not yet available.

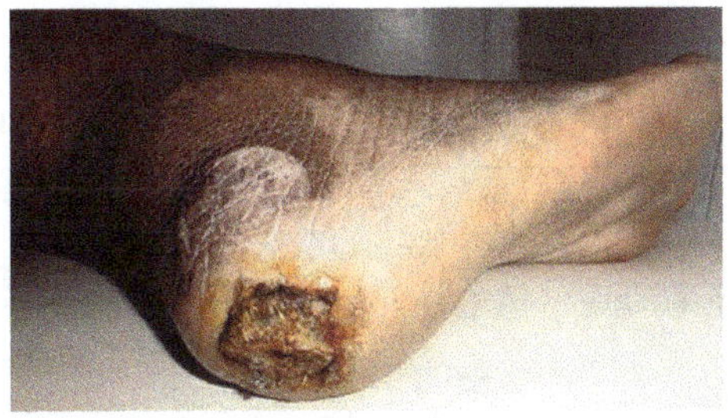

Figure 3: Ulcerous lesion of the right heel (archive of the Department of Dermatology, Joseph Raseta Befelatanana University Hospital, Antananarivo, Madagascar).

Table 1 shows some cases of Vitiligo associated with melanoma reported in the literature.

4. Conclusion

Our patient's case illustrates an occurrence of concomitant Vitiligo and melanoma, presumably the first reported case in Madagascar. Although the melanoma-Vitiligo association is an indication of an immunological response against normal melanocytes and melanoma antigens, the prognosis of melanoma is still fatal. In Madagascar the treatment of melanoma is difficult especially in case of metastatic forms. More attention should be given to the examination of melanocyte lesions in adult patients in order to detect melanoma at the onset stage. Malignant melanoma can be overlooked by patients, as in the case of our patient who was concerned about the presence of cosmetic disfiguring achromic lesions.

Table 1: Comparative analysis of some cases of melanoma associated with Vitiligo reported in the literature.

	Redondo and Del Olmo [14]	Alonso-Castro et al. [15]		Flores-Terry et al. [16]	Wang et al. [10]	Our case
Age	65	63	35	44	67	44
Gender	Woman	Woman	Woman	Woman	Man	Woman
Primary melanoma	Right leg	Not precised	Not precised	Left outer ear	Left sole	Rigth sole
Metastasis	Lymph nodes metastase	Pulmonary, bone, and axillary lymph nodes metastases	Lymph nodes metastases	Lymph nodes and pulmonary metastases	Lymph nodes	Lymph nodes and liver metastases
Vitiligo locations	Face and trunk	Face and neck	Face and neck	Face, scalp, trunk, and limbs	Face, trunk and limbs	Face, arms, trunk, and inguinal
Treatment	Surgical resection and chemotherapy	Target therapy vemurafenib	Target therapy vemurafenib	Target therapy dabrafenib	Chemotherapy	Palliative treatement
Delays of appearance of Vitiligo after the melanoma's discovery	2 months after the discovery of melanoma	After 2 weeks of treatment	After 8 weeks of treatment	After 2 months of treatment	4 months before the discovery of melanoma	2 years after the discovery of melanoma
Evolution	Death	Partial response	Complete response	Clinical regression	Death	Death

References

[1] B. Baghad, S. Belanouane, F. Elfatoiki, Z. Baline, K. F. Hali, and S. Chiheb, "Association mélanome et Vitiligo: quelle relation?" *Annales de Dermatologie et de Vénéréologie*, vol. 145, no. 4, pp. a72–a73, 2018.

[2] C. Raharisolo Vololonantenaina, J. L. Pécarrère, and J. F. Roux, "Le cancer à Madagascar. Expérience de l'Institut Pasteur de Madagascar de début septembre 1992 à fin juin 1996," http://www.pathexo.fr/documents/articles-bull/T91-1-MR96-120.pdf.

[3] K. Ezzedine, V. Eleftheriadou, M. Whitton, and N. van Geel, "Vitiligo," *The Lancet*, vol. 386, no. 9988, pp. 74–84, 2015.

[4] F. Rapelanoro Rabenja, F. M. P. Randrianasolo, L. S. Ramarozatovo, and C. Ratrimoarivony, "Therapeutic observation of Vitiligo," *International Journal of Dermatology*, vol. 44, no. S1, pp. 46–48, 2005.

[5] F. A. Sendrasoa, I. M. Ranaivo, M. Sata et al., "Treatment responses in patients with Vitiligo to very potent topical corticosteroids combined with vitaminotherapy in Madagascar," *International Journal of Dermatology*, vol. 58, no. 8, pp. 908–911, 2019.

[6] Y. Jin, M. Hayashi, P. Fain et al., "Major association of Vitiligo with HLA-A∗ 02: 01 in Japanese," *Pigment Cell & Melanoma Research*, vol. 28, no. 3, pp. 360–362, 2015.

[7] R. A. Spritz, "The genetics of generalized Vitiligo: autoimmune pathways and an inverse relationship with malignant melanoma," *Genome Medicine*, vol. 2, no. 10, p. 78, 2010.

[8] M. D. Saleem, E. Oussedik, J. J. Schoch, A. C. Berger, and M. Picardo, "Acquired disorders with depigmentation: a systematic approach to vitiliginoid conditions," *Journal of the American Academy of Dermatology*, vol. 80, no. 5, pp. 1215–1231, 2019.

[9] R. González and E. Torres-López, "Immunological basis of melanoma-associated Vitiligo-like depigmentation," *Actas Dermo-Sifiliográficas (English Edition)*, vol. 105, no. 2, pp. 122–127, 2014.

[10] J. R. Wang, K. J. Yu, W. H. Juan, and C. H. Yang, "Metastatic malignant melanoma associated with Vitiligo-like depigmentation," *Clinical and Experimental Dermatology*, vol. 34, no. 2, pp. 209–211, 2009.

[11] J. C. Becker, P. Guldberg, J. Zeuthen, E.-B. Bröcker, and P. thor Straten, "Accumulation of identical T cells in melanoma and Vitiligo-like leukoderma," *Journal of Investigative Dermatology*, vol. 113, no. 6, pp. 1033–1038, 1999.

[12] C. Hua, L. Boussermart, C. Mateus et al., "Association of Vitiligo with tumor response in patient with melanoma treated with pembrolizumab," *JAMA Dermatology*, vol. 152, no. 1, pp. 45–51, 2016.

[13] J. E. Lommerts, H.-E. Teulings, K. Ezzedine et al., "Melanoma-associated leukoderma and Vitiligo cannot be differentiated based on blinded assessment by experts in the field," *Journal of the American Academy of Dermatology*, vol. 75, no. 6, pp. 1198–1204, 2016.

[14] P. Redondo and J. Del Olmo, "Vitiligo and cutaneous melanoma," *New England Journal of Medicine*, vol. 359, no. 3, p. e3, 2008.

[15] L. Alonso-Castro, L. Rıos-Buceta, S. Vano-Galvan, C. Moreno, A. Soria-Rivas, and P. Jaén, "Vitiligo in 2 patients receiving vemurafenib formetastatic melanoma," *Journal of the American Academy of Dermatology*, vol. 69, no. 1, pp. e28–e29, 2013.

[16] M. A. Flores-Terry, A. Garrido-Martın, L. S. Sanchez-Mateos, M. P. Sánchez-Caminero, M. García-Arpa, and M. P. Cortina-de la Calle, "A case of Vitiligo-like depigmentation induced by dabrafenib in patients with metastatic melanoma," *Journal of the American Academy of Dermatology*, vol. 74, no. 5, p. AB184, 2016.

42

Metastatic Merkel Cell Carcinoma Masquerading as Multiple Immune-Related Adverse Events

Farees Saqlain,[1] Sophia Z. Shalhout,[1,2] Kevin S. Emerick,[1,3,4] Tomas G. Neilan,[1,5] Tatyana Sharova,[2] and David Michael Miller[1,2,6]

[1]*Harvard Medical School, Boston, MA, USA*
[2]*Department of Medicine, Division of Hematology/Oncology, Massachusetts General Hospital, Boston, MA, USA*
[3]*Department of Otolaryngology, Massachusetts Eye and Ear Infirmary, Boston, MA, USA*
[4]*Department of Otolaryngology, Harvard Medical School, Boston, MA, USA*
[5]*Department of Medicine, Division of Cardiology, Massachusetts General Hospital, Boston, MA, USA*
[6]*Department of Dermatology, Massachusetts General Hospital, Boston, MA, USA*

Correspondence should be addressed to David Michael Miller; dmiller4@mgh.harvard.edu

Academic Editor: Jacek Cezary Szepietowski

Merkel cell carcinoma is a rare cutaneous neuroendocrine carcinoma with a high rate of regional and distant metastasis and mortality. Here, we report a novel case of Merkel cell carcinoma which presented as a primary lesion to the left cheek with regional lymph node involvement and was treated with pembrolizumab and radiation. Widely metastatic disease eventually revealed on autopsy clinically mimicked immune-related organ insult leading to management with immunosuppressants. The patient also had a biopsy-confirmed immune-related cutaneous adverse event during admission. The case highlights a rare circumstance in which disease progression masqueraded as multiple immune-related end-organ adverse events. Contribution of on-target anti-PD-1 toxicity remains a possibility.

1. Introduction

Merkel cell carcinoma (MCC) is an aggressive primary cutaneous neuroendocrine carcinoma with risk factors including lighter complexion, age over 50, ultraviolet exposure, and immunosuppression [1]. The disease has a particularly high rate of locoregional and distant metastasis. A review of 9387 cases from the National Cancer Database showed that 65% of patients presented with local disease, 26% presented with nodal spread, and 8% presented with distant metastasis, with respective 5-year overall survival estimates of 51%, 35%, and 14% [2]. Common sites for distant metastasis include the distant lymph nodes, liver, lung, skin and subcutaneous tissue, and bone [3, 4]. Since 2017, immune checkpoint inhibitors have been approved by the FDA for medical management of metastatic disease, with the potential to cause a diverse array of immune-related adverse events (irAEs). Clinically significant hepatotoxicity, for example, is known to occur with pembrolizumab in a small subset of patients, typically 2 to 6 cycles after treatment initiation [5]. Here, we describe a novel case of regionally metastatic MCC managed with pembrolizumab and radiation, with distant, multisite progression initially masquerading as multiple end-organ immune-related adverse events. While biopsy supported attribution of concomitantly presenting dermatitis as an irAE, autopsy revealed metastatic disease to the liver, heart, muscle, and bone with little accompanying inflammation.

2. Case Presentation

A 77-year-old Caucasian female presented for multidisciplinary consult at our tertiary care center with a left cheek nodule growing over 4-5 months with more recent rapid growth. Shave biopsy of a 14 mm firm nodule 2 months prior to presentation to our clinic had shown MCC extending to peripheral and deep tissue edges with perinuclear dot-like positivity for CK20, positivity for synaptophysin, weak focal reactivity for AE1/AE2, and negative staining for TTF-1 (Figures 1 and 2).

Outside hospital (OSH) staging PET/CT scan revealed focal intense FDG avidity in the primary left cheek mass, as well as focal activity in multiple intraparotid lymph nodes, with no evidence of distant disease (Figure 3). Past medical history was notable for hypertension, hyperlipidemia, depression, and degenerative joint disease; there was no prior history of skin cancer or immunosuppression. Family history was negative for melanoma or nonmelanoma skin cancers.

Our examination revealed an exophytic, friable tumor measuring 27 mm × 22 mm on the left cheek and palpable mass in the left parotid and submandibular areas (Figure 4). Vitals were notable for a blood pressure of 168/78. ECOG performance status was 1. Initial labs were unremarkable. Her anti-Merkel cell polyomavirus oncoprotein antibody titer (AMERK test, University of Washington) was negative. She underwent core biopsy of the left submandibular mass which confirmed MCC infiltrating the connective tissue, with overt lymphatic invasion. She was staged as pathological stage IIIB disease (T2pN1bM0). Targeted next-generation sequencing (NGS) of her tumor revealed variants in TP53, RB1, FLT3, and PDGFRA. Due to the multifocality of her disease on presentation, coupled with the poor prognosis of patients with stage IIIB disease, the decision was made to proceed with bimodality therapy. She was initiated on pembrolizumab (200 mg, IV, q3 weeks) and radiation.

One week after her first dose of pembrolizumab and prior to initiation of radiotherapy, she presented to OSH emergency department with sudden-onset abdominal pain and nausea. Complete metabolic panel, complete blood count, troponin, and lipase were all within normal limits. Inpatient gastroenterology consultation concluded that the abdominal symptoms were likely pembrolizumab-related. Her symptoms resolved, and she was released after 1 day of inpatient supportive care with IV fluids, ondansetron, and prochlorperazine. She went on to complete a radiotherapy course of 60 gray to the left cheek and 54 gray to the left neck.

After approximately 2 months, and 3 doses, of immunotherapy and 1.5 months after commencing radiotherapy, the patient complained of oropharyngeal discomfort and was prescribed fluconazole and clotrimazole troches at OSH radiation oncology clinic for possible thrush.

A few days later, she presented to an OSH emergency room and was ultimately admitted with nausea, vomiting, fatigue, and more acute symptoms of somnolence, slurred speech, and shortness of breath. At presentation, her labs were remarkable for transaminitis (ALT of 213 U/L, ref: 0–40 U/L; AST of 252 U/L, ref: 0–37 U/L), conjugated hyperbilirubinemia (total bilirubin of 4.5 mg/dL, ref: 0.0–1.2 mg/dL; direct bilirubin of 4.0 mg/dL, ref: 0.0–0.3 mg/dL; indirect bilirubin of 0.5 mg/dL; ref: 0.0–1.5 mg/dL), alkaline phosphate (ALP) elevation (535 U/L, ref: 39–117 U/L), and PT-INR elevation to 1.3 (ref: 0.9–1.1). Labs were additionally notable for high-sensitivity troponin T elevation (67 ng/L, ref: 0–9 ng/L), creatinine elevation (2.70 mg/dL, ref: 0.5–1.5 mg/dL), leukocytosis, and lactatemia. She was managed with empiric broad-spectrum antibiotics and intravenous fluids with concern for sepsis. Multiorgan toxicity from pembrolizumab was also high on the differential. Her electrocardiogram showed normal sinus rhythm and anterior Q waves; transthoracic echocardiogram showed a left ventricular ejection fraction of 61% with no evidence of wall motion abnormality or pericardial effusion. A right upper quadrant ultrasound showed hepatomegaly with heterogeneous increased echotexture suggestive of fatty infiltration and cholelithiasis but no focal hepatic lesions or evidence of biliary obstruction.

Renal function and lactate readily responded to intravenous fluids. However, her liver function at the OSH continued to worsen, and on hospital day 3, she was started on intravenous methylprednisolone 80 mg daily for presumed autoimmune hepatitis and possible autoimmune myocarditis. She was then transferred to our hospital. Viral and autoimmune hepatitis panels were unremarkable. On hospital day 4, she was noted to have developed a nonpruritic eruption concentrated on the upper chest and back and upper extremities. A punch biopsy revealed an interface dermatitis with dyskeratosis and superficial perivascular lymphocytic infiltrate (Figure 5).

By hospital day 5, methylprednisolone was increased to pulse dose (1 g/day) in the setting of worsening bilirubinemia. High-sensitivity troponin T peaked at 143 ng/L before declining to 131 ng/L (ref: 0–9 ng/L), coinciding with escalation of pulse-dose steroids. Renal function precluded cardiac MRI, and coagulopathy was a relative contraindication for a myocardial biopsy. At this time, a repeat right upper quadrant ultrasound was obtained which was notable again for diffusely heterogeneous hepatic parenchyma, now interpreted as being suspicious for metastatic disease. An ultrasound-guided nonfocal liver biopsy was obtained, which confirmed extensive metastatic disease (Figures 6(a) and 6(b)). In the setting of progressive delirium and clinical decline, the patient was transitioned to symptom-directed therapy. She expired on hospital day 8.

At autopsy, 80% of the hepatic parenchyma was found to be replaced by tumor, with the remaining background tissue revealing steatosis, cholestasis, and necrosis with minimal inflammation (Figures 6(c) and 6(d)). Microscopic metastases were found in the left ventricular myocardium and the septum, the largest measuring 0.2 cm. Tumor cells were also found to be infiltrating representative sections of the bone marrow and psoas muscle. There was no evidence of autoimmune inflammation in any of the examined organs.

3. Discussion

We present here the case of a patient with regionally metastatic MCC treated with pembrolizumab and radiation, presenting acutely with symptoms and persistent lab abnormalities suggestive of checkpoint inhibitor therapy-(CIT-) related dermatitis, hepatitis, and myocarditis. This was managed in accordance with ASCO guidelines with high-dose systemic steroids [6]. Although a contemporaneous skin biopsy was consistent with a CIT-induced

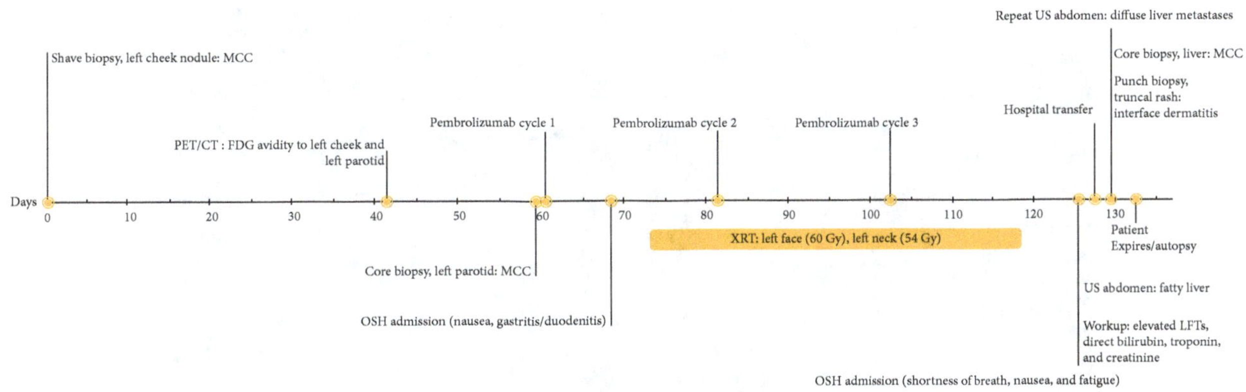

FIGURE 1: Patient clinical course. A timeline was provided beginning at day 0, set to the initial histological Merkel cell carcinoma diagnosis of the left cheek nodule. Abbreviations: MCC, Merkel cell carcinoma; PET/CT: positron emission tomography/computed tomography; FDG: fluorodeoxyglucose; OSH: outside hospital; XRT: radiation therapy; US: ultrasound; LFTs: liver function tests.

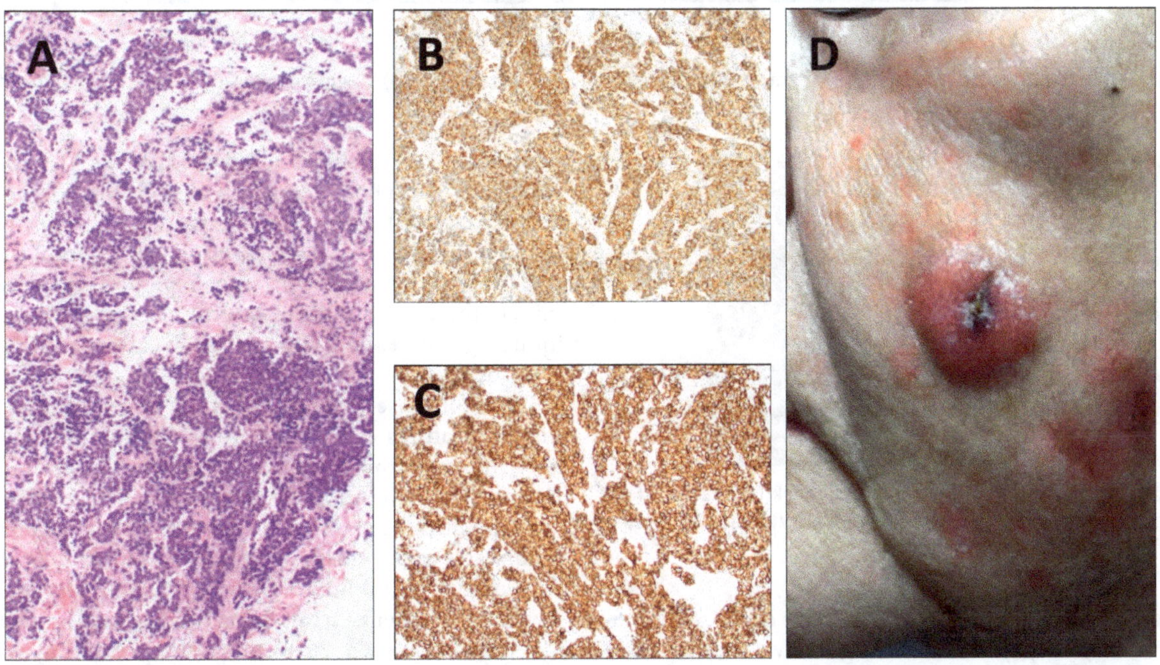

FIGURE 2: Shave biopsy pathology from the left cheek primary lesion. (a) Small purple cells consistent with neuroendocrine carcinoma. (b) Positivity for synaptophysin. (c) Perinuclear dot-like positivity for cytokeratin 20. (d) Primary lesion two weeks after initial confirmatory biopsy.

lichenoid eruption, liver biopsy, shortly prior to death, and autopsy were remarkable for diffuse replacement of liver parenchyma by disease, as well as metastatic deposits in the heart, skeletal muscle, and bone. Minimal signs of tissue inflammation were observed in those tissues, highlighting a novel circumstance in which metastatic MCC masqueraded as multiple distinct end-organ irAEs and presented concomitantly with confirmed irAE of the skin.

Though nonspecific on exam and histology, the patient's rash to the trunk and extremities was compatible with a pembrolizumab-mediated hypersensitivity irAE. 30–40% of patients treated with anti-PD-1 immunotherapy experience all-grade dermatologic irAEs, while the incidence of all-grade rash is 14–17% [7, 8]. The usual onset of rash is after the second cycle of therapy [7]. Anti-PD-1-mediated rash typically presents to the trunk or extremities as a maculopapular, often pruritic, eruption. While there is a wide range of possible histological presentations, the most commonly observed is an interface dermatitis, as was noted in this patient's case [7, 9, 10].

A retrospective study of 491 patients treated with pembrolizumab for solid organ tumors showed that 14.3% developed liver injury, as defined by lab abnormalities, at a median of 62 days from therapy initiation. Within this subset, only 29% of cases, 4.1% of the 491 cases overall, were adjudicated as likely to be drug-related on expert review (i.e., given Drug-Induced Liver Injury Network (DILIN) expert opinion scale scores of 1, definite, 2, highly likely, or 3, probable); most of the remainder were attributed to hepatic involvement by malignancy. The authors suggested an

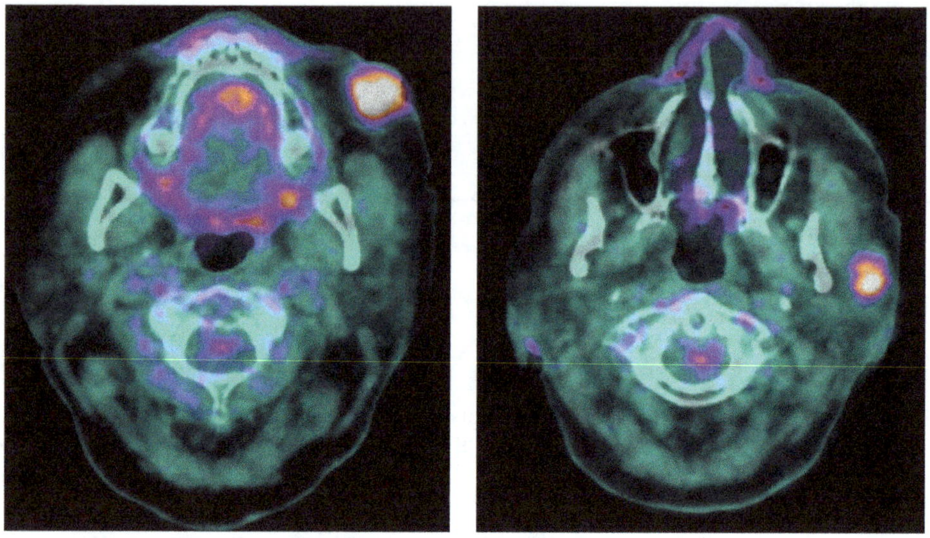

(a) (b)

Figure 3: Staging PET/CT scan. (a) Primary site of disease to the left cheek. (b) Regional metastasis to the left parotid.

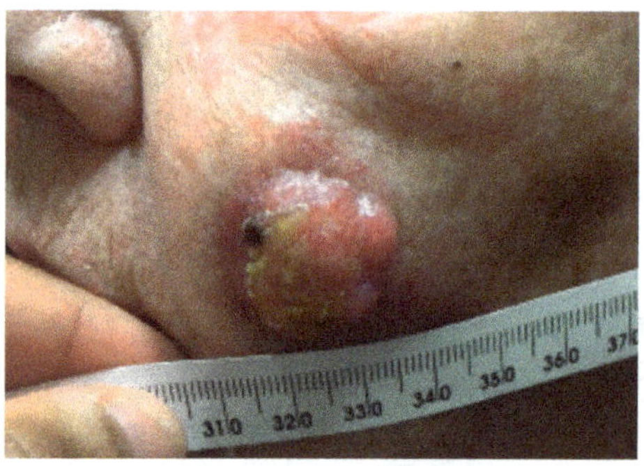

Figure 4: Primary site of disease to the left cheek (27 × 22 mm) at the time of presentation to our multidisciplinary clinic (7.5 weeks after confirmatory biopsy).

increased emphasis on contrast-enhanced cross-sectional scans and early biopsy in the setting of liver enzyme abnormalities as possible strategies to help reduce diagnostic uncertainty and avoid unnecessary empiric immunosuppression [11]. Proceeding with such a "prospectively obtained" liver biopsy in our case, where the patient could not undergo contrast-enhanced study due to acute kidney injury, might have expedited diagnosis of diffuse progression, prompting earlier goals of care discussion with the patient and family. In the setting of multiorgan insult, suspicion for hepatic metastasis in this case only developed when abdominal ultrasound was repeated at our institution with findings suspicious for malignancy. While neither conventional ultrasound nor noncontrast CT have been shown to be sensitive modalities for detection of hepatic metastases, interpretation at the outside hospital was likely complicated by the diffuse involvement of liver parenchyma, with absence of distinct focal lesions on ultrasound, as was noted in a case of MCC of the right lower eyelid diffusely metastatic to the liver reported in 2019 [12–15]. By the DILIN severity index definition, our patient's initial presentation would have been classified as moderate-severe (score 3; elevated ALT, ALP, bilirubin, and/or INR and hospitalization or prolongation of existing hospitalization). Labs were consistent with a cholestatic pattern of injury ($R = 1.2$). Although checkpoint inhibitors are more associated with the hepatocellular pattern of injury, there are multiple case reports of pembrolizumab inducing cholestatic injury, even after a single dose [11, 16, 17].

Multiple case reports and series have explored the histologic features associated with immunotherapy-related liver injury. Pathology for all of a series of seven patients treated with nivolumab or ipilimumab whose liver enzyme abnormalities responded to cessation of checkpoint inhibition and immunosuppression showed lobular hepatitis with milder portal inflammation [18]. Similarly, in another series of 8 patients treated with either pembrolizumab or nivolumab between 2016 and 2018 presenting with liver function abnormalities, again with clinical improvement on treatment cessation and immunosuppressive therapies, six out of eight cases were notable for histologic signs of acute lobular hepatitis, while 2 cases were characterized by varying degrees of steatotic and cholestatic changes [19]. Across both groups of patients, lobular scattered or spotty pattern necrosis was most frequently noted, although a few cases had more centrilobular and/or confluent patterns of necrosis. In contrast, liver histology for this case was remarkable for 80% replacement of hepatic parenchyma by tumor cells. The remaining parenchyma revealed nonspecific findings of patchy steatosis, cholestasis, and centrilobular necrosis with minimal inflammation. Significantly, the patient had already been initiated on steroids before tissue biopsy was performed. While the time course of histologic response of immune-related hepatitis to immunosuppression is not well characterized, a case report of pembrolizumab-induced cholestatic liver injury showed biopsy evidence of continued inflammation of the portal tract despite prior initiation of steroids [16].

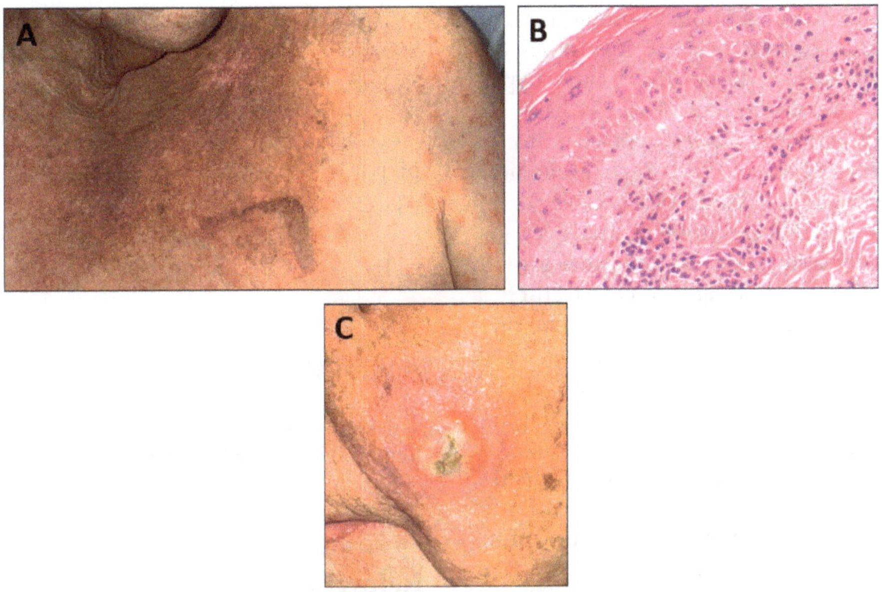

Figure 5: (a) Truncal eruption of pink macules and thin papules with minimal overlying scale coalescing centrally at the upper back and chest, with extension to the rest of torso and upper extremities, hospital day 4. (b) Biopsy revealed an interface dermatitis with dyskeratosis and superficial perivascular lymphocytic infiltrate. (c) Primary lesion to the left cheek showing significant recession on clinical examination after bimodality therapy, hospital day 4.

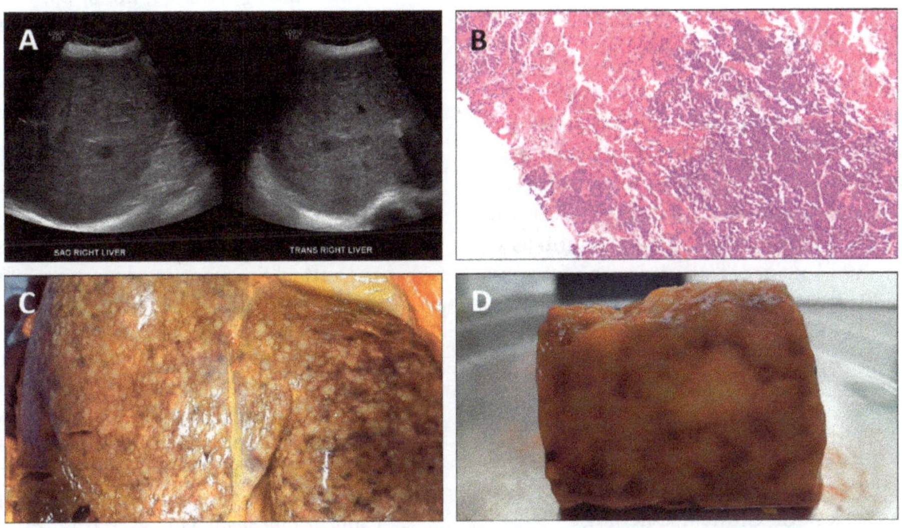

Figure 6: (a) Right upper quadrant ultrasound, hospital day 4, was notable for diffusely heterogeneous hepatic parenchyma with scattered hypoechoic lesions, suspicious for malignancy. No intrahepatic biliary ductal dilatation was observed. (b) Core liver biopsy revealed metastatic disease occupying roughly 60% of the total parenchyma. Background hepatic parenchyma was without signs of marked inflammation. (c) Gross inspection of the liver revealed replacement of the parenchyma by firm tan/yellow confluent nodules and punctate hemorrhagic areas. (d) Cross section of hepatic tissue recapitulated overwhelming tumor burden.

Myocarditis relating to CIT has an all-grade reported incidence ranging from 0.04% to 1.14%, with a mortality rate of up to 50% [20–22]. Cases of CIT-related myocarditis typically occur within 1-2 months of therapy initiation and may develop even after a single dose [22, 23]. This patient presented with presumed pembrolizumab-related myocarditis, ASCO grade 1-2 (abnormal cardiac biomarkers and electrocardiogram, possibly with mild symptoms) [6, 24]. EKG findings relating to myocarditis are diverse and nonspecific. While T-wave changes are the most common finding, Q-waves, as in this case, have also been documented [23, 25–27]. Echocardiogram for this patient was unremarkable; further cardiac workup was limited by renal and liver dysfunction. Ultimately, diagnosis of myocardial metastases was made on autopsy with no signs of inflammation in examined cell blocks, again with caveat of exposure to high-dose steroids during admission.

While infrequent overall, since 2001, many cases of cardiac metastasis of MCC have been reported in the literature, with clinical consequences including symptoms of chest pain and shortness of breath, various degrees of heart block, and malignant pericardial effusion with resultant tamponade [28–33]. With an additional complication of acute kidney injury, the scattered cardiac metastases observed on autopsy probably drove the acute hypertroponinemia observed in this patient's case, as has been observed in other head and neck cancers metastatic to the heart. A case of a 25-year-old woman with lingual squamous cell carcinoma with cardiac metastasis was notable for elevation in troponin-I and ST-elevation in leads V3–V6 attributed to metastatic infiltration of the myocardium rather than ischemic disease, although the case featured a much larger deposit of disease extending from the right ventricular free wall [34]. On-target toxicity from CIT may also have contributed. A 65-year-old woman treated with a single dose of nivolumab and experimental drug for stage IV squamous cell carcinoma of the lung presented with signs of myocarditis, including troponin-I elevation (0.12 ng/mL), LVEF of 25–30%, and enhancement on cardiac MRI, and was eventually discharged after improvement with immunosuppression. The patient later developed cardiogenic shock and was transitioned to comfort care in the setting of newly discovered hemorrhagic stroke. Notably, autopsy revealed widely metastatic squamous cell carcinoma, including metastatic deposits in both ventricles, the septum, and the right atrium [35].

4. Conclusions

Merkel cell carcinoma is an aggressive neuroendocrine cancer of the skin, with great propensity for regional and distant metastasis. Multisite progression of disease may mimic simultaneous presentation of multiple immune-related adverse events, especially if options for further workup are limited by clinical contraindications. Early diagnosis of progression may help avoid unnecessary immunosuppression and expedite curative or palliative therapy.

Abbreviations

ALP: Alkaline phosphatase
ALT: Alanine transaminase
AMERK: Merkel polyomavirus serology test
ASCO: American Society of Clinical Oncology
AST: Aspartate transaminase
CK: Cytokeratin
CT: Computed tomography
DILIN: Drug-Induced Livery Injury Network
DNR/DNI: Do not resuscitate/do not intubate
ECOG: Eastern Cooperative Oncology Group
EKG: Electrocardiogram
FDA: The United States Food and Drug Administration
FDG: Fluorodeoxyglucose
INR: International normalized ratio
IrAE: Immune-related adverse event
LFTs: Liver function tests
LVEF: Left ventricular ejection fraction
MCC: Merkel cell carcinoma
MRI: Magnetic resonance imaging
NCDB: National Cancer Database
NGS: Next-generation sequencing
OSH: Outside hospital
PET: Positron emission tomography
PT: Prothrombin time
US: Ultrasound
CIT: Checkpoint inhibitor therapy.

Acknowledgments

The Harvard Cancer Center Merkel Cell Carcinoma Patient Registry is funded by Project Data Sphere (DMM, FS, and SZS).

References

[1] B. D. Lemos, B. E. Storer, J. G. Iyer et al., "Pathologic nodal evaluation improves prognostic accuracy in Merkel cell carcinoma: analysis of 5823 cases as the basis of the first consensus staging system," *Journal of the American Academy of Dermatology*, vol. 63, no. 5, pp. 751–761, 2010.
[2] K. L. Harms, M. A. Healy, P. Nghiem et al., "Analysis of prognostic factors from 9387 Merkel cell carcinoma cases forms the basis for the new 8th edition AJCC staging system," *Annals of Surgical Oncology*, vol. 23, no. 11, pp. 3564–3571, 2016.
[3] T. L. Tello, K. Coggshall, S. S. Yom, and S. S. Yu, "Merkel cell carcinoma: an update and review," *Journal of the American Academy of Dermatology*, vol. 78, no. 3, pp. 445–454, 2018.
[4] M. Kouzmina, V. Koljonen, J. Leikola, T. Böhling, and E. Lantto, "Frequency and locations of systemic metastases in Merkel cell carcinoma by imaging," *Acta Radiologica Open*, vol. 6, no. 3, 2017.
[5] N. I. O. Health, "Livertox: clinical and research information on drug-induced liver injury," 2017.
[6] J. R. Brahmer, C. Lacchetti, B. J. Schneider et al., "Management of immune-related adverse events in patients treated with immune checkpoint inhibitor therapy: American society of clinical oncology clinical practice guideline," *Journal of Clinical Oncology*, vol. 36, no. 17, pp. 1714–1768, 2018.
[7] J. Naidoo, D. B. Page, B. T. Li et al., "Toxicities of the anti-PD-1 and anti-PD-L1 immune checkpoint antibodies," *Annals of Oncology*, vol. 26, no. 12, pp. 2375–2391, 2015.
[8] C. W. Lewis, J. Qazi, D. S. Hippe et al., "Patterns of distant metastases in 215 Merkel cell carcinoma patients: implications for prognosis and surveillance," *Cancer Medicine*, vol. 9, no. 4, pp. 1374–1382, 2020.
[9] V. R. Belum, B. Benhuri, M. A. Postow et al., "Characterisation and management of dermatologic adverse events to agents targeting the PD-1 receptor," *European Journal of Cancer*, vol. 60, pp. 12–25, 2016.
[10] D. Y. Wang, D. B. Johnson, and E. J. Davis, "Toxicities associated with PD-1/PD-L1 blockade," *The Cancer Journal*, vol. 24, no. 1, pp. 36–40, 2018.
[11] I. Tsung, R. Dolan, C. D. Lao et al., "Liver injury is most commonly due to hepatic metastases rather than drug hepatotoxicity during pembrolizumab immunotherapy,"

Alimentary Pharmacology & Therapeutics, vol. 50, no. 7, pp. 800–808, 2019.
[12] K. Kinkel, Y. Lu, M. Both, R. S. Warren, and R. F. Thoeni, "Detection of hepatic metastases from cancers of the gastrointestinal tract by using noninvasive imaging methods (US, CT, MR imaging, PET): a meta-analysis," *Radiology*, vol. 224, no. 3, pp. 748–756, 2002.
[13] H. B. Jee, "Is non-contrast CT adequate for the evaluation of hepatic metastasis in patients who cannot receive iodinated contrast media?" *PLoS One*, vol. 10, no. 7, e0134133 pages, 2015.
[14] W. J. Zwiebel, "Sonographic diagnosis of diffuse liver disease," *Seminars in Ultrasound, CT and MRI*, vol. 16, no. 1, pp. 8–15, 1995.
[15] L. S. Ana, "A rare cause of acute liver failure: diffuse liver metastization of Merkel cell carcinoma," *GE-Portuguese Journal of Gastroenterology*, vol. 27, no. 3, pp. 203–206, 2020.
[16] K. Kurokawa, M. Hara, S.-I. Iwakami et al., "Cholestatic liver injury induced by pembrolizumab in a patient with lung adenocarcinoma," *Internal Medicine*, vol. 58, no. 22, pp. 3283–3287, 2019.
[17] J. R. Penn and V. Rustgi, "An unusual case of cholestatic drug-induced liver injury following a single dose of pembrolizumab," *American Journal of Gastroenterology*, vol. 112, p. S1278, 2017.
[18] Y. Zen and M. M. Yeh, "Hepatotoxicity of immune checkpoint inhibitors: a histology study of seven cases in comparison with autoimmune hepatitis and idiosyncratic drug-induced liver injury," *Modern Pathology*, vol. 31, no. 6, pp. 965–973, 2018.
[19] D. Zhang, "Histologic patterns of liver injury induced by anti-PD-1 therapy," *Gastroenterology Report*, vol. 8, no. 1, pp. 50–55, 2019.
[20] S. S. Mahmood, M. G. Fradley, J. V. Cohen et al., "Myocarditis in patients treated with immune checkpoint inhibitors," *Journal of the American College of Cardiology*, vol. 71, no. 16, pp. 1755–1764, 2018.
[21] S. G. Al-Kindi and G. H. Oliveira, "Reporting of immune checkpoint inhibitor-associated myocarditis," *The Lancet*, vol. 392, no. 10145, pp. 382-383, 2018.
[22] J. J. Moslehi, J.-E. Salem, J. A. Sosman, B. Lebrun-Vignes, and D. B. Johnson, "Increased reporting of fatal immune checkpoint inhibitor-associated myocarditis," *The Lancet*, vol. 391, no. 10124, p. 933, 2018.
[23] L. Zhang, M Awadalla, S. S Mahmood et al., "Cardiovascular magnetic resonance in immune checkpoint inhibitor-associated myocarditis," *European Heart Journal*, vol. 41, no. 18, pp. 1733–1743, 2020.
[24] N. Palaskas, "Immune checkpoint inhibitor myocarditis: pathophysiological characteristics, diagnosis, and treatment," *Journal of the American Heart Association*, vol. 9, no. 2, 2020.
[25] S. Upadhrasta, H. Elias, K. Patel, and L. Zheng, "Managing cardiotoxicity associated with immune checkpoint inhibitors," *Chronic Diseases and Translational Medicine*, vol. 5, no. 1, pp. 6–14, 2019.
[26] H. Nakashima, Y. Honda, and T. Katayama, "Serial electrocardiographic findings in acute myocarditis," *Internal Medicine*, vol. 33, no. 11, pp. 659–666, 1994.
[27] C. C. Deluigi, P. Ong, S. Hill et al., "ECG findings in comparison to cardiovascular MR imaging in viral myocarditis," *International Journal of Cardiology*, vol. 165, no. 1, pp. 100–106, 2013.
[28] M. Conley, K. Hawkins, and D. Ririe, "Complete heart block and cardiac tamponade secondary to Merkel cell carcinoma cardiac metastases," *Southern Medical Journal*, vol. 99, no. 1, pp. 74–78, 2006.
[29] N. Y. Kazemi, C. Jain, M. C. Bois, A. Behfar, K. Olivier, and S. N. Markovic, "Heart block caused by cardiac metastasis from Merkel cell carcinoma: a case report," *Mayo Clinic Proceedings: Innovations, Quality & Outcomes*, vol. 3, no. 4, pp. 510–516, 2019.
[30] M. Di Loreto and R. Francis, "Merkel cell carcinoma cardiac metastasis causing cardiac tamponade," *BMJ Case Reports*, vol. 2017, 2017.
[31] N. Yamana, H. Sueyama, and M. Hamada, "Cardiac metastasis from Merkel cell skin carcinoma," *International Journal of Clinical Oncology*, vol. 9, no. 3, 2004.
[32] E. Page, "Cardiac metastasis from a Merkel cell skin carcinoma," *A case report. Archives des maladies du coeur et des vaisseaux*, vol. 94, no. 12, pp. 1423–1426, 2001.
[33] C. F. Suttie, G. Hruby, L. Horvath, and J. Thompson, "Cardiac metastasis in Merkel cell carcinoma," *Journal of Clinical Oncology*, vol. 32, no. 13, pp. e52–e53, 2014.
[34] H. Patel, M. Francke, H. Stahura, M. El-Hajjar, and J. Schulman-Marcus, "Solitary cardiac metastasis from primary oral squamous cell carcinoma presenting as ST-elevation MI," *BMJ Case Reports*, vol. 2018, 2018.
[35] N. Agrawal, A. Khunger, P. Vachhani et al., "Cardiac toxicity associated with immune checkpoint inhibitors: case series and review of the literature," *Case Reports in Oncology*, vol. 12, no. 1, pp. 260–276, 2019.

43

Cutaneous Pseudoepitheliomatous Hyperplasia from a Displaced Metallic Orthopedic Implant

Franklin R. Blum[1] **and Logan S. D'Souza**[2]

[1]*UNC Chapel Hill School of Medicine, Chapel Hill, NC, USA*
[2]*UNC School of Medicine Asheville, Asheville, NC, USA*

Correspondence should be addressed to Franklin R. Blum; franklin_blum@med.unc.edu

Academic Editor: Ravi Krishnan

While rare, cutaneous SCC in patients with darker Fitzpatrick skin types is essential to identify and investigate early and can have a myriad of clinical presentations. While clinical history-taking of suspicious skin lesions is often symptom-driven, other key patient history components, such as surgical history, are often overlooked. Differentiating, prioritizing, and risk-stratifying hyperkeratotic, verrucous papules in patients with darker Fitzpatrick skin types is an essential clinical skill for clinicians to develop to serve an increasingly diverse patient population. This original report presents the case of a displaced orthopedic screw causing pseudoepitheliomatous hyperplasia that was initially misdiagnosed as squamous cell carcinoma. This case highlights the importance of careful consideration of surgical history, choice of biopsy method, and skin type when examining lesions concerning for squamous cell carcinoma.

1. Introduction

The differential of a cutaneous verrucous lesion is broad, but includes verruca vulgaris, verrucous carcinoma, pseudoepitheliomatous hyperplasia (PEH), and squamous cell carcinoma (SCC). On physical exam, such lesions can have significant morphological overlap, requiring histologic differentiation for definitive diagnosis. This report presents the case of a metallic foreign body causing PEH that was initially misdiagnosed as squamous cell carcinoma.

Pseudoepitheliomatous hyperplasia is a benign proliferation of squamous epithelium that can extend into the dermis [1]; it is closely related to chronic inflammation of the underlying dermis. Identified causes of PEH include malignancy, wounds, retained foreign material, and even tattoo pigments [1, 2]. Considered benign, PEH can be difficult to distinguish from other hyperproliferative skin disorders on exam, especially SCC. The term pseudocarcinomatous hyperplasia is used by some for PEH for this malignant association [3]. Histologically, PEH and SCC can be difficult to differentiate, but factors that favor SCC include abundant mitoses, nuclear atypia, necrotic keratoses, and deep connective tissue invasion by epithelium [4]. Currently, there are no reports of cutaneous PEH being caused from a displaced metal orthopedic implant, the topic of this account, making this likely the first report.

Squamous cell carcinoma and PEH can be challenging to differentiate clinically in darker Fitzpatrick skin types. Nonmelanoma skin cancer is exceedingly rare in the Black population, with an estimated incidence of approximately 3 per 100,000 population [5], as compared to over 230 per 100,000 population in Whites [6]. Coupled with this low incidence, skin cancer appearance can also vary. In this case, the patient's young age, darker Fitzpatrick skin type, and the lesion's morphology and location of low sun exposure placed him at high concern for skin cancer, necessitating urgent dermatologic exploration.

2. Case Synopsis

A 22-year-old Fitzpatrick type 5 male presented to dermatology with a chief complaint of a growing and painful skin lesion on the left ankle for several months at the base of a fibular fracture scar from four years prior. As he was a college football player, the lesion was especially painful when moving laterally. Upon initial inspection by a physician assistant, a 1.6 cm × 1.6 cm hyperkeratotic, verrucous-appearing plaque was identified on the left lateral malleolus at the inferior end of a vertical linear scar (Figure 1(a)). A biopsy by shave method was performed (Figure 1(b)), which showed atypical squamous proliferation worrisome for invasive, well-differentiated squamous cell carcinoma (Figure 2(a)). He returned to clinic one week later, at which time electro-desiccation and curettage were performed. A timeline of events for his clinical care is listed in Table 1.

However, treatment was unsuccessful, as the patient returned to the clinic six months later reporting a one-month history of a similar lesion worrisome for recurrence. He was seen by a different provider from his initial evaluation. As the patient had professional football aspirations, the lesion was debulked and biopsied that same day. Biopsy could not exclude an atypical process (Figure 2(b)). A periodic acid–Schiff (PAS) stain was performed to exclude a fungal process and returned negative. Definitive treatment was set for the conclusion of the collegiate season a few weeks later. Further complicating his timeline was the upcoming National Football League (NFL) draft, an annual event during which professional football teams select new players for their rosters. He opted for Mohs surgery for a higher cure rate to minimize normal tissue removal and to prioritize his need to heal quickly for training. During evaluation on the day of his Mohs surgery, the recurrent lesion was visualized (Figure 3), and an operative plan was made. Upon shave debulking before the first stage of tumor extirpation, a shiny, somewhat mobile metal screw was visualized centrally (Figure 3).

The metallic object identified was most consistent with a displaced orthopedic surgical screw, concerning for pending implant failure. Mohs surgery was aborted given this new correlative clinical information. The patient verified that the linear scar on his lateral ankle was from a prior orthopedic surgical repair of a fibular fracture that was repaired with metal screws and plates approximately four years prior. It was posited that repetitive, forceful, high-intensity football training likely stressed the orthopedic fracture repair and contributed to failure, explaining the delayed lesion onset. The debulk was sent to dermatopathology for consultation and comparison with past biopsies. With additional tissue and clinical information, dermatopathology's findings were most consistent with cutaneous pseudoepitheliomatous hyperplasia. The patient was referred out of state to the original orthopedic surgeon who performed the corrective surgery four years prior before addressing the displaced metal implant, the underlying cause of his cutaneous proliferation. No adverse events were reported in the years following. The patient was subsequently lost to follow-up.

3. Discussion

While the underlying metallic foreign body and unique pathological features gave the definitive diagnosis, differentiating between benign and malignant causes of a verrucous papule requires a breadth of consideration. Lesion location, duration, and appearance as well as patient age, sex, race, and other demographic information influence a physician's clinical lens for diagnosis and management. However, one factor that infrequently plays a diagnostic role in dermatology is past surgical history. Reviewing a patient's prior surgical history, not just limited to dermatologic surgeries, should be performed preoperatively [7]. In this case, prior surgical history was vital to final diagnosis, and overlooking this fact was a fault in care that may have resulted in undue burden for the patient and medical system.

A limitation to our clinical approach that possibly resulted in unnecessary interventions and delayed diagnosis was inadequate lesion biopsy. Importantly, as described by Zayour et al., PEH may be misinterpreted as SCC in cases where the primary process localized in the dermis is not readily apparent or the biopsy is superficial and lacks a sufficient portion of the dermis [1]. A biopsy by shave method was performed at the initial evaluation, which may not have been sufficiently deep. Although guidelines of care published in the Journal of the American Academy of Dermatology (JAAD) do not indicate an optimal biopsy method for lesions concerning for SCC [8], National Comprehensive Cancer Network (NCCN) guidelines advise, when taking a biopsy, "if more than superficial lesion, inclusion of deep reticular dermis preferred" [9]. This case report challenges the JAAD guidelines and supports the more detailed NCCN guidelines. A biopsy by punch or surgical biopsy would have included the deeper reticular dermis.

Another important factor for consideration in this case was the patient's skin type. While rare, cutaneous SCC in patients with darker Fitzpatrick skin types is essential to identify and investigate early. The most important risk factor for SCC in this population is chronic scarring processes and areas of chronic inflammation [5], with common causes being leg ulcers, burn scars, radiation dermatitis, and discoid lupus [5, 10]. Of notable concern, cutaneous SCC in Black patients has been associated with a radically high mortality rate of around 18.4% [11]. Frequently, these tumors present at a more advanced stage and thus worse prognosis compared to patients with lighter skin types [12]. Additionally, cutaneous SCC arising from chronic scarring or inflammation in Black patients carries a metastatic risk of 20–40% compared to 1–4% metastatic risk of sun-induced SCC in Whites [5]. In general, nonhealing nodules adjacent to scarring necessitate biopsy to exclude malignancy [5]. As the lesion in this case was found within a previous surgical scar, urgent evaluation was merited. Although a benign case of PEH was identified, comparable lesion presentations should be treated with the same level of urgency in this patient population.

There is a paucity of literature describing cases of PEH in patients of darker skin types. Specifically, using combinations of the search terms "pseudo-epitheliomatous hyperplasia," "black," "skin," "African American," "Fitzpatrick 4," and "Fitzpatrick 5" on PubMed, only one pathology review had case descriptions of PEH in patients with darker skin

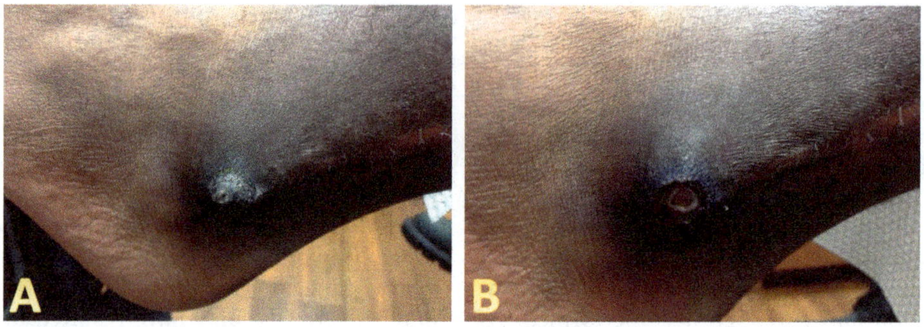

Figure 1: Initial clinic evaluation. 1.6 × 1.6 cm irregular, hyperkeratotic, verrucous-appearing papule distributed on the left lateral malleolus. A surgical scar is visualized, running vertically on the lateral ankle superior to the lesion (a). A biopsy by shave was performed (b).

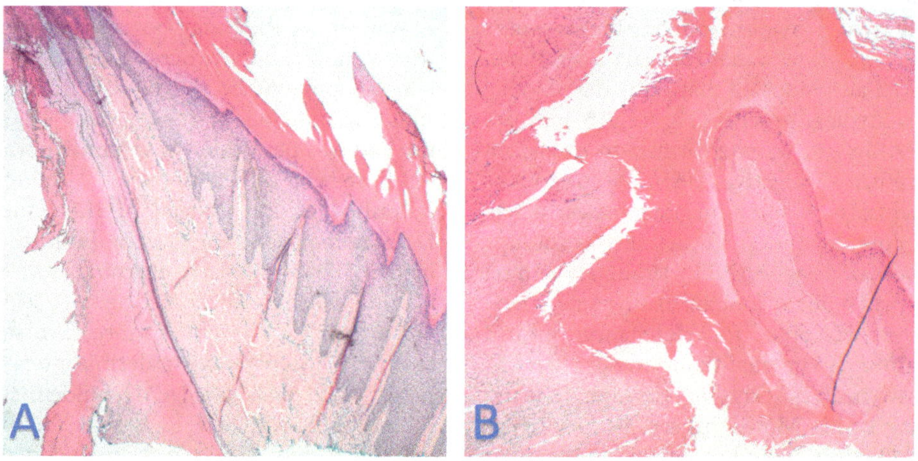

Figure 2: Histopathological imaging from initial biopsy (a) and 6-month recurrence (b). Papillomatous and endophytic squamous proliferation is present with keratin plug, parakeratin, and mild pleomorphism of keratinocytes extending to the base of the biopsy (a). 6 months later, the biopsy showed overlying thickened parakeratin alternating with parakeratin with serum accumulation (b). Collections of neutrophils were also observed in the stratum corneum (b), so a PAS stain was performed to evaluate for the presence of fungal organisms. No fungal organisms were noted. The adjacent *epidermis* displayed acanthosis and papillomatosis composed of suprabasilar keratinocytes without significant atypia (b).

Table 1: Timeline of events.

Event	Finding(s)	Intervention(s)
Initial evaluation by PA	Lesion identified on the left lateral malleolus	Shave biopsy performed
	1 week later	
Treatment with 1st MD	Biopsied lesion	ED&C* with pathology
	6 months later	
Reevaluation with 1st MD	Concern for recurrent lesion	Debulk with pathology performed definitive treatment scheduled
	3 weeks later	
Definitive treatment with 2nd MD	Recurrent lesion	Mohs surgery
	Intraoperation	
Surgery cessation	Discovery of displaced metallic orthopedic implant	Referral to orthopedics

*Electrodessication and curettage; PA = physician associate; MD = medical doctor.

types [13] and one discussed components of PEH in conjunction with verrucous sarcoidosis [14], but not from a metallic foreign body. Furthermore, using the search terms "metal," "screw," "foreign body," "pseudo-epitheliomatous hyperplasia," "orthopedic," "surgery," and "implant" on PubMed yielded reports of PEH from intentional mercery injection [15, 16] and unidentified mercury contact [17]. However, no reports were found of cutaneous PEH caused from a displaced metal orthopedic implant, making this likely the first report.

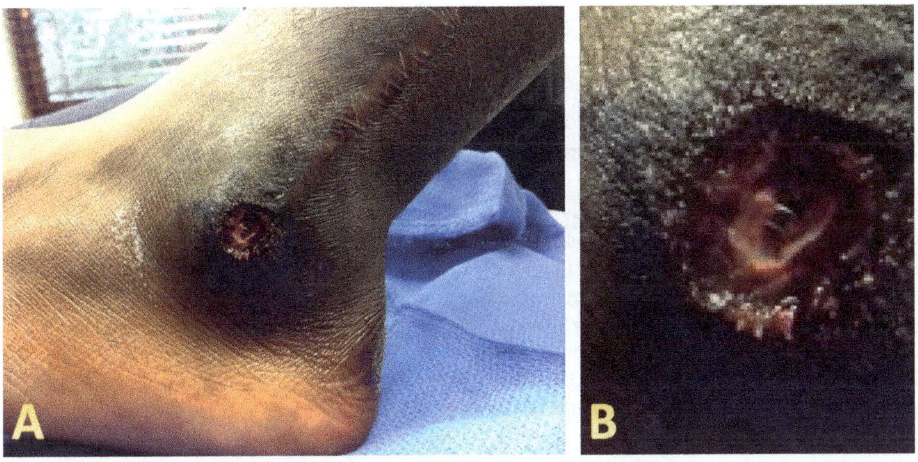

FIGURE 3: Mohs intraoperative imaging. After debulking, a metallic foreign body is present centrally (a), most consistent with a displaced orthopedic surgical screw. A closer view is appreciated (b).

Lastly, in patients with a verrucous papule presenting in close proximity to or within a known prior orthopedic surgical scar, considering preoperative imaging may reduce unnecessary patient and health system burden. This patient had a concerning lesion overlying previously placed metallic orthopedic implants. X-ray investigation may have revealed the underlying etiology of the lesion earlier than with dermatologic investigation alone.

4. Conclusion

This is likely the first report of PED caused from a displaced metal orthopedic implant, which occurred in a patient with Fitzpatrick type 5 skin. Differentiating between PEH and SCC in patients with darker Fitzpatrick skin types presents a clinical and histopathological challenge that carries significant risk if an incorrect diagnosis is made. This case highlights the importance of a careful consideration of a patient's surgical history, skin type, and choice of biopsy method when investigating lesions concerning for squamous cell carcinoma. Arriving at the correct diagnosis early in a lesion's treatment course can prevent undue burden on patients and the greater health system.

Abbreviations

PEH: Pseudoepitheliomatous hyperplasia
SCC: Squamous cell carcinoma.

Authors' Contributions

Mr. Franklin R. Blum gathered clinical images and wrote the entirety of the manuscript for review by the co-author. Dr. Logan D'Souza was responsible for patient care, obtained patient's informed verbal consent, and reviewed and edited the manuscript.

References

[1] M. Zayour and R. Lazova, "Pseudoepitheliomatous hyperplasia: a review," *The American Journal of Dermatopathology*, vol. 33, no. 2, pp. 112–126, 2011.

[2] E. Balfour, I. Olhoffer, D. Leffell, and T. Handerson, "Massive pseudo-epitheliomatous hyperplasia: an unusual reaction to a tattoo," *The American Journal of Dermatopathology*, vol. 25, no. 4, pp. 338–340, 2003.

[3] M. Valdebran, I. Neuhaus, and J. North, "Pseudocarcinomatous epithelial hyperplasia induced by imiquimod: a mimic of cutaneous squamous cell carcinoma," *Dermatologic Surgery*, vol. 43, no. 6, pp. 874–876, 2017.

[4] V. N. Nayak, K. Uma, H. C. Girish, S. Murgod, K. Shyamala, and R. B. Naik, "Pseudoepitheliomatous hyperplasia in oral lesions: a review," *Journal of International Oral Health*, vol. 7, no. 9, pp. 148–152, 2015.

[5] H. M. Gloster Jr. and K. Neal, "Skin cancer in skin of color," *Journal of the American Academy of Dermatology*, vol. 55, no. 5, pp. 741–760, 2006.

[6] J. Scotto, T. R. Fears, and J. F. Fraumeni Jr., *Incidence of Nonmelanoma Skin Cancer in the United States*, US Department of Health and Human Services, Washington, DC, USA, 1983.

[7] C. C. Otley, "Perioperative evaluation and management in dermatologic surgery," *Journal of the American Academy of Dermatology*, vol. 54, no. 1, pp. 119–127, 2006.

[8] J. Y. S. Kim, J. H. Kozlow, B. Mittal, J. Moyer, O. Thomas, and R. Phillip, "Guidelines of care for the management of cutaneous squamous cell carcinoma," *Journal of the American Academy of Dermatology*, vol. 78, no. 3, pp. 560–578, 2018.

[9] National Comprehensive Cancer Network, "Squamous cell skin cancer," 2022, https://www.nccn.org/professionals/physician_gls/pdf/squamous.pdf.

[10] S. K. T. Que, F. O. Zwald, and C. D. Schmults, "Cutaneous squamous cell carcinoma," *Journal of the American Academy of Dermatology*, vol. 78, no. 2, pp. 237–247, 2018.

[11] R. G. Mora and C. Perniciaro, "Cancer of the skin in blacks. I. A review of 163 black patients with cutaneous squamous cell

carcinoma," *Journal of the American Academy of Dermatology*, vol. 5, no. 5, pp. 535–543, 1981.
[12] S. Hu, R. M. Soza-Vento, D. F. Parker, and R. S. Kirsner, "Comparison of stage at diagnosis of melanoma among Hispanic, black, and white patients in Miami-Dade County, Florida," *Archives of Dermatology*, vol. 142, no. 6, pp. 704–708, 2006.
[13] J. M. Lynch, "Understanding pseudoepitheliomatous hyperplasia," *Pathology Case Reviews*, vol. 9, no. 2, pp. 36–45, 2004.
[14] M. E. Sussman, B. T. Pousti, S. K. Grossman, J. B. Lee, and S. Hsu, "Verrucous sarcoidosis: a rare clinical presentation of sarcoidosis," *Cureus*, vol. 13, no. 5, Article ID e15175, 2021.
[15] G. P. Lupton, G. F. Kao, F. B. Johnson, J. H. Graham, and E. B. Helwig, "Cutaneous mercury granuloma. A clinicopathologic study and review of the literature," *Journal of the American Academy of Dermatology*, vol. 12, no. 2 Pt 1, pp. 296–303, 1985.
[16] S. E. Vernon, "Case report: subcutaneous elemental mercury injection—clinical observations and implications for tissue disposal from the histopathology laboratory," *Annals of Clinical and Laboratory Science*, vol. 35, no. 1, pp. 86–90, 2005.
[17] K. Bothale, T. Dongre, S. Mahore, and S. Pande, "Cutaneous mercury granuloma," *Indian Journal of Occupational and Environmental Medicine*, vol. 17, no. 1, pp. 22–24, 2013.

Thyrotoxicosis Associated with Ustekinumab Treatment for Psoriasis

Bayanne Olabi [1] **and Shanti Ayob** [2]

[1]*Department of Dermatology, Lauriston Building, Edinburgh EH3 9EN, UK*
[2]*Department of Dermatology, NHS Treatment Centre, Nottingham NG7 2FT, UK*

Correspondence should be addressed to Bayanne Olabi; bayanne@doctors.org.uk

Academic Editor: Jacek Cezary Szepietowski

Biologic treatments have revolutionised the management of psoriasis in recent years; however, data on their safety profile in large populations and long-term effects are being gathered on an ongoing basis. Ustekinumab is a monoclonal antibody that targets interleukin-12/23 used in the treatment of moderate-to-severe psoriasis. Here, we report the case of a 32-year-old Caucasian gentleman who developed thyrotoxicosis following the commencement of ustekinumab treatment. Following control of thyroid status by the Endocrinology team, this recurred after recommencement of ustekinumab on two further occasions over a 5-year period. This is the second known reported association of this nature. Awareness of these possible adverse effects is imperative in managing patients and informing decision-making, and further long-term studies will help elucidate the precise safety profiles of biologic treatments.

1. Introduction

Psoriasis is a chronic immune-mediated skin condition driven by a complex interplay of effector cells and inflammatory cytokines [1]. Ustekinumab is a human $IgG1_K$ monoclonal antibody that targets interleukin-12/23 used in the treatment of moderate-to-severe plaque psoriasis in adults. This is a report of a patient who developed three distinct episodes of thyrotoxicosis over the course of 5 years, each episode following the commencement and recommencement of ustekinumab treatment for psoriasis.

2. Case Presentation

A 32-year-old Caucasian gentleman with severe plaque psoriasis was commenced on ustekinumab therapy in March 2011 (45 mg, 3 monthly), following failure of treatment with narrowband UVB phototherapy, methotrexate, cyclosporine, etanercept, and adalimumab due to side effects and/or secondary failure.

On review in June 2012, he was noted to have a tremor, lid lag, and a moderate goitre. Biochemistry revealed thyrotoxicosis, with a serum T3 level of 30 pmol/l (normal range: 3.5–6.7 pmol/l), a T4 level of 74.6 pmol/l (10–19.8 pmol/l), and a TSH level of <0.1 mU/l (0.27–4.2 mU/l). He was commenced on carbimazole by the Endocrinology team and ustekinumab was stopped.

However, the patient wanted good control of his psoriasis before his wedding and wished to recommence ustekinumab, despite understanding the risks of uncontrolled hyperthyroidism. It was restarted in August 2012. Whilst on ustekinumab, his hyperthyroidism remained difficult to control over the next 2 years, with weight loss (5 kg within 3 months of restarting ustekinumab) and clinical hyperthyroidism (tremors, palpitations, palpable goitre), requiring multiple uptitrations of carbimazole. Ustekinumab was eventually stopped in June 2014 due to persistent uncontrolled hyperthyroidism and he was switched to a fumaric acid ester (Fumaderm), followed by acitretin, both of which were ineffective at controlling his psoriasis. Radioiodine therapy was successfully administered

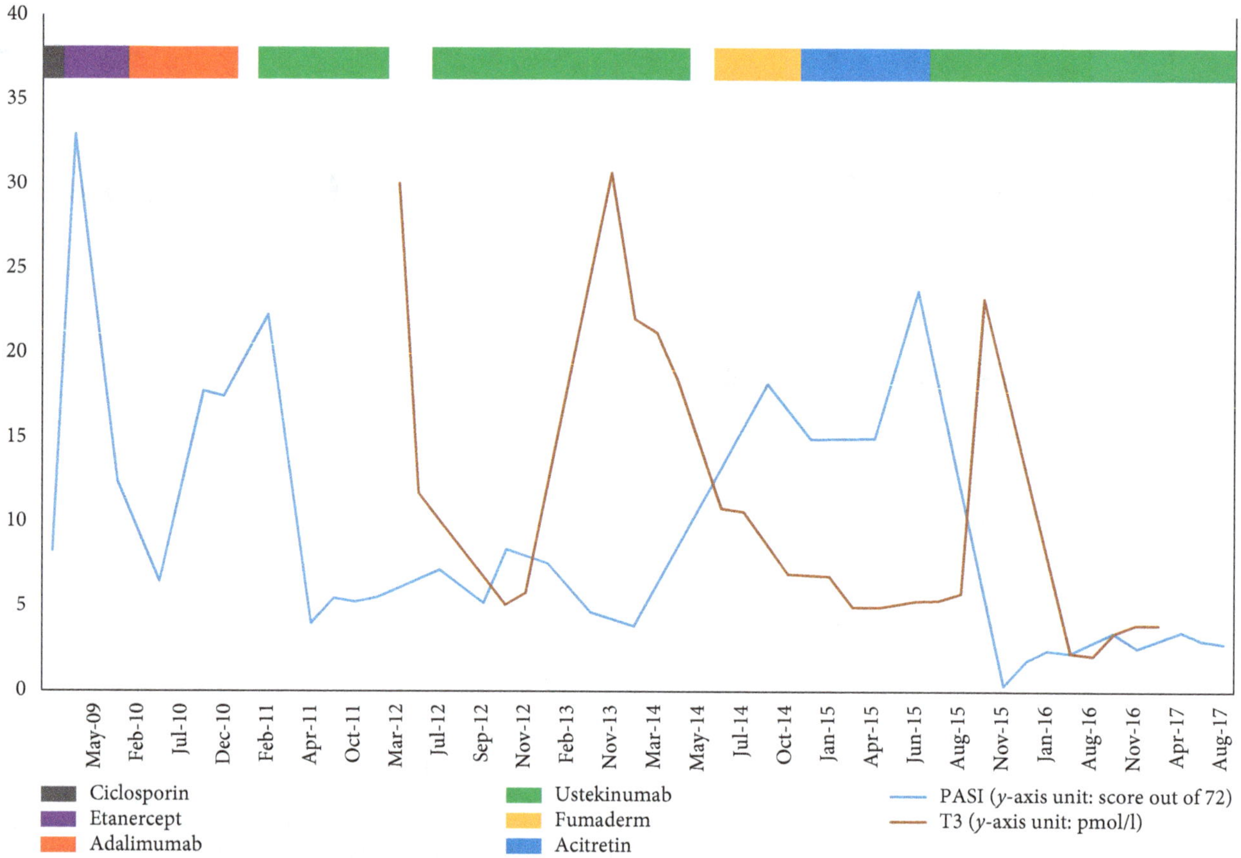

Figure 1: Graph to show PASI (blue solid line) and serum T3 level (solid pink line) during treatment with cyclosporine, etanercept, adalimumab, ustekinumab, Fumaderm, and acitretin between May 2009 and August 2017.

in June 2015, rendering him biochemically and clinically euthyroid.

The patient felt however that ustekinumab was the only treatment that satisfactorily controlled his psoriasis, and therefore after further discussion of potential risks this was restarted in August 2015. He developed hyperthyroidism again in November 2015, experiencing tremors and sweats with a serum T3 of 23.2 pmol/l, T4 of 43 pmol/l, and TSH of <0.1 mU/l. He required further treatment with carbimazole and eventually a second dose of radioiodine that caused hypothyroidism.

He remains on ustekinumab therapy to date and continues with long-term thyroxine replacement. The following chart displays the time-course of these events graphically (Figure 1).

3. Discussion

To our knowledge, this is the second reported case of ustekinumab treatment associated with thyrotoxicosis. In this case, the hyperthyroidism developed several months after first treatment with ustekinumab, and although the causative link was in question initially, recurrence of hyperthyroidism after recommencement of ustekinumab on two further separate occasions was more indicative of causality.

A previous case of autoimmune thyroiditis (Graves' disease) following ustekinumab treatment for psoriasis has recently been reported in a 68-year-old woman [2]. It was postulated that Graves' disease is mediated by Th2 pathways and that inhibition of Th1/Th17-mediated pathways by ustekinumab [3] may skew the Th1/Th2 balance, leading to the production of thyroid autoantibodies [4]. Other biologic treatments have been considered in this context, and two cases of autoimmune thyroid disease following treatment with anti-TNF-α agents have been previously reported in patients treated for rheumatoid arthritis [5, 6]. An article summarising 5-year single-centre experience with ustekinumab for psoriasis, which included 93 patients, reported a case of papillary thyroid cancer, but no reports of changes in thyroid state [7]. The British Association of Dermatologists Biologic Interventions Register (BADBIR) group collects data from most centres in the United Kingdom and Ireland and has also not reported any similar adverse reactions with ustekinumab in 450 patients [8]. There are no long-term data available about the safety profile of many biologic therapies in psoriasis as they have only been licensed relatively recently; therefore, awareness and reporting of these reactions are important in planning the management of these patients in the future.

References

[1] S. K. Mahil, F. Capon, and J. N. Barker, "Update on psoriasis immunopathogenesis and targeted immunotherapy," *Seminars in Immunopathology*, vol. 38, no. 1, pp. 11–27, 2016.

[2] S. Lee, J. An, D. Kim, M. Yoon, and H. Lee, "A case of interstitial lung disease and autoimmune thyroiditis associated with ustekinumab," *Acta Dermato Venereologica*, vol. 99, no. 3, pp. 331-332, 2019.

[3] N. Koutruba, J. Emer, and M. Lebwohl, "Review of ustekinumab, an interleukin-12 and interleukin-23 inhibitor used for the treatment of plaque psoriasis," *Therapeutics and Clinical Risk Management*, vol. 6, pp. 123–141, 2010.

[4] A. M. Ramos-Leví and M. Marazuela, "Pathogenesis of thyroid autoimmune disease: the role of cellular mechanisms," *Endocrinología y Nutrición*, vol. 63, no. 8, pp. 421–429, 2016.

[5] D. Vassilopoulos, K. Sialevris, S. Malahtari, M. Deutsch, S. Manolakopoulos, and A. J. Archimandritis, "Subacute thyroiditis presenting as fever of unknown origin in a patient with rheumatoid arthritis under etanercept treatment," *Journal of Clinical Rheumatology*, vol. 16, no. 2, pp. 88-89, 2010.

[6] A. W. Van Lieshout, M. C. Creemers, T. R. Radstake, L. D. Elving, and P. L. van Riel, "Graves' disease in a patient with rheumatoid arthritis during treatment with anti-tumor necrosis factor-alpha," *The Journal of Rheumatology*, vol. 35, pp. 938-939, 2008.

[7] T. Vergou, A. E. Moustou, and C. Antoniou, "Five-year experience with ustekinumab for psoriasis: real-life data of a single centre," *Journal of the European Academy of Dermatology and Venereology*, vol. 31, no. 1, pp. e40–e41, 2017.

[8] R. B. Warren, C. H. Smith, Z. Z. N. Yiu et al., "Differential drug survival of biologic therapies for the treatment of psoriasis: a prospective observational cohort study from the British Association of Dermatologists Biologic Interventions Register (BADBIR)," *Journal of Investigative Dermatology*, vol. 135, no. 11, pp. 2632–2640, 2015.

45

Isotretinoin-Induced Delusional Disorder, Somatic Subtype

Katharine V. Jensen[1] **and Adam Abba-Aji**[1,2]

[1]*Department of Psychiatry, Faculty of Medicine and Dentistry, University of Alberta, Edmonton, Alberta, Canada*
[2]*Young Adult Evaluation, Treatment & Reintegration Service, Alberta Hospital Edmonton, Alberta, Canada*

Correspondence should be addressed to Adam Abba-Aji; abbaaji@ualberta.ca

Academic Editor: Jacek Cezary Szepietowski

Isotretinoin, an active form of vitamin A, is the drug of last resort for the treatment of severe acne. Depression, suicidal ideation, and psychosis are among the most well-documented psychiatric side effects. Here, we report a case of isotretinoin-induced psychosis, which was diagnosed as delusional disorder somatic subtype, in a young male in the absence of any prodromal symptoms, previous psychiatric history, or family history of mental illness. The onset of psychosis was in the context of a dosage increase from 40 mg/day to 80 mg/day. Isotretinoin was discontinued, and the patient showed improvement on low-dose quetiapine.

1. Introduction

Isotretinoin is the drug of last resort for the treatment of severe nodular acne. It is the 13-cis isomer of retinoic acid, the active form of vitamin A [1, 2]. Isotretinoin is being increasingly prescribed for severe acne, as well as moderate acne and other skin conditions, including seborrhea, seborrheic dermatitis, and scarring [1, 3, 4]. Isotretinoin inhibits the growth of the bacterium *Propionibacterium acnes*, diminishes the size of sebaceous glands resulting in decreased sebum secretion, and hinders new comedone formation. It is also thought to have anti-inflammatory properties [1, 3]. Isotretinoin needs to be administered for approximately 2 months to take effect, and the treatment is usually continued for a minimum of 4 months.

Isotretinoin is one of the most well-known teratogenic drugs [2, 5]. It is notorious for its ability to cause serious birth defects, including heart, craniofacial, and nervous system malformations [5]. Other common side effects include dry eyes, mouth, lips, nose, or skin. Other less frequent, but more serious side effects include inflammatory bowel disease, elevated triglycerides, bone loss, vision impairment, increased intracranial pressure, sensitivity to the sun, diabetes, anemia, leukopenia, and organ damage including the liver, pancreas, intestine, and esophagus [1, 2, 6].

Despite many documented psychiatric side effects, including depression, suicide, and psychosis [7–13], the topic remains controversial as a causal relationship has not been established. Psychiatric side effects are included as a "Black Box" warning by the U.S. Food and Drug Administration (FDA). In 2002, isotretinoin received widespread media attention after a 15-year-old boy taking isotretinoin who was believed to be acutely psychotic and suicidal, stole, and flew an airplane into a building in Florida. The family filed a wrongful death lawsuit against the manufacturer of isotretinoin [14].

Compared with all drugs in the FDA's Adverse Event Reporting System (FAERS) database up to December 31, 2019, isotretinoin ranked within the top 3 for number of reports of depression [15, 16]. In the FAERS Public Dashboard for isotretinoin, depression was listed as the number 1 suspected side effect, and it was reported in 12.22% of cases. Suicidal ideation was reported in 4.05% of cases [16].

In this report, we present a unique case of a patient who developed somatic delusions after an isotretinoin dosage increase.

2. Case Report

Mr. C was a 24-year-old university-educated single male with no prior history of psychosis and no family history of mental illness. He presented to the emergency department accompanied by his parents due to multiple worsening somatic delusions. According to his parents, he became preoccupied with his physical appearance following an increase in the dosage of his isotretinoin from 40 mg/day to 80 mg/day. Mr. C believed that his face was disfigured after using Tobradex eye drop. He believed the eye drop had pooled in his nose, damaged his throat, and disfigured his face. He alleged that his forehead and teeth had shifted and that his tongue had atrophied. He denied spending a lot of time in front of a mirror; although, when he looked in the mirror, he saw a distorted face. He later complained of further symptoms including muscle atrophy, weakness, and trouble walking, despite a normal gait.

He denied symptoms of depression or anxiety. He denied auditory, visual, and tactile hallucinations as well as suicidal and homicidal ideations. There was no history of substance use, including cannabis and alcohol. All of the investigations, including complete blood count, electrolytes, blood glucose, thyroid function tests, liver enzymes, and renal function tests, were normal. His drug urine screen was negative for illicit substances, including benzodiazepines. Computed tomography (CT) of the head was normal. The electroencephalogram (EEG) was reported within normal limits as no focal abnormalities nor epileptic activities were identified.

In Mr. C's case, the absence of any prodromal symptoms, previous psychiatric history, or family history of mental illness made a primary psychotic disorder unlikely. Furthermore, the temporality of his symptoms coincided with the doubling of the isotretinoin dose from 40 mg to 80 mg daily. Additionally, there is a biological gradient or dose-response relationship, meaning that as the dose of isotretinoin increases, so does the potential of developing psychiatric symptoms, such as psychosis.

Based on his symptoms, he was given a diagnosis of delusional disorder, somatic subtype, as he had multiple somatic delusions for longer than 1 month, but his functioning was not markedly impaired, and his behaviour was not obviously bizarre. Somatic symptom disorder was considered as a differential diagnosis; however, Mr. C's concern about his somatic symptoms did not reflect a fear of underlying illness. The isotretinoin was discontinued, and he was started on quetiapine 100 mg orally at bedtime and was compliant with medication. Patient's symptoms resolved two weeks following the discontinuation of the isotretinoin, and the quetiapine was similarly discontinued after two months. Patient was discharged from psychiatric care to his family physician following a four-month period of sustained remission from the date of his discharge from his index psychiatric admission.

3. Discussion

Isotretinoin, a retinoid derivative of vitamin A, is widely considered an effective treatment for severe nodular acne [1]. It is being increasingly prescribed for severe acne, as well as other skin conditions. Despite many documented psychiatric side effects [1, 7–13], the etiology of isotretinoin-induced psychosis remains poorly understood. Though, it has been previously reported that an excess of dietary vitamin A induces psychosis [17]. Furthermore, in patients with psychosis, isotretinoin is contraindicated as it worsens the course of the disease [18].

To the best of our knowledge, this is the first case report of isotretinoin-induced delusional disorder, somatic type. It is a unique case, as it was an increase in the dosage of isotretinoin that triggered the psychotic episode and not the initiation of isotretinoin therapy. In the majority of case reports, the patients had a past psychiatric history or a family history of mental illness. Whereas the patient presented here had no prodromal symptoms, no previous psychiatric history, and no family history of mental illness. In this case, isotretinoin was considered the precipitant of psychosis as the onset of psychotic symptoms followed an increase in the dosage of isotretinoin from 40 mg/day to 80 mg/day.

The general treatment principles for drug-induced psychosis were followed, and isotretinoin was discontinued; a low dose of the antipsychotic, quetiapine 100 mg, was started, and adjunct sedatives were used for short-term agitation. Subsequently, the patient's somatic complaints diminished, and he settled. Approximately two weeks after discontinuing isotretinoin and starting quetiapine, the psychotic symptoms had resolved. The patient continued to take quetiapine for approximately two months prior to it being discontinued. He was followed by psychiatry for a total of 4 months prior to being discharged back to the care of his family physician. He had no relapses following the discontinuation of isotretinoin.

Psychiatrists are familiar with the physical side effects, such as extrapyramidal symptoms and metabolic syndrome, that can occur in patients on psychotropic drugs. However, it is pertinent to consider that nonpsychotropic drugs commonly prescribed by other medical specialties may cause psychiatric side effects. Although no causal relationship between isotretinoin and psychopathology has been established, the numerous case reports, including the one presented here, support the association. Therefore, physicians must be aware of this relationship and monitor patients on isotretinoin for psychiatric symptoms and consider stopping the drug and providing appropriate psychiatric treatment as soon as possible. Furthermore, any psychiatric side effect from isotretinoin treatment should be reported to permit better understanding of the incidence of psychotic symptoms with this treatment.

4. Conclusion

Isotretinoin is being increasingly prescribed due to its effectiveness for acne. It is likely that we are going to see more isotretinoin-induced psychiatric side effects as a result of its frequent use. It is important that all patients taking isotretinoin be screened regularly by the prescribing physician for signs of depression, suicidal ideation, and psychosis. It is also important that psychiatrists take a detailed history, including a medication history, so that a diagnosis of medication-induced psychosis, such as the one presented in this report, is not overlooked.

References

[1] C. S. Costa, E. Bagatin, A. L. C. Martimbianco et al., "Oral isotretinoin for acne," *Cochrane Database of Systematic Reviews*, vol. 11, no. 11, 2018.
[2] P. Brzezinski, K. Borowska, A. Chiriac, and J. Smigielski, "Adverse effects of isotretinoin: a large, retrospective review," *Dermatologic Therapy*, vol. 30, no. 4, Article ID e12483, 2017.
[3] E. Bagatin, "Oral isotretinoin: the most promising dermatological off-label uses," *Expert Review of Dermatology*, vol. 5, no. 6, pp. 617–626, 2010.
[4] C. De Souza Leão Kamamoto, A. Sanudo, K. M. Hassun, and E. Bagatin, "Low-dose oral isotretinoin for moderate to severe seborrhea and seborrheic dermatitis: a randomized comparative trial," *International Journal of Dermatology*, vol. 56, no. 1, pp. 80–85, 2017.
[5] D. Henry, C. Dormuth, B. Winquist et al., "Occurrence of pregnancy and pregnancy outcomes during isotretinoin therapy," *Canadian Medical Association Journal*, vol. 188, no. 10, pp. 723–730, 2016.
[6] V. P. Kontaxakis, D. Skourides, P. Ferentinos, B. J. Havaki-Kontaxaki, and G. N. Papadimitriou, "Isotretinoin and psychopathology: a review," *Annals of General Psychiatry*, vol. 8, no. 1, 2009.
[7] J. D. Bremner, K. D. Shearer, and P. J. McCaffery, "Retinoic acid and affective disorders: the evidence for an association," *The Journal of Clinical Psychiatry*, vol. 73, no. 1, pp. 37–50, 2012.
[8] T. Deniz and C. Emeksiz, "Isotretinoin intoxication in attempted suicide: a case report," *Marmara Medical Journal*, vol. 21, no. 3, pp. 269–272, 2008.
[9] D. K. Wysowski, M. Pitts, and J. Beitz, "An analysis of reports of depression and suicide in patients treated with isotretinoin," *Journal of the American Academy of Dermatology*, vol. 45, no. 4, pp. 515–519, 2001.
[10] S. J. Enders and J. M. Enders, "Isotretinoin and psychiatric illness in adolescents and young adults," *Annals of Pharmacotherapy*, vol. 37, no. 7-8, pp. 1124–1127, 2003.
[11] Y. Barak, Y. Wohl, Y. Greenberg et al., "Affective psychosis following Accutane (isotretinoin) treatment," *International Clinical Psychopharmacology*, vol. 20, no. 1, pp. 39–41, 2005.
[12] A. Suuberg, "Psychiatric and developmental effects of isotretinoin (retinoid) treatment for acne vulgaris," *Current Therapeutic Research-Clinical and Experimental*, vol. 90, pp. 27–31, 2019.
[13] J. O'Donnell, "Overview of existing research and information linking isotretinoin (accutane), depression, psychosis, and suicide," *American Journal of Therapeutics*, vol. 10, no. 2, pp. 148–159, 2003.
[14] R.. Acne, *Drug Maker Sued over Florida Suicide*, The New York Times, New York, NY, USA, 2002.
[15] K. B. Hoffman, A. R. Demakas, M. Dimbil, N. P. Tatonetti, and C. B. Erdman, "Stimulated reporting: the impact of US food and drug administration-issued alerts on the adverse event reporting system (FAERS)," *Drug Safety*, vol. 37, no. 11, pp. 971–980, 2014.
[16] FDA's adverse event reporting system (FAERS) database, ," 2020, https://fis.fda.gov/sense/app/d10be6bb-494e-4cd2-82e4-0135608ddc13/sheet/33a0f68e-845c-48e2-bc81-8141c6aaf772/state/analysis%0D%0A.
[17] K. O'Reilly, S. J. Bailey, and M. A. Lane, "Retinoid-mediated regulation of mood: possible cellular mechanisms," *Experimental Biology and Medicine*, vol. 233, no. 3, pp. 251–258, 2008.
[18] A. Kepska, M. Majtyka, M. Kowman, I. Kłoszewska, E. Kwiecińska, and A. Zalewska-Janowska, "Dermatitis artefacta as a symptom of schizophrenia?" *Advances in Dermatology and Allergology*, vol. 4, pp. 277–279, 2014.

46

A Unique Presentation of Cutaneous Diffuse Large B-Cell Lymphoma

Mary Awad, Erik Holzwanger, and Sandeep Jubbal

University of Massachusetts Medical School, Worcester, MA, USA

Correspondence should be addressed to Mary Awad; maryeawad@gmail.com

Academic Editor: Alireza Firooz

Cutaneous B-cell lymphomas (CBCL) are rare heterogeneous neoplastic diseases composing about 22.5% of all cutaneous lymphomas. These diseases can be divided into primary and secondary cutaneous variants with primary cutaneous B-cell lymphoma (PCBCL) divided into three distinct entities including primary cutaneous marginal zone lymphoma, primary cutaneous follicle center lymphoma, and primary cutaneous diffuse large B-cell lymphoma, leg type (PCDLBCL, LT). Secondary cutaneous diffuse large B-cell lymphoma (CDLBCL) and PCDLBCL, LT are more aggressive neoplasms compared to the aforementioned CBCL with survival rates of 37% and 50% after 5 years, respectively. CDLBCL can present as cutaneous or subcutaneous nodules, papular lesions, or indurated plaques. Here, we present a case of CDLBCL of an 88-year-old female that was mistaken for lower extremity cellulitis with phlegmon. Our patient failed two courses of antibiotic therapy as an outpatient and received a third as an inpatient before a cutaneous biopsy clinched the diagnosis.

1. Introduction

Diffuse large B-cell lymphoma (DLBCL) comprises one-third of all non-Hodgkin's lymphomas (NHL). DLBCL is composed of multiple diverse neoplasms involving both primary extranodal and nodal types. Epidemiologically, DLBCL is most common in Caucasians and men and the incidence increasing with older age. Of the extranodal subtypes, gastrointestinal, head and neck, and skin and soft tissue comprise the majority of primary sites. The distinction between primary cutaneous diffuse large B-cell lymphoma (PCDLBCL) and DLBCL with secondary cutaneous involvement is based on extracutaneous involvement at the time of diagnosis. PCDLBCL can metastasize to extracutaneous sites, as is seen in 40% of patients with PCDLBCL, leg type (PCDLBCL, LT), often making it difficult to establish a primary cutaneous diagnosis [1]. Prognosis of DLBCL is variable based on subtype with 5-year survival rates ranging from 30–80%; however, prognosis of secondary cutaneous DLBCL and PCDLBCL, LT are both poor with 5-year disease specific survival rates at 37% and 50%, respectively [2]. It is therefore critical to diagnose cutaneous diffuse large B-cell lymphoma (CDLBCL) early on in its pathogenesis [3].

2. Case

An 88-year-old woman with a history of type II diabetes mellitus, chronic deep venous thrombosis (DVT) of right femoral vein, and atrial fibrillation on coumadin presented to her primary care physician (PCP) with right lower leg extremity swelling, erythema, and pain. A week prior to presentation, there was development of a sore on her right posterior ankle that began to crust over. The patient's leg became increasingly edematous, painful, warm, and erythematous throughout the week. Her primary care physician prescribed cephalexin for 10 days followed by doxycycline for four days. She continued to have progression of her symptoms while on these antibiotics (Figure 1(a)). She then developed intermittent purulent drainage from the sore behind the ankle concurrently with severe pain radiating down the leg (Figure 1(c)). She was then hospitalized and assessed for a deep soft tissue infection, abscess, and deep vein thrombosis. Cefazolin was given with subsequent

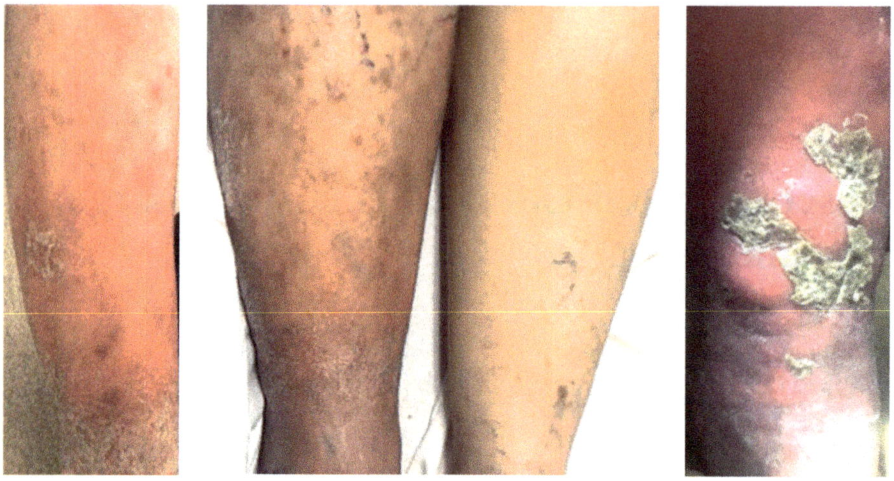

(a) (b) (c)

Figure 1: (a) Photograph of right lower extremity anterior view taken 4 days prior to admission following 10 days of cephalexin therapy. (b) Photograph of bilateral lower extremities anterior view taken on hospital day 4; on day 4 of cefazolin therapy prior to biopsy and diagnosis. (c) Photograph taken on hospital day 10 after 3 failed treatments of antibiotic therapy and after diagnosis of DLBCL.

improvement in the degree of erythema, though she continued to endorse significant pain. As the erythema receded to the mid-shin, the patient had persistent scattered papules and macules along the upper calf (Figure 1(b)). Blood cultures were negative and over the course of her illness, she remained afebrile without night sweats or chills. Laboratory workup revealed an elevated CRP (11.4 mg/L), which was felt to be secondary to an active infection. At presentation, a complete blood count with differential was within normal limits (white blood cell count 6.0 thousand cells/μL). On hospital day 3, she underwent a CT lower extremity with contrast due to continued pain, which was significant for diffuse heterogeneity in the calf muscle, notably a $1.8 \times 1.3 \times 3.8$ cm lesion in the gastrocnemius without evidence of a drainable fluid collection or air within the soft tissue. The leading differential at this time was myositis with phlegmon leading to persistent pain and continued erythema and edema. She proceeded to have a skin biopsy for culture and histochemistry, which displayed an atypical mononuclear infiltrate, and previous imaging was reinterpreted as possible malignancy. Immunohistochemical staining done was negative for CD10 and positive for CD20, MUM1, BCL-2, and BCL-6 consistent with primary cutaneous diffuse large B-cell lymphoma, leg type; however, secondary cutaneous nongerminal DLBCL was not ruled out.

Of note, during hospitalization LDH was found to be elevated to 506 U/L. Following discharge, there was an overall increase in LDH value with slight fluctuations from 694 U/L to 616 U/L and ultimately reaching a maximum value of 737 U/L when last assessed. Patient's complete blood count remained unremarkable throughout hospitalization besides for mild normocytic anemia (hemoglobin approximately 11.5 g/dL). CT abdomen and pelvis with contrast revealed an enlarged right inguinal lymph node 1.6×1.8 cm. There was no intra-abdominal or retroperitoneal lymphadenopathy. CT chest with contrast did not show new nodules nor did it show mediastinal or hilar adenopathy. PET/CT scan performed 2 weeks after discharge and 1 month following presentation showed extensive intensely FDG-avid muscular, soft tissue, and dermal lymphomatous involvement in lower extremities, right greater than left. There were additionally discrete soft tissue nodules and lymph nodes in the lower extremities, left buttock, right inguinal region, and right external iliac. The patient was diagnosed with advanced stage IV nongerminal DLBCL. The patient was later started on rituximab to polychemotherapy (R-CHOP) but was transitioned to hospice care after developing sepsis, DIC, and a new DVT.

3. Discussion

DLBCL typically presents in males in the 7th decade of life with a median age of 64 years old, though DLBCL can present at any age, accounting for 20% of NHL in children under 14 years old [4]. In a study comparing cutaneous lymphomas, it was found that 22.5% of cases of cutaneous lymphoma were of B-cell lymphomas with 44.4% constituting primary cutaneous disease [5]. Primary cutaneous lymphomas are divided into 3 subtypes according to the 2008 World Health Organization-European Organization for Research and Treatment of Cancer (EORTC) including primary cutaneous marginal zone lymphoma, primary cutaneous follicle center lymphoma, and primary cutaneous diffuse large B-cell lymphoma, leg type [6].

PCDLBCL, LT in contrast to the aforementioned CBCL and other DLBCL commonly affects females and has a poor prognosis. The median age for PCDLBCL, LT at presentation is 70–82 years old [1, 6]. Most cases involve the lower legs; however, around 10% of cases can involve other cutaneous sites and extracutaneous dissemination is common. Most cases are MUM-1/IRF-4, BCL-2, and BCL-6 positive as was seen with our patient [6].

A study assessing presentations of DLBCL secondary cutaneous disease found that secondary cutaneous disease most commonly involves the legs and most frequently presents as cutaneous nodules, but in 16% of cases, it presents with papular lesions, as was seen with our patient [3]. There is scarce literature detailing the course of secondary cutaneous DLBCL. The prognosis and clinical course is much more aggressive in secondary cutaneous DLBCL compared to the indolent PCBCL in what has been reported. A patient diagnosed with secondary cutaneous DLBCL qualifies for stage IV disease per Ann Arbour staging giving an unfavorable diagnosis to those with the disease. Other unfavorable factors include age > 60, ECOG > 2, involvement of more than 2 extranodal sites, and elevated LDH [4].

Our patient's case was complex due to her comorbidities, partial response to antibiotic therapy, and lack of constitutional symptoms which led to a difficult diagnosis. Initially, we believed her underlying type II diabetes mellitus, peripheral vascular diseases, and chronic lower extremity edema predisposed her to an infectious etiology. Therefore, we continued to treat as if this patient had a cellulitis with phlegmon in the setting of supportive radiographic evidence. Ultimately, minimal improvement in symptoms led to a biopsy leading to a diagnosis of CDLBCL. This case highlights the difficulty in diagnosing patients with CDLBCL given the rarity and unusual presentation of this illness. At the time of diagnosis, our patient had extracutaneous involvement including the gastrocnemius and, on PET-scan, surrounding lymph nodes therefore limiting our confidence in diagnosing primary cutaneous disease.

Survival rates for CDLBCL have improved with the addition of rituximab to polychemotherapy (R-CHOP); however, up to 40% of disease becomes refractory to this treatment or relapses [4]. Unfortunately, our patient was unable to complete R-CHOP therapy after developing DIC, sepsis, and a new DVT. Given the late age of onset of this disease, aggressive polychemotherapy may not be feasible, and therefore more targeted or localized therapies are required. Exciting developments in CD19 targeted chimeric antigen receptor T-cell (CAR-T) therapy show promise in treating B-cell malignancies expressing the CD19 transmembrane glycoprotein, as is seen in many DLBCL. However, these treatments are costly and can have consequential side effects such as cytokine release syndrome and neurotoxicity [7]. Gaps do remain in our understanding of this disease process, specifically in secondary cutaneous disease. Research must focus on understanding the microenvironment of this neoplasm as a means of better targeting the cells driving this process.

References

[1] C. B. Hope and L. B. Pincus, "Primary cutaneous B-cell lymphomas with large cell predominance-primary cutaneous follicle center lymphoma, diffuse large B-cell lymphoma, leg type and intravascular large B-cell lymphoma," *Seminars in Diagnostic Pathology*, vol. 34, no. 1, pp. 85–98, 2017.

[2] J. J. Castillo, E. S. Winer, and A. J. Olszewski, "Sites of extranodal involvement are prognostic in patients with diffuse large B-cell lymphoma in the rituximab era: an analysis of the surveillance, epidemiology and end results database," *American Journal of Hematology*, vol. 89, no. 3, pp. 310–314, 2014.

[3] W. Lee, K. Won, C. Won et al., "Secondary cutaneous diffuse large B-cell lymphoma has a higher international prognostic index score and worse prognosis than diffuse large B-cell lymphoma, leg type," *Acta Dermato Venereologica*, vol. 96, no. 2, pp. 245–250, 2016.

[4] J. W. Suh, "Aggressive B-cell lymphomas: how many categories do we need?" *Modern Pathology*, vol. 26, no. 1, pp. S42–S56, 2012.

[5] S. H. Tan, C. S. Sim, and B. H. Ong, "Cutaneous lymphomas other than mycosis fungoides in Singapore: a clinicopathological analysis using recent classification systems," *British Journal of Dermatology*, vol. 149, no. 3, pp. 542–553, 2003.

[6] R. A. Wilcox, "Cutaneous B-cell lymphomas: 2019 update on diagnosis, risk stratification, and management," *American Journal of Hematology*, vol. 93, no. 11, pp. 1427–1430, 2018.

[7] R. Havard and D. M. Stephens, "Anti-CD19 chimeric antigen receptor T cell therapies: harnessing the power of the immune system to fight diffuse large B cell lymphoma," *Current Hematologic Malignancy Reports*, vol. 13, no. 6, pp. 534–542, 2018.

47

Cutaneous Effects of Notch Inhibitor Therapy: A Report of Two Cases

Claire J. Wiggins[1,2] **and Susan Y. Chon**[1]

[1]*MD Anderson Cancer Center, Department of Dermatology, 1515 Holcombe Blvd, Houston, TX 77030, USA*
[2]*Baylor College of Medicine, 1 Baylor Plaza, Houston, TX 77030, USA*

Correspondence should be addressed to Claire J. Wiggins; claire.wiggins@bcm.edu

Academic Editor: Sergio A. Cuevas Covarrubias; sergioa@servidor.unam.mx

As aberrant Notch signaling has been linked to cancerous growth, Notch inhibitors represent a novel category of targeted oncological therapy. Notch pathways in tumor cells may contribute to proliferation or limit apoptosis and differentiation. Healthy skin differentiation and homeostasis are reliant on normal Notch expression, and disruption of this signaling has been implicated in dermatological conditions such as hidradenitis suppurativa, psoriasis, atopic dermatitis, and lichen planus. Here, we describe two cases of patients with cutaneous side effects from Notch inhibitor treatment for adenoid cyst carcinoma (ACC) and review the role of Notch signaling in skin disease. By illuminating connections between medication side effects and disease pathogenesis, our goal is to increase awareness of the cutaneous side effects of Notch inhibitor treatment.

1. Introduction

Targeted cancer therapies have brought about a paradigm shift in the field of oncology by honing in on the biochemical pathways relevant to common oncogenic mutations. Notch signaling is a highly conserved transduction pathway that is implicated in many cancers, *NOTCH* genes acting as either an oncogene or tumor suppressor depending on the cellular context [1]. Unregulated Notch signaling has been linked to hematological malignancies such as T-ALL, Hodgkin's lymphoma, and multiple myeloma, as well as solid tumors including breast, renal, lung, ovarian, prostate, and head and neck [2]. Notch may contribute to cancerous growth by preventing apoptosis and differentiation or by promoting cell proliferation [2]. Due to its role in a variety of cancers, the Notch signaling pathway represents a promising therapeutic target.

In the epidermis, Notch plays a critical role in skin development and homeostasis, with Notch activity required during the entire lifespan [1]. Mammals possess 4 different receptors, Notch 1–4, and each has demonstrated expression in the epidermis. Although the ablation of Notch 2–4 does not cause any phenotypic changes in the skin, deletion of Notch 1 receptor leads to abnormalities in the interfollicular epidermis (IFE) and hair follicle (HF), although the evidence does indicate overlap in each receptor's function [3, 4]. Notch 1 has been shown to induce differentiation of keratinocytes as well as arrest the growth of mature keratinocytes through the calcineurin-NFAT pathway [5]. The Notch pathway stimulates epidermal differentiation and promotes barrier formation [3, 6]. Retinoic acid (RA) signaling in the skin has also been directly linked to Notch 1 activity [4, 7].

When normal Notch signaling is disrupted, a number of pathologies have been documented. Inflammatory skin conditions such as hidradenitis suppurativa (HS), psoriasis, atopic dermatitis, and lichen planus have been linked to Notch dysfunction [6, 8, 9]. Notch-deficient skin has been associated with myeloproliferative disorders and *B*-lymphoproliferative disorders [6, 10]. Interestingly, a high frequency of Notch 1 receptor mutations has been identified in cutaneous squamous cell carcinoma (cSCC), indicating that Notch mutation plays an early role in skin carcinogenesis, similar to adenomatous polyposis coli mutation in colon cancer [11]. However, in head and neck SCC, over expression of Notch, rather than under expression in cases of cSCC, was linked with poorer prognosis [12, 13]. Notch 1 has been established as a tumor suppressor for both basal cell carcinoma (BCC) and cSCC [1].

Notch signaling plays a variety of roles in cutaneous tissue and contrasting roles in various tissues that warrant further study, especially as Notch inhibitor therapies for cancer are being developed. Here, we describe two cases of patients with cutaneous side effects from Notch inhibitor treatment for adenoid cyst carcinoma (ACC). We aim to draw attention to important management issues for this targeted therapy as well as gain insight into the pathogenesis of these side effects through the mechanisms of this therapy.

2. Case Report

2.1. Case #1. A 49-year-old woman receiving Notch signaling inhibitor treatment for metastatic ACC bearing activating Notch mutations presented with a rash thought to be caused by her treatment regimen with AL 101 (BMS-906024).

These erythematous hyperkeratotic papules and plaques were first noted on her antecubital fossae and bilateral lower legs. A biopsy of one of these lesions on the lower leg revealed actinic keratosis (AK), which was treated with Efudex BID for 2 weeks with good inflammatory response but without complete resolution. Over the next several weeks, she continued to develop new similar scaly papules and plaques on her legs. Patient was then treated with acitretin 10 mg daily, which led to near complete resolution of the growths.

Additionally, several months after initiation of the primary growths, she then developed erythematous subcutaneous cystic nodules on the buttock area and antecubital fossae, which were occasionally painful and pruritic. Several lesions between the buttocks drained a thick white fluid. She was prescribed doxycycline and sitz baths to treat these HS-like lesions, which helped reduce but not entirely resolve the lesions. The patient was also found to have milia on left antecubital fossa and forehead and eczematous dermatitis on the back: both likely are additional adverse effects of Notch signaling inhibitor treatment, as once the treatment was discontinued, the cutaneous symptoms abated.

2.2. Case #2. A 39-year-old woman presented with painful "whelps" under her breasts, axilla, and groin, which appeared in association with the initiation of treatment with a notch signaling inhibitor AL 101 (BMS-906024) for metastatic ACC bearing activating Notch mutations.

These erythematous nodules were very painful and pruritic, and several in the groin drained white fluid. She was subsequently diagnosed with HS as well as folliculitis and was prescribed oral doxycycline, topical clindamycin, and topical chlorhexidine.

Upon follow-up several weeks later, new lesions had appeared in the groin area, but the lifespan of each lesion was decreased. Patient was additionally recommended to utilize dilute bleach baths. After discontinuation of her Notch inhibitor treatment, her hidradenitis has stabilized and has been under control with a topical regimen of clindamycin and chlorhexidine.

3. Discussion

Our patients, both on a Notch signaling inhibitor for treatment of ACC, suffered from new onset cutaneous conditions, which were potentially caused by Notch inhibition. Neither patient had a history of skin cancer nor other significant dermatologic history. Our first patient was diagnosed with AK, HS, milia, and eczematous dermatitis. The latter patient was diagnosed with HS and folliculitis. All of these dermatologic conditions first occurred within 2 months of the initiation of Notch signaling inhibitor therapy. Of note, both patients were receiving the AL101 medication as a part of the ACCURACY clinical trial (ID: NCT03691207). NOTCH1 has been shown to control propagation and differentiation in aggressive ACC subtypes, prompting the investigation into Notch inhibiting therapies for ACC [14–16].

Due to Notch's central role in supporting the inner and outer root sheath of the HF, it is unsurprising that blockade of Notch could contribute to inflammatory diseases of the HF such as HS and folliculitis, in addition to the mechanisms of immunological dysregulation that contribute to the inflammatory reaction, fibrosis, and scarring [17]. The proposed biochemical pathogenesis of familial HS involves Notch dysfunction due to sequence variants in portions of the gamma secretase complex [17, 18]. These upstream changes result in altered HF keratinization, which causes blockage and dilation of the HF. Follicular hyperkeratosis leads to inflammation, keratin-filled epidermal cysts, abscess, and sinus tract formation [19]. In studies of Notch-deficient mice where components of the gamma secretase complex are knocked out, HFs are replaced by epidermal cysts [20]. Dysfunction of Notch has been noted in other inflammatory conditions, such as psoriasis and atopic dermatitis; however, the development of dermal cysts and follicular occlusion found in these animal knockout models lend evidence to a more specific connection between HS and Notch signaling [18].

Although data support the role of defective Notch signaling in the pathogenesis of HS, whether or not it is the driving factor of HS is still in question [17]. Importantly, knockout models with dysfunctional Notch signaling do present with HS-like lesions, but they also swiftly develop cSCC as well. This deviates from the classic HS presentation, making dysregulated Notch signaling perhaps a secondary, rather than primary, driver of HS [18]. Interestingly, in accordance with the results from animal knockout models, our patients on Notch inhibiting therapy presented here developed HS-like lesions, and one also presented with AK lesions or precursors to cSCC.

Cutaneous squamous cell carcinoma (cSCC) is the most common skin cancer with metastatic potential, representing about 20% of epithelial skin tumors. Notch 1 mutation has been established as a gatekeeper event in the development of cSCC in humans [11]. In areas of photoexposed skin, invasive cSCC lesions have been found to have decreased expression on Notch 1 [21]. Given this established connection, the development of AK in our patient on a Notch inhibiting treatment could be reasonable to expect. Although highly treatable in early stages, advanced cSCC carries a 5-year survival rate below 30%, indicating the importance of timely intervention [22, 23]. Therefore, in populations at increased risk for cSCC, proper management of these patients must include vigilant cutaneous surveillance.

Increasing clinical awareness of these potential side effects of Notch inhibitor medication can help guide safe patient management, which is important if this treatment is approved for widespread use. Currently, reports of mild gastrointestinal upset are the only documented side effects of Notch inhibitors, but our observations indicate that significant cutaneous side effects may also emerge [24]. Informing patients of potential diverse cutaneous side effects and treating them in a timely fashion will help improve overall outcomes. Learning about these side effect profiles can additionally shed light on the mechanisms of these adverse effects and open up the possibility for more rigorous studies of causation. Although the roles of Notch signaling in HS and cSCC, for example, are not fully understood, reviewing patient symptoms in the context of new therapies can continue to help describe these pathogeneses. In the case of AK and cSCC in particular, early treatment will remain central to the management of these sequelae. Here, our Notch-inhibitor patient with AK was treated successfully with acitretin, an important clinical pearl. Notch and retinoic acid signaling are interrelated, and both contribute to epidermal differentiation, so this form of side-effect management could be a logical and effective treatment for similar patients in the future [7]. This report aims to raise awareness of potential clinical effects of a treatment currently in phase II clinical trial and to encourage future study of the discussed skin lesion pathogeneses.

References

[1] C. Nowell and F. Radtke, "Cutaneous Notch signaling in health and disease," *Cold Spring Harbor Perspectives in Medicine*, vol. 3, no. 12, Article ID a017772, 2013.

[2] I. Espinoza and L. Miele, "Notch inhibitors for cancer treatment," *Pharmacology & Therapeutics*, vol. 139, no. 2, pp. 95–110, 2013.

[3] M. Nicolas, A. Wolfer, K. Raj et al., "Notch 1 functions as a tumor suppressor in mouse skin," *Nature Genetics*, vol. 33, no. 3, pp. 416–421, 2003.

[4] S. Vauclair, F. Majo, A.-D. Durham, N. B. Ghyselinck, Y. Barrandon, and F. Radtke, "Corneal epithelial cell fate is maintained during repair by Notch1 signaling via the regulation of vitamin A metabolism," *Developmental Cell*, vol. 13, no. 2, pp. 242–253, 2007.

[5] C. Mammucari, A. T. Di Vignano, A. A. Sharov et al., "Integration of Notch1 and calcineurin/NFAT signaling pathways in keratinocyte growth and differentiation control," *Developmental Cell*, vol. 8, no. 5, pp. 665 676, 2005.

[6] A. Dumortier, A.-D. Durham, M. Di Piazza et al., "Atopic dermatitis-like disease and associated lethal myeloproliferative disorder arise from loss of Notch signaling in the murine skin," *PLoS One*, vol. 5, no. 2, Article ID e9258, 2010.

[7] C. A. Collins and F. M. Watt, "Dynamic regulation of retinoic acid-binding proteins in developing adult and neoplastic skin reveals roles for β-catenin and Notch signalling," *Developmental Biology*, vol. 324, no. 1, pp. 55–67, 2008.

[8] C. Marasca, E. Scala, R. Di Caprio et al., "Notch dysregulation and hidradenitis suppurativa, psoriasis, atopic dermatitis, and lichen planus: let us talk about numb," *British Journal of Dermatology*, vol. 180, no. 4, pp. 950-951, 2019.

[9] E. Scala, A. Balato, C. Marasca et al., "New insights into mechanism of Notch signalling in hidradenitis suppurativa," *Giornale Italiano di Dermatologia e Venereologia*, vol. 10, 2018.

[10] S. Demehri, Z. Liu, J. Lee et al., "Notch-deficient skin induces a lethal systemic *B*-lymphoproliferative disorder by secreting TSLP, a sentinel for epidermal integrity," *PLoS Biology*, vol. 6, no. 5, p. e123, 2008.

[11] A. P. South, K. J. Purdie, S. A. Watt et al., "Notch1 mutations occur early during cutaneous squamous cell carcinogenesis," *Journal of Investigative Dermatology*, vol. 134, no. 10, pp. 2630–2638, 2014.

[12] B. Yu, J. Wei, X. Qian, D. Lei, Q. Ma, and Y. Liu, "Notch1 signaling pathway participates in cancer invasion by regulating MMPs in lingual squamous cell carcinoma," *Oncology Reports*, vol. 27, no. 2, pp. 547–552, 2012.

[13] J.-T. Lin, M.-K. Chen, K.-T. Yeh et al., "Association of high levels of jagged-1 and Notch1 expression with poor prognosis in head and neck cancer," *Annals of Surgical Oncology*, vol. 17, no. 11, pp. 2976–2983, 2010.

[14] A. Panaccione, M. T. Chang, B. E. Carbone et al., "Notch1 and SOX10 are essential for proliferation and radiation resistance of cancer stem-like cells in adenoid cystic carcinoma," *Clinical Cancer Research*, vol. 22, no. 8, pp. 2083–2095, 2016.

[15] W. Chen, G. Cao, X. Yuan et al., "Notch1 knockdown suppresses proliferation, migration, and metastasis of salivary adenoid cystic carcinoma cells," *Journal of Translational Medicine*, vol. 13, no. 1, p. 167, 2015.

[16] R. Ferrarotto, Y. Mitani, L. Diao et al., "Activating Notch1 mutations define a distinct subgroup of patients with adenoid cystic carcinoma who have poor prognosis, propensity to bone and liver metastasis, and potential responsiveness to Notch1 inhibitors," *Journal of Clinical Oncology*, vol. 35, no. 3, pp. 352–360, 2017.

[17] B. C. Melnik and G. Plewig, "Impaired Notch-MKP-1 signalling in hidradenitis suppurativa: an approach to pathogenesis by evidence from translational biology," *Experimental Dermatology*, vol. 22, no. 3, pp. 172–177, 2013.

[18] J. W. Frew and K. Navrazhina, "No evidence that impaired Notch signalling differentiates hidradenitis suppurativa from other inflammatory skin diseases," *British Journal of Dermatology*, vol. 182, no. 4, pp. 1042-1043, 2020.

[19] S. Fismen, G. Ingvarsson, D. Moseng, D. Nathalie Dufour, and L. Jørgensen, "A clinical-pathological review of hidradenitis suppurativa: using immunohistochemistry one disease becomes two," *APMIS*, vol. 120, no. 6, pp. 433–440, 2012.

[20] S. Demehri and R. Kopan, "Notch signaling in bulge stem cells is not required for selection of hair follicle fate," *Development*, vol. 136, no. 6, pp. 891–896, 2009.

[21] J. Panelos, F. Tarantini, M. Paglierani et al., "Photoexposition discriminates notch 1 expression in human cutaneous squamous cell carcinoma," *Modern Pathology*, vol. 21, no. 3, pp. 316–325, 2008.
[22] R. E. Kwa, K. Campana, and R. L. Moy, "Biology of cutaneous squamous cell carcinoma," *Journal of the American Academy of Dermatology*, vol. 26, no. 1, pp. 1–26, 1992.
[23] B. S. Cherpelis, C. Marcusen, and P. G. Lang, "Prognostic factors for metastasis in squamous cell carcinoma of the skin," *Dermatologic Surgery*, vol. 28, no. 3, pp. 268–273, 2002.
[24] P. Rizzo, D. Mele, C. Caliceti et al., "The role of Notch in the cardiovascular system: potential adverse effects of investigational Notch inhibitors," *Frontiers in Oncology*, vol. 4, p. 384, 2015.

48

IVIG and under Burn Unit Care Yield Favorable Outcomes in Pediatric Patients with Toxic Epidermal Necrolysis: A Case Report and Literature Review

Tareq Z. Alzughayyar,[1] Wasim Noureddin Ibrahim Hamad,[1] Eman A. S. Abuqweider,[1] Bilal Nabeel Mohammad Alqam,[1] Sadi A. Abukhalaf,[1] Rami A. Misk,[2] Fawzy M. Abunejma,[3] Jihad Samer Zalloum,[1] Mohanad Saleh,[4] Ali A. Abumunshar,[2] and Yousef I. M. Zatari[2]

[1]*Al-Quds University, Faculty of Medicine, Jerusalem, State of Palestine*
[2]*An-Najah National University, Faculty of Medicine & Health Sciences, Nablus, State of Palestine*
[3]*Al-Ahli Hospital, Hebron, State of Palestine*
[4]*Intensive Care Unit Al-Ahli Hospital, Hebron University, Hebron, State of Palestine*

Correspondence should be addressed to Tareq Z. Alzughayyar; tareq-20007@hotmail.com

Academic Editor: Tak-Wah Wong

Body reactions to drugs can manifest as Stevens–Johnson syndrome (SJS) and toxic epidermal necrolysis (TEN). TEN is the most severe form of cutaneous reactions with an incidence rate of 1-2 per million cases per year. Despite TEN being a critical and life-threatening condition, there is little to no evidence of clear management protocol. We reported a 5-year-old male child who presented with lamotrigine-induced TEN and was successfully treated with intravenous immune globulin (IVIG) with a burn unit care level, while TEN treatment with IVIG is an appropriate approach with predictable good outcomes, burn unit care is also effective in creating highly favorable effects. Upon reviewing the literature, several studies indicate that TEN patients treated with the combination of IVIG and burn unit care lead to decreased levels of morbidity and mortality than when treated with IVIG or burn unit care alone. Therefore, treatment involving both IVIG and burn unit care should be considered for TEN patients.

1. Introduction

Toxic epidermal necrolysis (TEN) is a severe cutaneous reaction to drugs or their metabolites with multisystem involvement. With a high mortality rate that is greater than 30% [1], low annual incidence of 1-2 cases per million people [2, 3], and largely unknown pathogenesis—TEN is identified as a cutaneous hypersensitivity reaction and is regarded as the most severe of its type, capable of affecting more than 30% of the total body surface area (TBSA). It is advocated that TEN patients are treated in major burn centers that oversee specialized care in protecting vital organs, dressing care, and infection prevention during the process of re-epithelialization [4]. Furthermore, the largest trial to date showed a decreased mortality rate from 51.4% to 29.8% after transfer to a burn unit within 7 days [5].

Despite the significant acute and chronic morbidity associated with the disease, recent advances of treatment protocols are limited in regard to quantity and adequate efficacy. Optimal therapies for patients with TEN remain unclear. Primarily, the treatment of TEN poses itself as a challenge due to the rarity of the condition and the limited number of studies that discuss alternative or varying options for TEN treatment.

In our paper, our suggested method of approach is distinguished by the application of both burn care and IVIG, which would be working in tandem on the premises of combatting and treating TEN. In response to our TEN-patient case, this course of action proved to be highly effective. While reviewing the literature, we also found that this method decreases mortality in other cases that used the same approach.

2. Case Presentation

A 5-year-old male with one week of decreased activity was admitted due to fever and diffuse rash. A known case of Fragile X syndrome was in his usual state of health until the age of 3 years when he had drop attacks which were managed with valproic acid prescribed by a neurologist. Two weeks before admission, lamotrigine was added to control his symptoms. Two days before admission, the patient developed fever and papular skin rash on his hands, feet, and oral cavity which was treated by an external doctor as hand-foot-mouth disease (Figure 1). On the day of admission, he was brought to the hospital due to worsening in his symptoms with difficulty in feeding. As soon as he arrived, lamotrigine was stopped.

On examination, the patient looked ill and toxic. His temperature, heart rate, blood pressure were, respectively, 39°C, 125 bpm, and 117/81, and his weight was 18 kg. He had extensive bullous skin lesions on his face, hands, feet, oropharynx, and trunk along with hemorrhagic crusting of the lips and bilateral oral conjunctivitis and presented with Nikolsky sign positive (Figure 2). No genital and perianal blisters were found. No splenomegaly, hepatomegaly, and lymphadenopathy were observed.

Laboratory examination results were WBC 6.8 cells/mm, and the differential count was normal. Platelet 180, hemoglobin 12.4, SGPT 18, SGOT 46, creatinine 0.6, BUN 14, NA+ 142, CRP 36, ESR 9, and both INR and aPTT were normal, and SCORTEN score was calculated (Table 1). Eye swap showed *Staphylococcus aureus* growth, and skin biopsy revealed full-thickness epidermal necrosis.

Due to the relatively normal workup and previous medication history, toxic epidermal necrolysis was considered. Due to the large area of involvement (more than 50%), the patient was managed in the burn unit by a multidisciplinary team with strict isolation including isolated room and barrier isolations (gloves and gown), daily wound dressing with local Bactroban application, IV ceftriaxone stopped after negative blood culture, and good hydration (3 times the maintenance; maintenance was 1400 ml/day). Besides that, IVIG (1 mg/kg/day) for 3 days—unfortunately, IVIG is very expensive (3000 USD daily) and not covered by governmental health insurance—and methylprednisone (1.5 mg/kg/day) for 3 days were given. Eye lubrication and antibiotics were considered, and IV paracetamol was used to manage his pain. On the 4th day, improvement was seen by the peeling of skin over his hands, feet, and trunk. His lab workup was normal, and CRP was 26. Upon discharge on the 8th day, the patient was active, his skin was completely recovered (Figure 3), and CRP was 3.

3. Discussion

TEN is a rare mucocutaneous hypersensitivity reaction involving greater than 30% of the total body surface area (TBSA) and is most commonly triggered by medication. Even though it is a rare disorder, it is considered a significant concern due to its high mortality rate that reaches 30% [6]. Since its major cause of death is sepsis [7] followed by acute respiratory distress, cardiac arrest, and renal failure, early diagnosis and management are very critical.

TEN is a systemic disease that affects multiple organs. Hence, its management requires that of a multidisciplinary team composed of physicians for both wound and medical management. Although there is no evidence-based protocol for the management of TEN, many studies are acknowledging and affirming the survival benefits for TEN patients when treated in a burn unit [8–10] despite the variation among burn centers in relation to their systemic interventions applied to TEN patients. It is also possible that some survivors of TEN may develop severe, chronic, and often debilitating complications that can permanently impair activities of daily living and quality of life [11].

In a comprehensive compilation and analysis of the literature and data gathered from multiple TEN-focused studies, Table 2 reviews 39 reported cases for TEN patients who are less than 18 years. From these 39 patients, 29 patients were treated in a burn unit and had a mortality rate of 10.3%, whereas the 17 patients that were treated with IVIG had a mortality rate of 5.8%. Based on the literature, the application of both approaches in this age group may cause improvement in mortality. Unfortunately, limited data due to the rarity of the disease prevent us from proving this result (Table 2).

In addition to stopping culpirt trigger(lamotrigine in our case), the main principles of supportive care are the same as major burns and include wound care, fluid and electrolyte management, nutritional support, temperature management, pain control, and monitoring and treating superinfections [19, 20]. Several studies indicate a better prognosis for patients transferred promptly to a burn care unit or intensive care unit. In a retrospective multicenter review of 199 TEN patients treated at burn care centers, the overall mortality was 32% as compared with 51% among patients initially cared for in other settings but were then transferred to a burn center more than one week after disease onset [21].

According to the literature, a high dose of IVIG (2 gm\kg) improved the efficacy of patient recovery as opposed to the patients who did not receive it [8, 9]. Furthermore, a recent meta-analysis of IVIG use in SJS\TEN showed decreased mortality amongst pediatric patients [9]. Studies supporting the rapid recovery after administration of IVIG suggest that the pathophysiology of TEN is related to the abnormal interaction between the cell-surface death receptor Fas and its respective ligand (FasL), which leads to keratinocyte apoptosis and detachment. IVIG has immunomodulatory properties by causing FcR blockade as well as providing anti-idiotypic antibodies to auto-antibodies. Despite there not being a standard management protocol in SJS\TEN, IVIG is still considered a key treatment based on the supporting evidence of many studies that report beneficial outcomes and reduced mortality of using IVIG in SJS\TEN patients [17, 22–25].

Furthermore, corticosteroid was used in the reported patient even though the benefit is controversial. Some studies

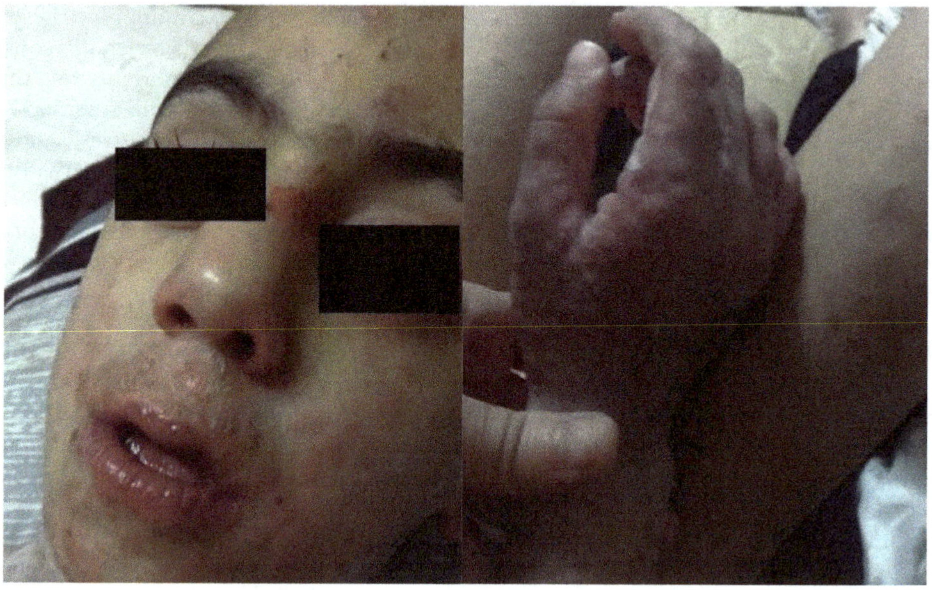

Figure 1: The vesicular lesion involves the hand and mouth of the patient.

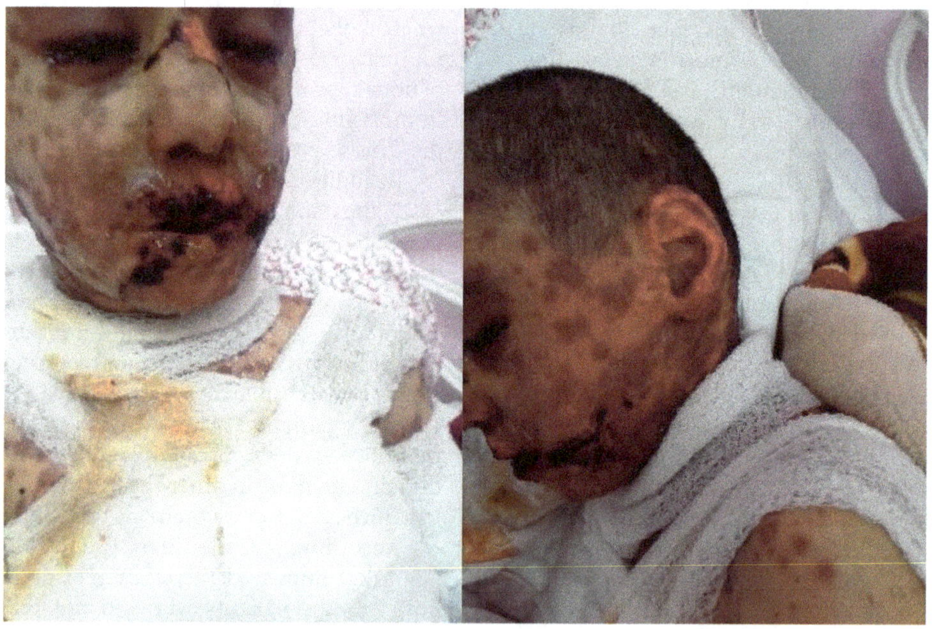

Figure 2: Lesions involving the whole head and face including eyes.

Table 1: SCORTEN score 3.

Prognostic factor	Value in index case	Score
Age	5	0
Malignancy	No	0
Heart rate	125	1
BUN	14	0
BSA	50%	1
HCO_3	18	1
Blood glucose	88	0

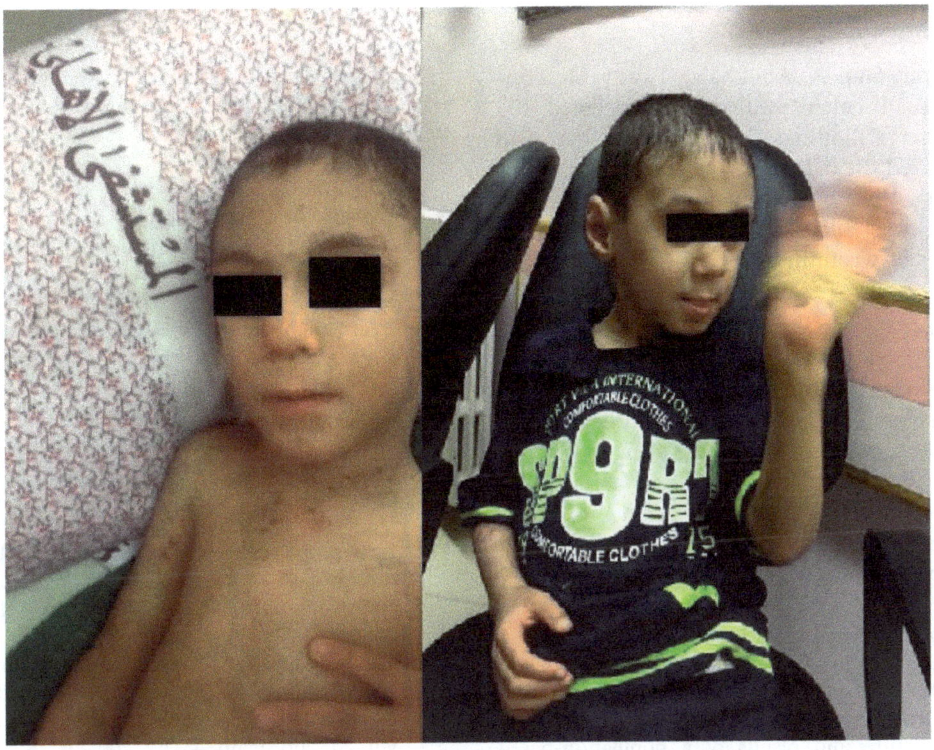

Figure 3: Lesion resolves completely after treatment.

Table 2: Literature review of 39 cases of TEN (treatment approaches and mortality rate).

Study	Number of patients	TEN : SJS	M : F	IVIG (n)	IVCS (n)	Another drug modality	TBSA% (mean ± SD)	BU/ ICU (n)	Mortality (n)
Adzick et al. [12]	4	4 : 0	2 : 2	0	0	—	86.25 ± 10.23	4	1
Inamo et al. [13]	3	2 : 1	3 : 0	0	0	Ulinastatin	N/A	0	0
Zahra and Soror [14]	1	1 : 0	0 : 1	1	0	—	90%	1	0
Moudgil et al. [15]	2	0 : 2	1 : 1	2	0	—	N/A	0	0
Prais et al. [16]	4	N/A	0 : 4	4	4	—	N/A	0	0
Spies et al. [11]	15	15 : 0	9 : 6	0	0	—	76 ± 5	15	1
Stella et al. [17]	9	9 : 0	4 : 5	9	9	LMWH	61	9	1
Straussberg et al. [18]	1	0 : 1	0 : 1	1	1	—	N/A	0	0

TEN: toxic epidermal necrolysis, SJS: Stevens–Johnson syndrome, IVIG: intravenous immunoglobulin, IVCS: intravenous corticosteroid, TBSA: total body surface area affected, BU: burn unit, ICU: intensive care unit, LMWH: low molecular weight heparin, and N/A: not available.

report an increase in the risk of infection and a higher mortality rate with steroid administration [10, 26]. However, other studies advocate using short-term yet high-dose corticosteroids for drug hypersensitivity reactions [19]. In addition, two retrospective studies suggested that using steroids at an early stage of the disease might be beneficial in decreasing the mortality rate without affecting healing time [23, 24].

4. Conclusion

Treatment of TEN is still a challenge due to rarity of disease and limited number of studies about the best treatment approach, and we suggest a new approach in patients less than 18 years which includes IVIG and burn care as mentioned in the case presentation to be considered in the future case-control study because it shows decrease in mortality by reviewing the literature of the previous case report and series which use the same approaches in this age group.

Consent

The patient and family consent was obtained by the patient himself and patient's family.

Authors' Contributions

Tareq Z. Alzughayyar, Sadi A. Abukhalaf, Fawzy M. Abuniejma, and Mohanad Saleh studied and designed the concept, Jihad Samer Zalloum, Ali A. Abumunshar, and Rami A. Misk collected the data, and Tareq Z. Alzughayyar, Yousef I. M. Zatari, Wasim Noureddin Ibrahim Hamad, Eman A. S. Abuqweide, Bilal Nabeel Mohammad Alqam, and Sadi A. Abukhalaf wrote the paper.

Acknowledgments

Special thanks to Sherin Johnson, a Biology (Bachelors of Science) and Journalism (Bachelors of Arts) student at the University of Houston, for her awesome editing.

References

[1] F. A. Pereira, A. V. Mudgil, and D. M. Rosmarin, "Toxic epidermal necrolysis," *Journal of the American Academy of Dermatology*, vol. 56, no. 2, pp. 181–200, 2007.

[2] B. Rzany, M. Mockenhaupt, S. Baur et al., "Epidemiology of erythema exsudativum multiforme majus, Stevens-Johnson syndrome, and toxic epidermal necrolysis in Germany (1990–1992): structure and results of a population-based registry," *Journal of Clinical Epidemiology*, vol. 49, no. 7, pp. 769–773, 1996.

[3] P. Saiag, E. Caumes, O. Chosidow, J. Revuz, and J.-C. Roujeau, "Drug-induced toxic epidermal necrolysis (Lyell syndrome) in patients infected with the human immunodeficiency virus," *Journal of the American Academy of Dermatology*, vol. 26, no. 4, pp. 567–574, 1992.

[4] C.-Y. Wei, T.-M. Ko, C.-Y. Shen, and Y.-T. Chen, "A recent update of pharmacogenomics in drug-induced severe skin reactions," *Drug Metabolism and Pharmacokinetics*, vol. 27, no. 1, pp. 132–141, 2012.

[5] R. A. Schwartz, P. H. McDonough, and B. W. Lee, "Toxic epidermal necrolysis: part I: introduction, history, classification, clinical features, systemic manifestations, etiology, and immunopathogenesis," *Journal of the American Academy of Dermatology*, vol. 69, no. 2, pp. 173.e1–173.e13, 2013.

[6] P. D. Mahar, J. Wasiak, B. Hii et al., "A systematic review of the management and outcome of toxic epidermal necrolysis treated in burns centres," *Burns*, vol. 40, no. 7, pp. 1245–1254, 2014.

[7] E. Letko, D. N. Papaliodis, G. N. Papaliodis, Y. J. Daoud, A. R. Ahmed, and C. S. Foster, "Stevens-Johnson syndrome and toxic epidermal necrolysis: a review of the literature," *Annals of Allergy, Asthma & Immunology*, vol. 94, no. 4, pp. 419–436, 2005.

[8] D. R. Yarbrough, "Experience with toxic epidermal necrolysis treated in a burn center," *Journal of Burn Care & Rehabilitation*, vol. 17, no. 1, pp. 30–33, 1996.

[9] T. McGee and A. Munster, "Toxic epidermal necrolysis syndrome: mortality rate reduced with early referral to regional burn center," *Plastic and Reconstructive Surgery*, vol. 102, no. 4, pp. 1018–1022, 1998.

[10] S. L. Engelhardt, M. J. Schurr, and R. B. Helgerson, "Toxic epidermal necrolysis," *Journal of Burn Care & Rehabilitation*, vol. 18, no. 6, pp. 520–524, 1997.

[11] M. Spies, A. P. Sanford, J. F. A. Low, S. E. Wolf, and D. N. Herndon, "Treatment of extensive toxic epidermal necrolysis in children," *Pediatrics*, vol. 108, no. 5, pp. 1162–1168, 2001.

[12] N. S. Adzick, S. H. Kim, C. C. Bondoc et al., "Management of toxic epidermal necrolysis in a pediatric burn center," *Archives of Pediatrics & Adolescent Medicine*, vol. 139, no. 5, pp. 499–502, 1985.

[13] Y. Inamo, T. Okubo, M. Wada et al., "Intravenous ulinastatin therapy for Stevens-Johnson syndrome and toxic epidermal necrolysis in pediatric patients," *International Archives of Allergy and Immunology*, vol. 127, no. 1, pp. 89–94, 2002.

[14] S. S. Zahra and I. Soror, "Intravenous immunoglobulin in the treatment of lamotrigine-induced toxic epidermal necrolysis," *Iranian Journal of Allergy, Asthma and Immunology*, vol. 7, no. 4, pp. 239–241, 2008.

[15] A. Moudgil, S. Porat, P. Brunnel, and S. C. Jordan, "Treatment of Stevens-Johnson syndrome with pooled human intravenous immune globulin," *Clinical Pediatrics*, vol. 34, no. 1, pp. 48–51, 1995.

[16] D. Prais, R. Straussberg, J. Amir, M. Nussinovitch, and L. Harel, "Treatment of anticonvulsant hypersensitivity syndrome with intravenous immunoglobulins and corticosteroids," *Journal of Child Neurology*, vol. 21, no. 5, pp. 380–384, 2006.

[17] M. Stella, P. Cassano, D. Bollero, A. Clemente, and G. Giorio, "Toxic epidermal necrolysis treated with intravenous high-dose immunoglobulins: our experience," *Dermatology*, vol. 203, no. 1, pp. 45–49, 2001.

[18] R. Straussberg, L. Harel, D. Ben-Amitai, D. Cohen, and J. Amir, "Carbamazepine-induced Stevens-Johnson syndrome treated with IV steroids and IVIG," *Pediatric Neurology*, vol. 22, no. 3, pp. 231–233, 2000.

[19] J.-C. Roujeau, O. Chosidow, P. Saiag, and J.-C. Guillaume, "Toxic epidermal necrolysis (Lyell syndrome)," *Journal of the American Academy of Dermatology*, vol. 23, no. 6, pp. 1039–1058, 1990.

[20] R. A. Schwartz, P. H. McDonough, and B. W. Lee, "Toxic epidermal necrolysis: part II: prognosis, sequelae, diagnosis, differential diagnosis, prevention, and treatment," *Journal of the American Academy of Dermatology*, vol. 69, no. 2, pp. 187–e1, 2013.

[21] T. L. Palmieri, D. G. Greenhalgh, J. R. Saffle et al., "A multicenter review of toxic epidermal necrolysis treated in U.S. burn centers at the end of the twentieth century," *Journal of Burn Care & Rehabilitation*, vol. 23, no. 2, pp. 87–96, 2002.

[22] S. Walsh and D. Creamer, "IVIg in TEN: time to re-evaluate the efficacy of intravenous immunoglobulin in the management of toxic epidermal necrolysis," *British Journal of Dermatology*, vol. 167, no. 2, pp. 230-231, 2012.

[23] Y.-C. Huang, Y.-C. Li, and T.-J. Chen, "The efficacy of intravenous immunoglobulin for the treatment of toxic epidermal necrolysis: a systematic review and meta-analysis," *British Journal of Dermatology*, vol. 167, no. 2, pp. 424–432, 2012.

[24] C. Prins, F. A. Kerdel, R. S. Padilla et al., "Treatment of toxic epidermal necrolysis with high-dose intravenous immunoglobulins," *Archives of Dermatology*, vol. 139, no. 1, pp. 26–32, 2003.

[25] P. Tristani-Firouzi, M. J. Petersena, J. R. Saffle, S. E. Morris, and J. J. Zone, "Treatment of toxic epidermal necrolysis with intravenous immunoglobulin in children," *Journal of the American Academy of Dermatology*, vol. 47, no. 4, pp. 548–552, 2002.

[26] H. Saeed, I. S. Mantagos, and J. Chodosh, "Complications of Stevens-Johnson syndrome beyond the eye and skin," *Burns*, vol. 42, no. 1, pp. 20–27, 2016.

49

Kaposi Varicelliform Eruption in a Patient with Pemphigus Vulgaris: A Case Report and Review of the Literature

Bibisha Baaniya and Sudha Agrawal

Department of Dermatology and Venerology, B.P. Koirala Institute of Health Sciences, Dharan, Nepal

Correspondence should be addressed to Bibisha Baaniya; cul.bibisha@gmail.com

Academic Editor: Jacek Cezary Szepietowski

Haemorrhagic crusted lesions over pre-existing pemphigus vulgaris erosions should arouse suspicion of Kaposi varicelliform eruption (KVE). Immediate treatment with antivirals helps to prevent mortality and morbidities. Here, we report a case of a 67-year-old male who developed haemorrhagic crusted lesions on pre-existing pemphigus lesions during his hospital stay and obtained almost 90% resolution of cutaneous lesions of Pemphigus vulgaris as well as Kaposi varicelliform eruption within 2 weeks of acyclovir treatment along with the continuation of systemic steroids. We also highlight the review of the literature of other reported cases with its management.

1. Introduction

Pemphigus vulgaris (PV) is an autoimmune intraepidermal blistering disorder of the skin and mucous membrane caused due to damage to intercellular adhesion structures, i.e., desmogleins resulting in acantholysis [1]. Kaposi varicelliform eruption (KVE) is a rare and potentially fatal viral infection typically due to herpes simplex virus (HSV) 1 or 2, rarely by coxsackie A16 virus and vaccinia virus over a pre-existing dermatosis [2]. This phenomenon has been well studied in atopic dermatitis; hence, alternatively, KVE is also called eczema herpeticum. However, it is only rarely known to occur in patients with pemphigus vulgaris [3].

The mechanisms underlying the pathogenesis of KVE remain incompletely understood. It is assumed that the defective skin barrier, acting in conjunction with immune deficiencies (both cell-mediated and humoral immunity), is implicated [4]. Furthermore, treatment of these patients with systemic immunosuppressants also compromises the integrity of the immune system [3].

Antiviral therapy with acyclovir is the treatment of choice, which is usually combined with a systemic antibiotic to control heavy bacterial colonization [5]. Before the advent of acyclovir therapy, the mortality in cases of KVE was as high as 50%; now with specific acyclovir treatment, it is around 10% [6]. Here, a case of pemphigus vulgaris with KVE is being presented along with the review of the literature of other reported cases with its management.

2. Patient Information

A 67-year-old male had presented to Dermatology OPD of our hospital 8 months back with a history of oral erosions for 2 months and cutaneous erosions for 1 month and was diagnosed as pemphigus vulgaris (Figure 1). The patient was advised to take an oral steroid 60 mg daily along with other supportive treatments. In spite of proper counselling of the prognosis and long-term follow-up of pemphigus, he was taking prednisolone on and off and was unable to come for the follow-up because of the COVID-19 pandemic.

2.1. Investigations and Treatment. The patient presented again 5 weeks before the admission with multiple erosions that extended to the anterior chest and was advised to continue prednisolone 50 mg once daily, azathioprine (100 mg once daily), doxycycline (100 mg once daily), and nicotinamide (500 mg daily) for 5 weeks.

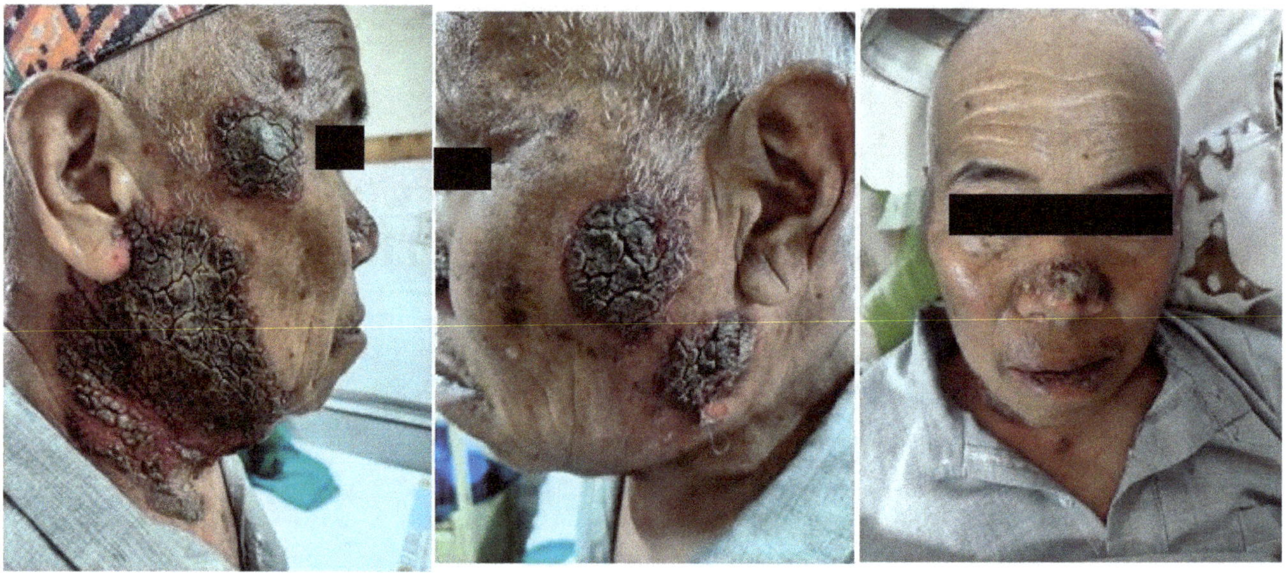

Figure 1: 8 months prior to admission: hyperkeratotic plaque and erosions.

However, he failed to show satisfactory improvement (Figure 2), and his swab for bacterial culture and sensitivity revealed *Pseudomonas aeruginosa* sensitive to piperacillin; hence, he was admitted to the dermatology ward and started on the same antibiotic and intravenous, dexamethasone 8 mg once daily along with skin care. After receiving these medications for 2 weeks, once the pseudomonas infection resolved, dose of dexamethasone was increased to 16 mg over the next 2 weeks, and the patient got significant improvement. However, 1 week after initiating steroid dose escalation, the patient developed few monomorphic haemorrhagic crusts on the cheeks overlying the pre-existing lesions (Figure 3), which progressed over the next week to involve bilateral cheeks, malar region, and bridge of the nose with few lesions in the forehead, bilateral ears, and chest. These lesions were associated with extensive cutaneous pain and myalgia (Figure 4).

Although he denied past history of herpes infection, his HSV-1 IgM and IgG also came out to be positive and hence was diagnosed as KVE. Then, he was immediately started on oral acyclovir 400 mg thrice daily, and dexamethasone was tapered rapidly to 9 mg from 16 mg once daily over a week (Figure 5). Further ophthalmological consultation was done, and herpes keratitis was ruled out. Within 1 week of the treatment, the crusts decreased significantly, and treatment was continued. The erosions also healed rapidly thereafter.

His comorbidities were type 2 diabetes mellitus, grade 2 benign prostatic enlargement, right nephrolithiasis, and osteopenia.

2.2. Outcome and Follow-Up. Once there was 90% resolution in the haemorrhagic crust, the patient was discharged on 60 mg prednisolone and oral acyclovir 400 mg thrice daily (Figure 6). Oral acyclovir was continued with the same dose for a total of 4 weeks until almost 100% improvement was achieved (Figure 7). After that, monthly tapering of the dose of oral prednisolone was done, and the patient was instructed to follow up via teledermatology consultation during the COVID-19 pandemic as he came from remote hilly area.

3. Discussion

Austrian dermatologist Moriz Kaposi first described KVE or eczema herpeticum. Some authors, however, define these two terms differently: eczema herpeticum as disseminated HSV infection over pre-existing eczematous skin disease and KVE as any disseminated cutaneous infection with HSV type 1 or 2 [5].

After an incubation period of about 3–10 days, KVE presents with disseminated eruption of closely grouped, painful, monomorphic, umbilicated vesicles, accompanied by fever, malaise, and regional lymphadenopathy. The vesicles tend to evolve rapidly to pustules or dry out, forming crusts over eroded areas during the course of the disease. The eruption is frequently located on the head, neck, and the upper part of the trunk and usually heals within 2 to 6 weeks [2]. In our case, one week prior to developing haemorrhagic crusts over pre-existing erosions, another patient residing next to our patient had developed herpes labialis and was started on oral acyclovir 400 mg thrice daily. On inquiring, our patient denied any previous herpes infection; hence, we concluded it to be the primary infection he had acquired from the nearby patient. We could not keep our patient in isolation due to logistic constraints secondary to ongoing COVID-19 pandemic.

Recurrent episodes of KVE may occur [7]. Secondary bacterial infection, viremia, and multiorgan involvement are the important causes for mortality; and hence, KVE is a dermatological emergency. Ocular complications such as keratitis, conjunctivitis, blepharitis, uveitis, and loss of vision can also occur [2]. In our patient, herpes keratitis was ruled out after ophthalmological consultation. Here, we list the case series and reports of KVE with pemphigus vulgaris (Table 1).

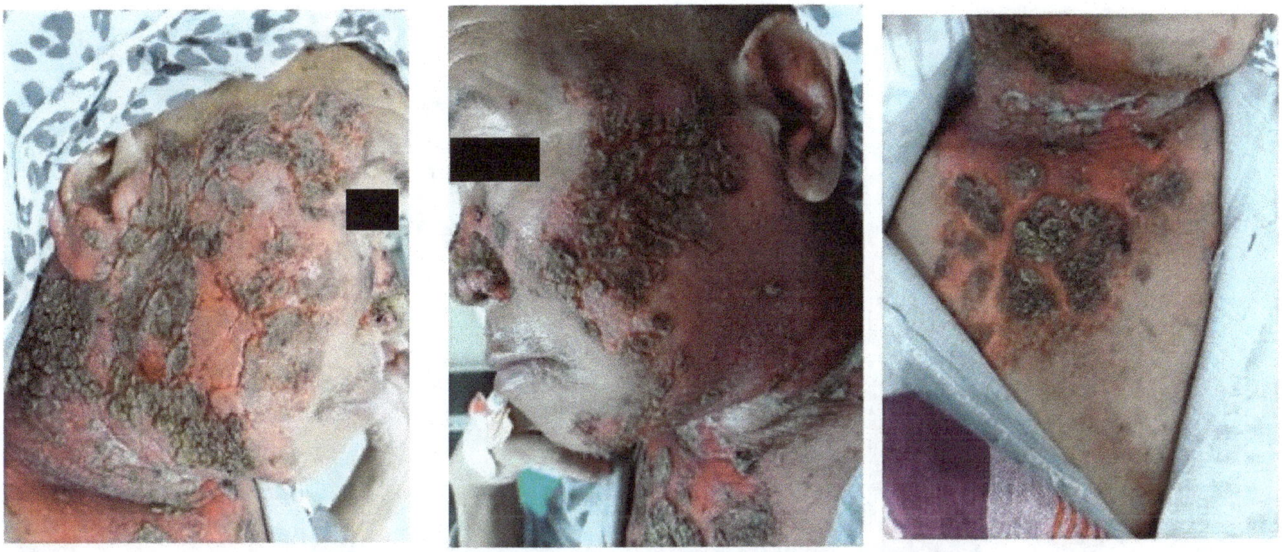

FIGURE 2: Day 1 of admission: extension of erosions despite high-dose oral steroids.

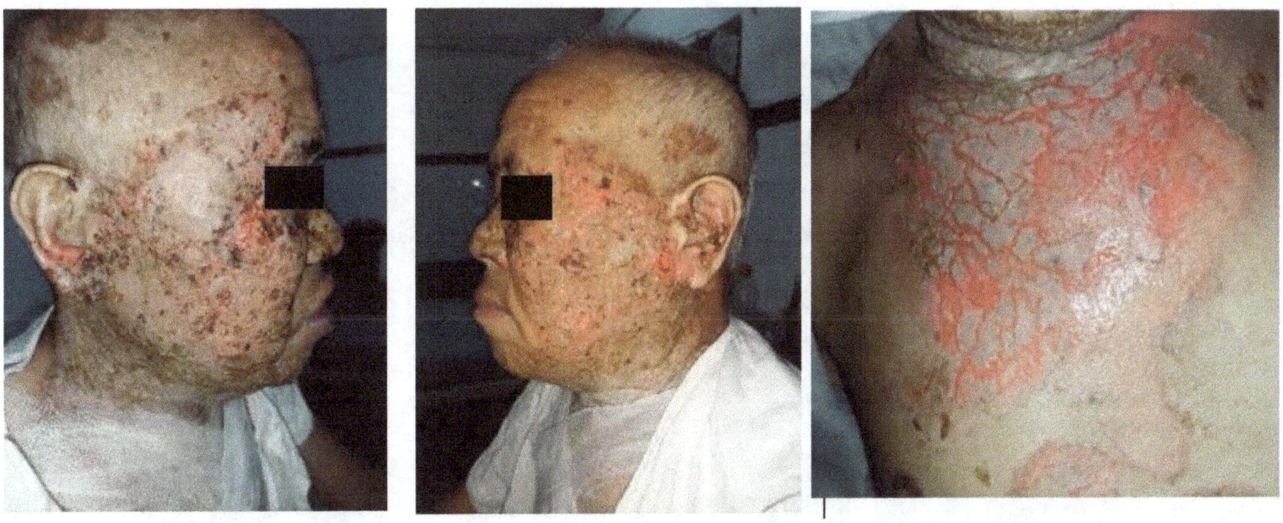

FIGURE 3: Day 20 of admission: improvement of erosions but appearance of haemorrhagic crusts.

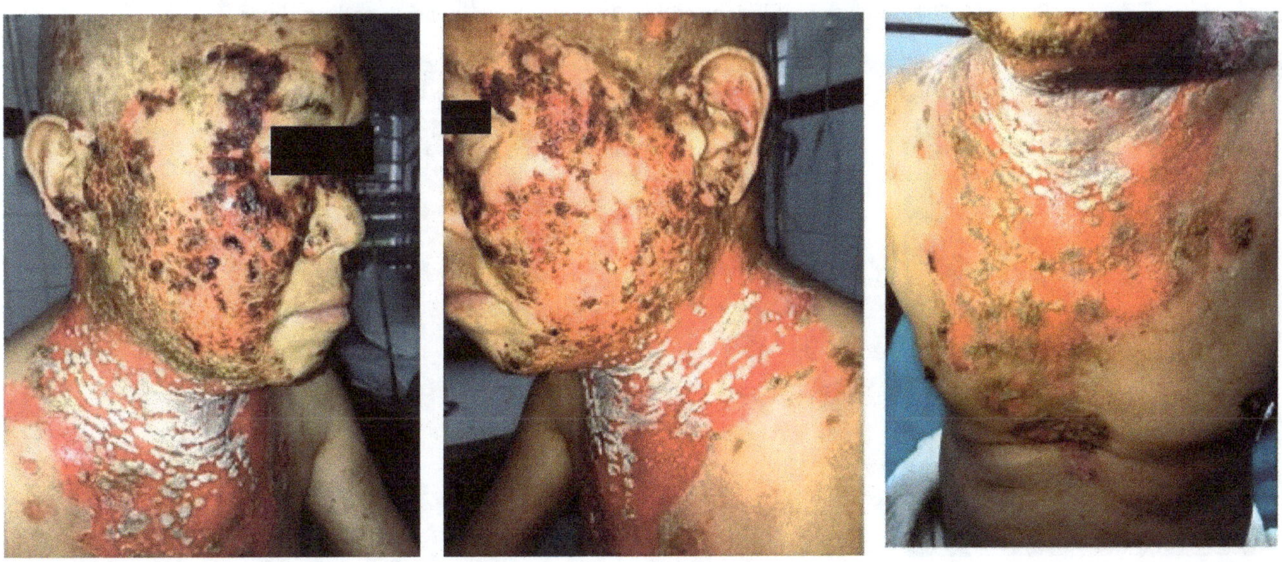

FIGURE 4: Day 23 of admission: extensive haemorrhagic crusts in the face and few in the periphery of erosions in the chest.

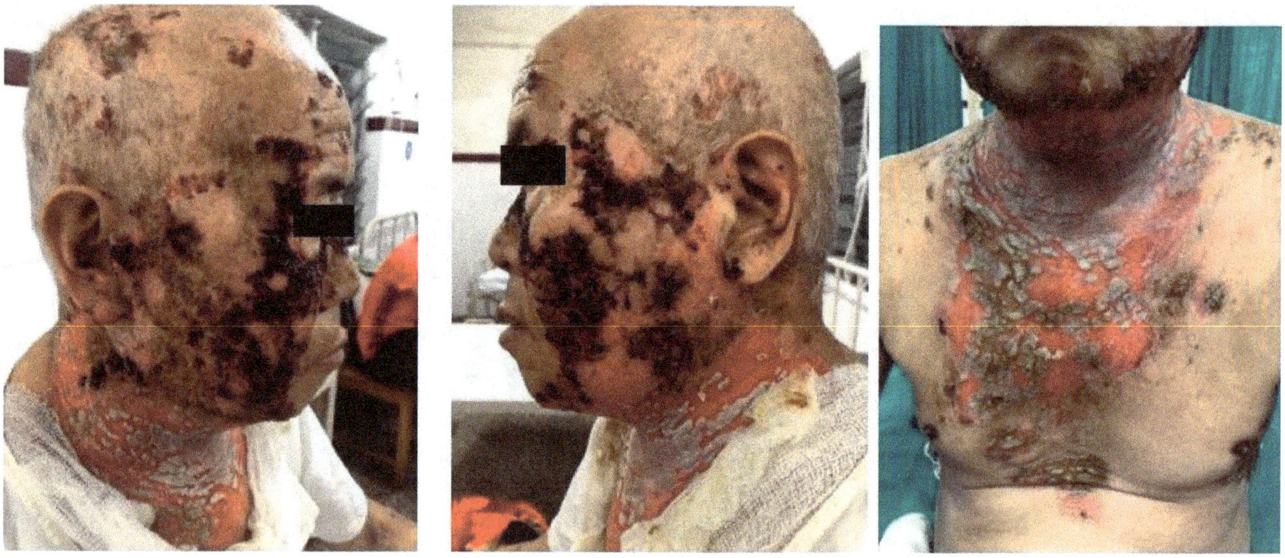

Figure 5: Day 27 of admission: further extension of haemorrhagic crusts.

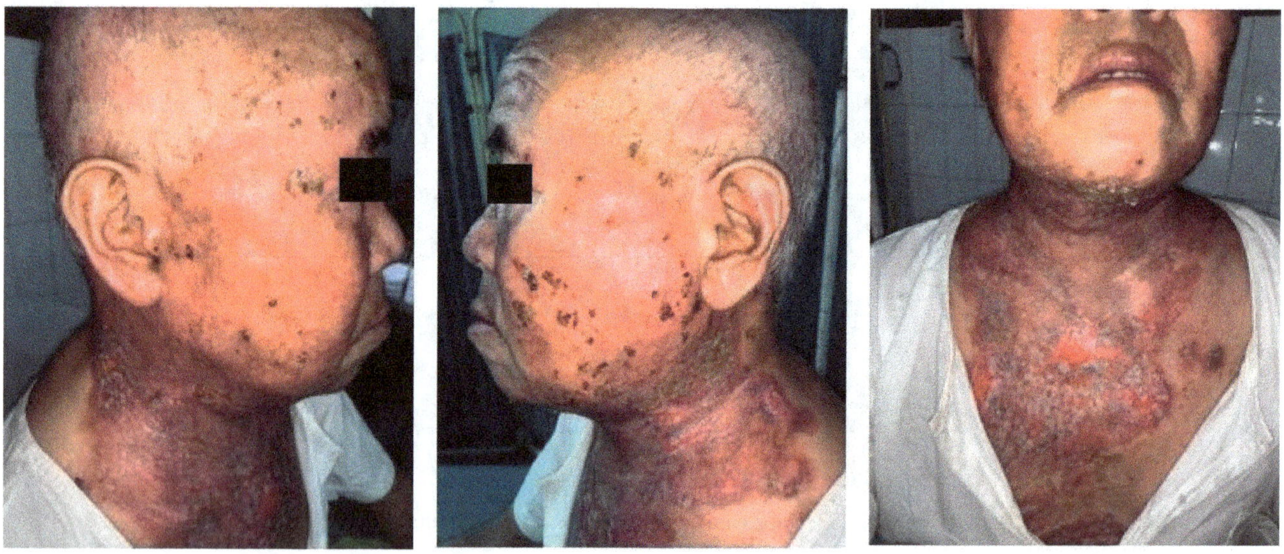

Figure 6: 90% resolution of lesions within 2 weeks of commencing oral acyclovir.

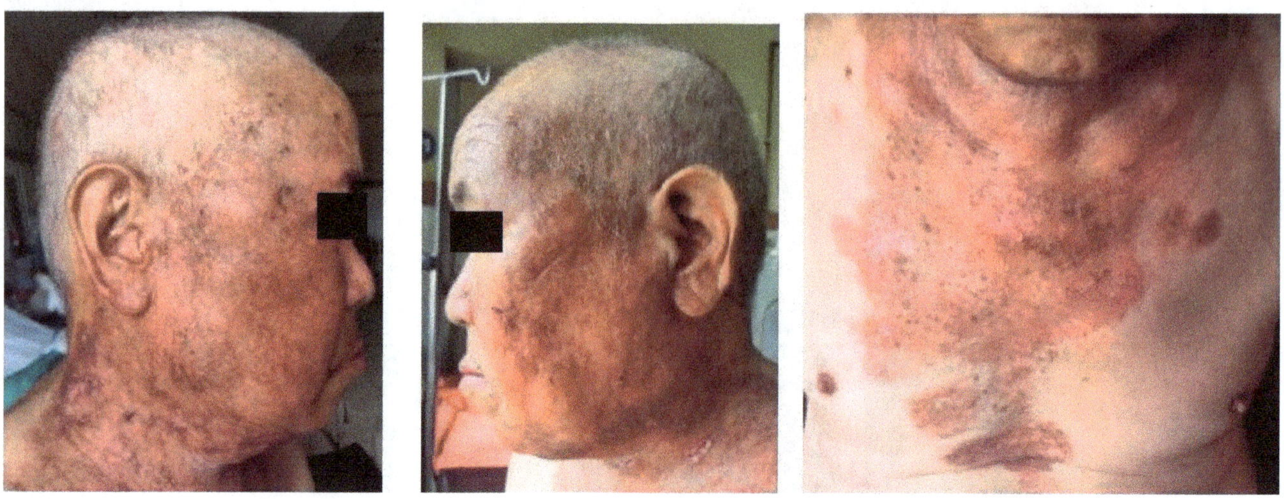

Figure 7: Almost 100% improvement within 4 weeks of commencing antiviral treatment.

Table 1: Case series and reports of KVE with pemphigus vulgaris.

SN	Author/year	Age (years)/sex	Morphology of pemphigus vulgaris	Morphology of KVE	Investigations	Treatment of KVE	Treatment of pemphigus vulgaris	Outcome of KVE
1	Lehman and el-Azhary [3]	44.1/male	Focal lesions with oral involvement	Not mentioned	Polymerase chain reaction (PCR), skin swabs, viral culture, direct immunofluorescence	Ganciclovir (PO) (dose and duration not mentioned)	Mycophenolate mofetil, prednisone (modification not mentioned)	Resolved (time to resolution not mentioned)
		51.6/female	Widespread lesions with oral involvement	Not mentioned	PCR, skin swabs, viral culture, direct immunofluorescence	Acyclovir (IV) (dose and duration not mentioned)	Intramuscular corticosteroids (modification not mentioned)	Resolved (time to resolution not mentioned)
		70.2/female	Focal lesions with oral, conjunctival, perianal involvement	Not mentioned	PCR, skin swabs, viral culture, direct immunofluorescence	Valacyclovir hydrochloride 1 gm PO BD ×10 days	Azathioprine, prednisone (modification not mentioned)	Resolved (time to resolution not mentioned)
		39.3/female	Focal lesions with oral involvement	Not mentioned	PCR, skin swabs, viral culture, direct immunofluorescence	Acyclovir (IV) (dose and duration not mentioned)	Mycophenolate mofetil, azathioprine, prednisone (modification not mentioned)	Resolved (time to resolution not mentioned)
		45.9/female	Oral erosions only	Not mentioned	PCR, skin swabs, viral culture, direct immunofluorescence	Valacyclovir hydrochloride 1 gm PO BD × 10 days	None	Resolved (time to resolution not mentioned)
		85.7/female	Focal lesions with oral involvement	Not mentioned		Acyclovir (IV) (dose and duration not mentioned)	Rituximab (modification not mentioned)	Resolved (time to resolution not mentioned)
2	Nath et al. [8]	40/female	Not mentioned	Lesions in the face, neck, trunk, upper limbs, and thighs	Tzanck smear positive	Acyclovir 400 mg PO TDS × 5 days	DCP (phase 1, 1st cycle) (modification not mentioned)	KVE not healed and PV worsened, the patient left the hospital in critical condition
		27/female	Not mentioned	Lesions in breasts	Tzanck smear positive	Acyclovir 400 mg PO TDS × 10 days	Dexamethasone cyclophosphamide pulse (DCP) (phase 1, 3rd cycle), prednisolone, cyclophosphamide (modification not mentioned)	KVE resolved, PV unaltered (time to resolution not mentioned)
		26/female	Not mentioned	Lesions in the trunk, upper limbs, and thighs	Tzanck smear positive	Acyclovir 500 mg IV TDS × 18 days	Dexamethasone azathioprine pulse (DAP) (phase 1, 1st cycle), prednisolone, azathioprine (modification not mentioned)	KVE partially healed, the patient left the hospital
		40/female	Not mentioned	Lesions in the trunk	Tzanck smear positive	Acyclovir 400 mg PO TDS × 13 days	DCP (phase 1, 3rd cycle), prednisolone, cyclophosphamide (modification not mentioned)	KVE resolved, PV unaltered (time to resolution not mentioned)

Table 1: Continued.

SN	Author/year	Age (years)/sex	Morphology of pemphigus vulgaris	Morphology of KVE	Investigations	Treatment of KVE	Treatment of pemphigus vulgaris	Outcome of KVE
3	Rao et al. [9]	30/male	Not mentioned	Umbilicated grouped vesicular eruption around the eyes, mouth, and axilla	Tzanck smear positive, IgM positive	Acyclovir 800 mg PO 5 times a day × 14 days	DCP (modification not mentioned)	Resolved (time to resolution not mentioned)
		45/female	Not mentioned	Umbilicated grouped vesicular eruption around the eyes, mouth, and axilla	Tzanck smear positive, IgM positive	Acyclovir 800 mg PO 5 times a day × 14 days	DCP (modification not mentioned)	Succumbed to multiorgan failure
4	Vora et al. [7]	26/male	Old crusted lesions of PV over the scalp with patchy hair loss	Umbilicated vesicular lesions over the face, chest, back, and limbs	Tzanck smear positive, histopathology suggestive of KVE	Acyclovir 10 mg/kg IV every 8 hours × 10 days	Prednisolone 10 mg, azathioprine 50 mg BD (no modification)	Healed with varicelliform scars (time to resolution not mentioned)
5	Marfatia et al. [10]	30/male	Erosions in the oral cavity, genitals, and trunk	Not mentioned	HIV positive, chest X-ray suggestive of pulmonary TB	Acyclovir (PO) (dose and duration not mentioned)	Dexamethasone IM TDS, treatment of tuberculosis and HIV (modification not mentioned)	KVE resolved (time to resolution not mentioned)
6	Corral et al. [1]	33/male	Not mentioned	Painful bullous lesions on the scalp, oral cavity, and trunk	Not mentioned	Acyclovir (IV) (dose and duration not mentioned)	Intravenous immunoglobulin, followed by a second pulse therapy with methylprednisolone, mycophenolate mofetil was held	KVE resolved (time to resolution not mentioned)
7	Feldmeyer et al. [11]	71/male	Not mentioned	Refractory vegetating skin lesions, especially of the centrofacial area	Nasal smear was positive for HSV2 by direct immunostaining, culture negative	Valacyclovir 500 mg PO BD × 10 days	Prednisone, and cyclosporine, intravenous immunoglobulin (modification not mentioned)	KVE resolved in 10 days and PV also remitted
8	Chiu et al. [12]	66/female	Not mentioned	Generalized painful lesions over the lower trunk, buttocks, bilateral popliteal, and inguinal areas	Histopathology and immunohistochemistry for herpes virus were positive; HSV IgG increased	Famciclovir 750 mg PO OD × 10 days	Discontinued the systemic steroid	KVE showed remarkable improvement in 10 days
9	Mackley et al. [13]	72/female	Not mentioned	Innumerable deep, punched-out erosions scattered over the existing geographic erosions	Tzanck smear positive, direct fluorescent antibody test positive for HSV-1	Acyclovir 15 mg/kg IV OD (duration not mentioned); discharged on chronic prophylactic acyclovir	Prednisone, mycophenolate mofetil, and cyclosporine (modification not mentioned)	Significant improvement (time to resolution not mentioned)
10	Ortiz [14]	66/male	Not mentioned	Lesions in the chin, cheeks, and neck	Tzanck negative, biopsy suggestive of KVE	Not mentioned	Prednisone, gold salts (modification not mentioned)	Not mentioned
11	Our case (2020)	67/male	Erosions in the face, neck, chest, and oral cavity	Haemorrhagic crusts in the face, neck, and chest over pre-existing erosions	HSV-1 IGM and IgG positive	Acyclovir 400 mg PO TDS × 4 weeks	Dexamethasone decreased from 16 mg to 9 mg, azathioprine continued	Almost 100% resolution in both KVE and PV within 4 weeks

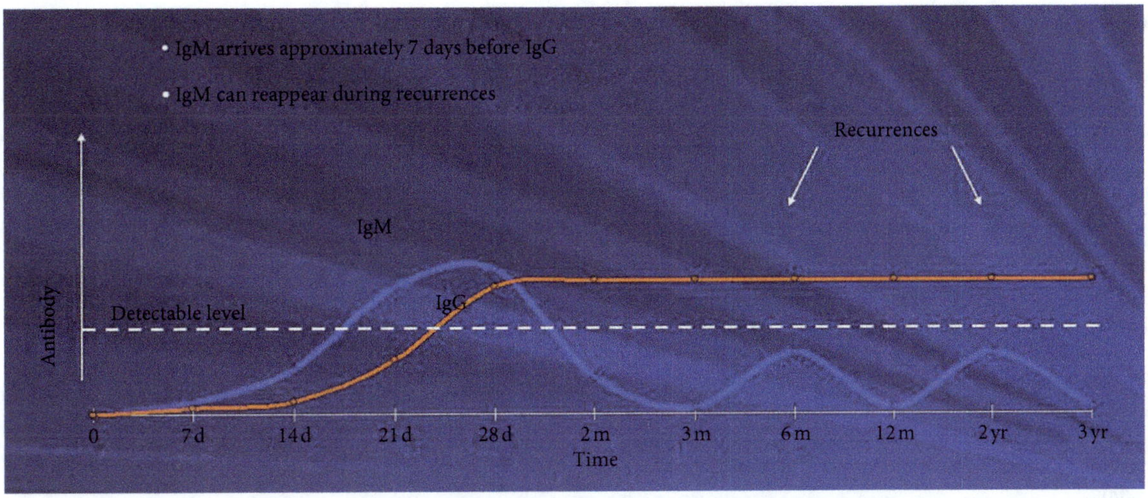

Figure 8: Graph of IgM and IgG response in HSV infection [15].

Kaposi's varicelliform eruption is diagnosed clinically, and investigations such as Tzanck smear and HSV serology are only supportive [2, 3]. Viral culture, direct fluorescence antibody staining, and polymerase chain reaction are the most reliable techniques for herpes simplex virus detection. Histological findings such as intraepidermal blister, acantholysis, ballooning degeneration of the keratinocytes, and multinuclear giant cells with intranuclear inclusion help in diagnosis of HSV infection [7]. In our patient, HSV-1 IgG and IgM both were positive which further supported diagnosis, but other investigations were not done due to logistic constraints.

A positive serology indicates present or past infection; IgM antibody testing cannot discriminate primary versus recurrent episodes of HSV infection, and a positive HSV IgG antibody serology cannot be used for diagnosis of an active infection (Figure 8). If both HSV IgM and IgG are positive, then it implies that infection date is indeterminate [15]. Thus, HSV serology only contributes as a supportive diagnostic tool [2]. In our patient, HSV-1 IgG and IgM both were positive on the 3rd week of exposure with the nearby patient which further supported the fact that he had primary infection.

Treatment of KVE must be initiated with antivirals as soon as possible since it is a potentially life-threatening disease. No formal guidelines for antiviral treatment are established for treatment of KVE in immunobullous diseases, and different authors have followed different guidelines (Table 1). In a study by Lehman and el-Azhary, they used valacyclovir 1 g PO BD for 10 days or acyclovir 400 mg PO TDS for 10 days or ganciclovir during the first episode. In recurrent episodes, they initiated valacyclovir 1 g PO OD or acyclovir 400 mg PO BD as chronic suppressive therapy [3]. Zouhair et al. continued oral acyclovir until complete lesion resolution in herpetic superinfection of the pemphigus patient, and they observed relief in 5 to 20 days [16]. Similarly, our case achieved almost 100% resolution of lesions with 4-week acyclovir therapy. On the contrary, Rao et al. treated their patients with oral acyclovir 800 mg 5 times a day for 10 to 14 days [9]. The prodrug valacyclovir is converted into acyclovir during 1st-pass metabolism in the liver but has a better oral bioavailability than acyclovir [17].

Lehman and el-Azhary also considered reducing the dose of systemic immunosuppressants and claimed that patients with severe skin disease or with additional complications from the viral infection may require intravenous antiviral therapy [3]. In our patient, we continued oral acyclovir 400 mg thrice daily until complete resolution, i.e., 4 weeks, and dose of the systemic steroid was also decreased with significant improvement in patient's symptoms.

Although we have tried our best to manage our patient, lack of PCR and immunological tests such as direct immunofluorescence, indirect immunofluorescence, and ELISA due to logistic constraints are the major limitations.

3.1. Patient's Perspective. When I developed oral and skin erosions, I immediately consulted the doctors and was prescribed some oral and topical medications. However, they failed to improve the lesions which really made me frustrated. Nevertheless, I always had trust in my doctor, and as per their suggestion, I got admitted to ward. After that, my lesions healed significantly, and now, I am happy that almost all of my erosions are gone.

4. Conclusion

The diagnosis of Kaposi varicelliform eruption is usually made clinically. Appearance of umbilicated vesicular rash is the usual presentation, but haemorrhagic crusts over preexisting lesions are an uncommon presentation as in our case. Investigations such as PCR, viral culture, histopathology, HSV serology, and Tzanck smear have only supportive value. It is also important to diagnose it in time and start antiviral treatment immediately as it is associated with significant morbidity and mortality. Acyclovir 400 mg PO TDS or 10 mg/kg IV or valacyclovir 500 mg PO BD until resolution of KVE is usually recommended. Similarly, the dose of corticosteroids can be decreased or stopped depending on the clinical status of pemphigus vulgaris and other immunosuppressants such as mycophenolate mofetil can be deferred until resolution of KVE.

Consent

Written informed consent for patient information and images to be published were obtained.

References

[1] I. S. Corral, T. H. P. D. Freitas, R. T. R. D. Aquino, D. A. S. Koller, M. E. R. Magliari, and H. Muller, "Severe multi-resistant pemphigus vulgaris: prolonged remission with a single cycle of rituximab," *Anais Brasileiros de Dermatologia*, vol. 88, no. 4, pp. 639–642, 2013.

[2] I. Kucukyilmaz, E. Alpsoy, and S. Yazar, "Kaposi's varicelliform eruption in association with rosacea," *Journal of the American Academy of Dermatology*, vol. 51, no. 5, pp. S169–S172, 2004.

[3] J. S. Lehman and R. A. el-Azhary, "Kaposi varicelliform eruption in patients with autoimmune bullous dermatoses," *International Journal of Dermatology*, vol. 55, no. 3, pp. e136–e140, 2016.

[4] E. Sato, K. Hiromatsu, K. Murata, and S. Imafuku, "Loss of ATP2A2 allows herpes simplex virus 1 infection of a human epidermis model by disrupting innate immunity and barrier function," *Journal of Investigative Dermatology*, vol. 138, no. 12, pp. 2540–2549, 2018.

[5] A. Wollenberg, C. Zoch, S. Wetzel, G. Plewig, and B. Przybilla, "Predisposing factors and clinical features of eczema herpeticum: a retrospective analysis of 100 cases," *Journal of the American Academy of Dermatology*, vol. 49, no. 2, pp. 198–205, 2003.

[6] C. E. Wheeler and D. C. Abele, "Eczema herpeticum, primary and recurrent," *Archives of Dermatology*, vol. 93, no. 2, pp. 162–173, 1966.

[7] R. Vora, A. Pilani, N. Jivani, and R. Kota, "Kaposi varicelliform eruption," *Indian Dermatology Online Journal*, vol. 6, no. 5, pp. 364–366, 2015.

[8] A. K. Nath, T. Sori, and D. M. Thappa, "A case series of kaposi's varicelliform eruption in dermatology in-patients in a tertiary care centre," *Indian Journal of Dermatology*, vol. 56, no. 1, pp. 110–115, 2011.

[9] G. Rao, K. Chalam, G. Prasad, M. Sarnathan, and H. Kumar, "Mini outbreak of Kaposi's varicelliform eruption in skin ward: a study of five cases," *Indian Journal of Dermatology, Venereology and Leprology*, vol. 73, no. 1, pp. 33–35, 2007.

[10] Y. Marfatia, S. Patel, S. Makrandi, and P. Sharma, "Human immunodeficiency virus and pemphigus vulgaris: an interesting association," *Indian Journal of Dermatology, Venereology and Leprology*, vol. 73, no. 5, pp. 354-355, 2007.

[11] L. Feldmeyer, R. M. Trüeb, L. E. French, and J. Hafner, "Pitfall: pemphigus herpeticatus should not be confounded with resistant pemphigus vulgaris," *Journal of Dermatological Treatment*, vol. 21, no. 5, pp. 311–313, 2010.

[12] S.-H. Chiu, Y.-C. Su, and C.-C. E. Lan, "Pemphigus vulgaris complicated with atypical Kaposi varicelliform eruption," *Dermatologica Sinica*, vol. 36, no. 4, p. 254, 2018.

[13] C. L. Mackley, D. R. Adams, B. Anderson, and J. J. Miller, "Eczema herpeticum: a dermatologic emergency," *Dermatology Nurses' Association*, vol. 14, no. 5, 2002.

[14] K. Ortiz, "Erupción variceliforme de kaposi en una serie de 8 pacientes," *Medicina Cutánea Ibero-Latino-Americana*, vol. 42, no. 4–6, pp. 97–103, 2014.

[15] https://www.pulse-clinic.com/herpes/.

[16] K. Zouhair, T. el Ouazzani, S. Azzouzi, S. Sqalli, and H. Lakhdar, "Surinfection herpétique du pemphigus: six cas [herpetic superinfection of pemphigus: 6 cases]," *Annales de Dermatologie et de Vénéréologie*, vol. 126, no. 10, pp. 699–702, 1999.

[17] C. M. Perry and D. Faulds, "Valaciclovir," *Drugs*, vol. 52, no. 5, pp. 754–772, 1996.

50

Epidemic, Endemic, or Stewart–Bluefarb? When Several Forms of Kaposi Seem to Dispute Paternity

Hugues Adegbidi,[1] Bérénice Dégboé,[1] Fabrice Akpadjan,[1] Nadège Agbessi-Mekoun,[2] Christiane Koudoukpo,[2] Alida Kouassi,[1] and Félix Atadokpede[1]

[1]*Dermatology and Venereology Service, National University Hospital CNHU-HKM, University of Abomey-Calavi, Cotonou, Benin*
[2]*Dermatology and Venereology Service, Department University Hospital of Parakou (CHUD-Parakou), University of Parakou, Parakou, Benin*

Correspondence should be addressed to Bérénice Dégboé; kebdegboe@yahoo.fr

Academic Editor: Ioannis D. Bassukas

The role of human herpes virus 8 (HHV8) is demonstrated in the occurrence of Kaposi's disease, but the role of cofactors is still hardly known. We report a case of Kaposi's disease which occurred 10 years after a local trauma in an HIV-positive patient from Central Africa. A 38-year-old female, from and living in Central Africa, consulted for angiomatous papulo-nodules associated with purple-colored macules and painful lymphoedema of the right leg and foot that had been developing for 6 months. She reported a history of posttraumatic lymphoedema of the affected limb as a result of a road accident that occurred ten years earlier. The mucous were healthy. There was no sign of systemic lesions. The diagnosis of Kaposi's disease was evoked with, in differential, a Stewart–Bluefarb syndrome-type of pseudo-Kaposi and an epidemic Kaposi disease. Retroviral serology was positive to HIV1 with a CD4 count of 600 cells/mm^3. Histopathology of the lesions and duplex ultrasonography could not be performed. The rest of the biological assessment was without particularity. The diagnosis of epidemic Kaposi's disease associated with cofactors involved in endemic Kaposi's disease and Stewart–Bluefarb syndrome was retained. An antiretroviral treatment (emtricitabine, tenofovir, and efavirenz) allowed to obtain after 6 months a noticeable improvement of the lesions and a disappearance of the pain with however the persistence of a residual lymphoedema. This is a special case of Kaposi's disease that seems to involve several factors. The role of cofactors in Kaposi's disease remains to be elucidated.

1. Introduction

Kaposi's disease (KD), previously named Kaposi's sarcoma, was first described in 1872 by Moritz von Kaposi. It is characterized by cutaneous and/or visceral tumor lesions following after the proliferation of fusiform cells and dermal vessels. It is caused by an infection with HHV8 (human herpes virus 8) also called KSHV (Kaposi's sarcoma-associated herpes virus). Depending on the context, there are currently four forms of KD: classical, endemic, epidemic, and iatrogenic [1–3].

Since the advent of the HIV-AIDS (human immunodeficiency virus-acquired immunodeficiency syndrome) pandemic, it has experienced an epidemiological outbreak. The risk of developing KD is higher in areas where there is a high prevalence of HHV8 infection and HIV infection: Central, West, and South Africa [4–8].

Stewart–Bluefarb syndrome is a form of pseudo-Kaposi corresponding to reactional posttraumatic angiodysplasia. It is clinically and histologically similar to MK [9].

Although the role of HHV8 in KD is demonstrated in the occurrence of KD, cofactors remain poorly understood [1–3]. We report here a case of KD occurring after a 10-year-old vascular trauma on a patient from Central Africa with HIV infection.

2. Observation

A 38-year-old woman who is from and lives in Central Africa consulted for solid lesions and purple-colored patches on her right leg and foot that had been evolving for six months. The patient's interview revealed a notion of pain of the affected limb, an antecedent of trauma of the same limb in a road accident that had occurred ten years before and that resulted in a leg lymphoedema. The physical examination found the patient in good general condition, without fever. Locally, there were infiltrated purple macula associated with angiomatous papulo-nodules and lymphoedema of the right leg. The external part of the lower third of the same leg is the seat of an unsightly and atrophic scar and erosion of the external malleolus (Figure 1). At palpation of the pulse, there was no thrill or associated breath at auscultation. The mucous were unharmed. There was no sign of impairment of other organs. So, the diagnosis of endemic KD was evoked in view of the geographical origin of the patient, with a pseudo-Kaposi of Stewart–Bluefarb and an epidemic KD being differentially diagnosed. Hemogram revealed nothing particular. C-reactive protein was positive at 35 mg/L. The histopathology of the lesions and the ultrasonography of the affected limb have not been performed. HIV serology was positive to HIV1. The CD4 count was 600 cells/mm3. The diagnosis of epidemic KD on an anteriorly traumatized leg in a patient from Central Africa was retained.

The patient was put on a combination of antiretrovirals including two nucleoside reverse transcriptase inhibitors (emtricitabine-tenofovir) and a non-nucleoside reverse transcriptase inhibitor (efavirenz). The development was marked by the complete disappearance of the pain and an important regression of the lesions after six months of treatment, with however the persistence of residual lymphoedema (Figure 2).

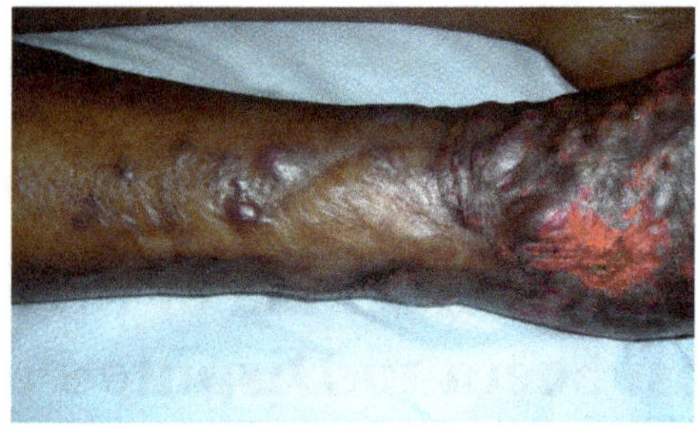

Figure 1: Kaposi's disease showing angiomatous papulo-nodules on lymphoedema of the right leg and foot.

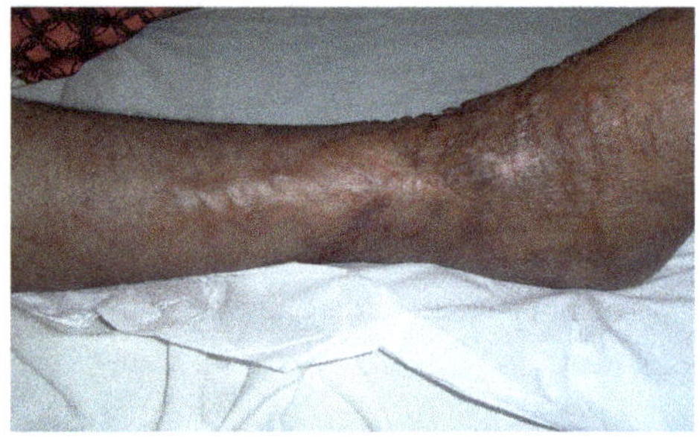

Figure 2: Kaposi's disease showing fewer papulo-nodules on residual lymphoedema of the right leg and foot after 6 months of antiretroviral treatment.

3. Discussion

Our clinical case poses a real diagnostic problem. Despite the positivity of retroviral serology, endemic KD and Stewart–Bluefarb syndrome could not be formally eliminated.

The responsibility of the HHV8 is no longer to be demonstrated in the occurrence of the KD. Anti-HHV8 antibodies are found in at least 95% of all forms of KD cases. However, prevalence and clinical forms differ according to geographic areas and underlying terrain [1–3, 10, 11]. The presence of HHV8 therefore appears to be necessary but not a sufficient condition for the onset of KD. Genetic, immune, and environmental cofactors were referred to [1, 2]. With the case of our patient, we also suggest local cofactors such as microtrauma or tissue remodeling in the stimulation of the virus and the proliferation of fusiform cells.

With the influence of the environment, endemic KD occurs in several forms: indolent cutaneous, acral aggressive, disseminated, and generalized lymphadenopathy in children with bad prognosis. The regions of high endemicity are Latin America, South Africa, and West and Central Africa, the region of origin of our patient. Seroprevalence to HHV8 is around 40–90% compared to 3–5% in the countries of Europe (north, south, and west), Asia, and North America [2, 11, 12]. Endemic KD affects adults as well as children. Its transmission is more probably horizontal (child-child) or vertical (mother-child and parents-children) [1, 3, 6–8]. It is diagnosed most often between 30 and 40 years with a marked predominance with males. However, in these areas there is no parallelism between the frequency of seroprevalence with HHV8 and that of endemic KD [4–6].

With the advent of HIV infection, the once rare KD has experienced a real outbreak. Its prevalence among HIV-positive patients varied between 15% and 29% with a clear male predominance during the 1980s. Its sexual transmission is demonstrated in homosexuals. Currently, its incidence has decreased considerably with the introduction of antiretroviral combinations (ARVs) [1–5].

KD associated with epidemic HIV is particularly aggressive with bilateral or profuse cutaneous involvement, mucosal, and systemic involvement all in the context of severe immunosuppression [1, 11, 12]. Indeed, the Th1-type cytokines secreted during HIV infection potentiate the activation of HHV8 resulting in an increase of viral load and higher risk of occurrence of KD. Also, the activating protein "Tat" which intervenes during the replication of HIV type 1 stimulates the secretion of proangiogenic chemokines, which will in turn induce the development of KD through the release of fibroblastic growth factors. This latter mechanism may account for the fact that KD is more common with HIV1 than with HIV2 infection [1, 3, 4, 11].

Immunosuppression plays a key role. For example, in areas with high seroprevalence of HIV and HHV8, the prevalence of epidemic KD is often higher. Central Africa's countries range among the most affected by this coinfection. In these countries, the prevalence of epidemic KD varies between 8% and 18% [1–3, 5, 6].

The positive retroviral serology in our patient was a strong argument in favor of an epidemic KD. However, the absence of severe immunodepression and the unilateral character also pointed to an endemic localized KD more than epidemiological factors, or a pseudo-Kaposi type Stewart–Bluefarb, due to previous trauma.

Stewart–Bluefarb pseudo-Kaposi is a rare condition that affects young adults between 20 and 30 years, with predominance in males. It is secondary to a reactive angiodysplasia affecting the blood vessels. Its pathogenesis is not clearly elucidated, but it suggests that any condition favoring the increase of venous pressure produces a retrograde blood flow that can stimulate, especially in fragile anatomical areas, the proliferation of endothelial and fibroblastic cells under the action of the vascular endothelium growth factor (VEGF). The contributing factors may be trauma, as is the case in our patient, an arteriovenous fistula during hemodialysis, vascular surgery, or a significant hormonal period such as puberty or pregnancy [9, 13].

The diagnosis of the Stewart–Bluefarb syndrome with Kaposi's disease is clinically and histologically difficult. The labeling of perivascular cells by CD34 antigen, the detection of HHV8 viral DNA, the presence of crystalloid intracytoplasmic inclusions, or the positivity of factor VIII R antigen were put forward as elements that enable the distinction between a pseudo-Kaposi and a KD [1, 14]. In its classic form, Stewart–Bluefarb syndrome occurs as purple, infiltrated, well-defined, firm, and sometimes sensitive plaques. Sometimes, it is purple-colored nodules associated with brown spots and localized oedema as is the case in our patient. The lesions are unilateral acral or hanging, of sudden appearance. The duplex ultrasound of the limb associated with arteriography reveals the arteriovenous fistula [9, 13, 14].

The treatment of epidemic KD is different from that of other forms. In other forms, immunosuppressive chemotherapy or radiotherapy is often used for the treatment of diffuse forms. In epidemic KD, combined ARV treatment is recommended [3, 10]. The action of ARVs is very probably indirect. By inhibiting the replication of HIV, they induce the restoration of the immune system, which results in the decrease of the HHV8 viral load and thus the partial or total regression of KD, thus confirming the opportunistic nature of this tumor [10]. Moreover, it is shown that early ARV treatment and limited forms of epidemic KD allow remission in at least 80% of patients [12]. Additional chemotherapy or radiotherapy may be necessary to better control of the tumor [1, 3].

Given the therapeutic and prognostic implications and subject to the exact date of the HIV infection, we have retained the diagnosis of epidemic KD precipitated by the cofactors implicated in the endemic KD and the Stewart–Bluefarb-type of pseudo-Kaposi. The evolution was favorable with an important regression of the tumor under ARV combination.

4. Conclusion

Our observation poses a diagnostic problem of a unilateral localized form of KD in an HIV seropositive patient living in a HHV8 seroprevalence zone. It has allowed us to draw attention to the fact that KD can be multifactorial and can lead to an intricate clinical picture. It could also involve for a given clinical form the combination of genetic, immunological, environmental, and local cofactors. Could KD, then, be a continuum in which the weight of one of the factors involved could predispose to a particular clinical form?

Authors' Contributions

H. Adegbidi was involved in collection of clinical information. H. Adegbidi and B. Degboe were involved in conception of the draft of this work, writing the article, and researching references. F. Akpadjan, N. Agbessi-Mekoun, C. Koudoukpo, F. Atadokpede, and A. Kouassi reviewed the manuscript.

References

[1] P. Curtiss, L. C. Strazzulla, and A. E. Friedman-Kien, "An update on Kaposi's sarcoma: epidemiology, pathogenesis and treatment," *Dermatology and Therapy*, vol. 6, no. 4, pp. 465–470, 2016.

[2] E. Ruocco, V. Ruocco, M. L. Tornesello, A. Gambardella, R. Wolf, and F. M. Buonaguro, "Kaposi's sarcoma: etiology and pathogenesis, inducing factors, causal associations, and treatments: facts and controversies," *Clinics in Dermatology*, vol. 31, no. 4, pp. 413–422, 2013.

[3] J. W. Schneider and D. P. Dittmer, "Diagnosis and treatment of kaposi sarcoma," *American Journal of Clinical Dermatology*, vol. 18, no. 4, pp. 529–539, 2017.

[4] A. C. De-Araujo, R. C. Rafael Manuel, R. Del Bianco et al., "Seroprevalence of human herpesvirus 8 infection in individuals from health care centers in Mozambique: potential for endemic and epidemic kaposi's sarcoma," *Journal of Medical Virology*, vol. 82, pp. 1216–1223, 2010.

[5] R. Dupre, E. Kassa-Kelembho, S. Plancoulaine et al., "Human herpesvirus 8 serological markers and viral load in patients with AIDS-associated kaposi's sarcoma in central african republic," *Journal of Clinical Microbiology*, vol. 43, no. 9, pp. 4840–4843, 2005.

[6] K. Stolka, P. Ndom, J. Hemingway-Foday et al., "Risk factors for kaposi's sarcoma among HIV-positive individuals in a case control study in Cameroon," *Cancer Epidemiology*, vol. 38, no. 2, pp. 137–143, 2014.

[7] N. K. El-Mallawany, J. Villiera, W. Kamiyango et al., "Endemic kaposi sarcoma in HIV-negative children and adolescents: an evaluation of overlapping and distinct clinical features in HIV-related disease," *Infectious Agents and Cancer*, vol. 13, p. 33, 2018.

[8] N. K. El-Mallawany, C. L. McAtee, L. R. Campbell, and P. N. Kazembe, "Pediatric kaposi sarcoma in context of the HIV epidemic in sub-Saharan Africa: current perspectives," *Pediatric Health, Medicine and Therapeutics*, vol. 9, pp. 35–46, 2018.

[9] Z. Alioua, H. Lamsyah, M. Sbai et al., "Pseudomaladie de kaposi secondaire à une malformation artérioveineuse superficielle : syndrome de stewart-bluefarb," *Annales De Dermatologie Et De Vénéréologie*, vol. 135, no. 1, pp. 44–47, 2008.
[10] A. B. Steuer, J. M. Cohen, M. P. Christman, L. A. Penn, N. Brinster, and A. Femia, "Acquired immunodeficiency syndrome-related kaposi sarcoma," *Dermatology Online Journal*, vol. 24, no. 12, p. 7, 2018.
[11] F. Buonaguro, M. Tornesello, L. Buonaguro et al., "Kaposi's sarcoma: aetiopathogenesis, histology and clinical features," *Journal of the European Academy of Dermatology and Venereology*, vol. 17, no. 2, pp. 138–154, 2003.
[12] M. Fatahzadeh, "Kaposi sarcoma: review and medical management update," *Medical Management and Pharmacology Update*, vol. 113, no. 1, 2012.
[13] S. B. Verma and R. Vasani, "Stewart-Bluefarb syndrome revisited," *Clinical and Experimental Dermatology*, vol. 41, no. 5, pp. 522–525, 2016.
[14] A. C. Renkl, J. M. Weiss, K. Scharffetter-Kochanek, and T. Weiss, "Pseudo-kaposi-sarkom oder kaposi-sarkom?" *Der Hautarzt*, vol. 59, no. 3, pp. 233–236, 2008.

51

Halo Nevi are not Trivial: About 2 Young Patients of Regressed Primary Melanoma that Simulates Halo Nevi

S. De Schrijver,[1] I. Theate,[2] and O. Vanhooteghem[1]

[1]*Dermatology Department, CHU UCL Namur, Site Sainte Elisabeth, Place Louise Godin 15, 5000 Namur, Belgium*
[2]*Institute of Pathology and Genetics (IPG), Avenue George-Lemaître 25, 6041 Gosselies, Belgium*

Correspondence should be addressed to O. Vanhooteghem; ovanhooteghem@hotmail.com

Academic Editor: Jacek Cezary Szepietowski

Background. Halo nevi are often considered benign, and the possibility of malignancy is not always clear to practitioners. We present two case reports suggesting that a halo nevus appearance can be seen in melanoma, even in young adults. A literature search for halo nevi revealing melanoma shows that this is a very rare condition. *Case presentation.* This report of two young patients indicates the importance of obtaining a detailed history to detect warning signs such as itching, pain, spontaneous bleeding, and previous alterations according to the patient, including a previously totally black colour in an already fully regressed melanoma. *Conclusions.* The risk of a halo nevus being malignant is higher if there is only one unique halo nevus and no personal or familial history of vitiligo. We postulate that a regressing atypical nevus or a regressing melanoma may be induced by an immunologic reaction as halo nevus type of clinical picture.

1. Introduction

Halo nevus, also called Sutton's nevus, is a melanocytic nevus surrounded by a halo of depigmentation, which is usually symmetrically round or oval. Halo nevi affect up to 5% of Caucasian children six to fifteen years old [1, 2] in an equal sex distribution and are more common in patients with an increased number of nevi and/or a personal or familial history of vitiligo. Halo nevus is seen in common acquired nevi, though it may be seen in a congenital nevus, blue nevi, Spitz nevi, and even, but rarely, in melanoma. The most common location is the back, and multiple lesions are present in approximately half of all cases [2–4]. This regression of pigmentation is believed to present a T-cell mediated immune response to nevus antigens [3]. There are four clinical stages in the life of a halo nevus, with the duration of the process ranging from months to decades [4, 5]. Starting as a pigmented nevus surrounded by a halo of depigmentation (stage 1), a pink nevus surrounded by a halo of depigmentation then develops (stage 2), followed by a circular area of depigmentation with total or partial disappearance of the nevus (stage 3) and finally normal-appearing skin after repigmentation of the halo (stage 4). It is important to assess the clinical features of the halo nevus [6]. A biopsy is not indicated if the pigmented part is regular in appearance; however, biopsy might be justified in the presence of atypical or worrisome features, as a halo appearance can be seen in dysplasia or, rarely, in melanoma.

2. Case Presentation 1

A 43-year-old man without medical history presented with an existing irregular halo and depigmented macule on the left upper arm for two and a half years that had changed according to the patient (Figure 1). He mentioned that the lesion was first a dark black colour and then, all of a sudden, started to disappear, with currently only a light shadow remaining centrally around a further fully depigmented lesion. Clinical assessment did not reveal other halo nevi or clinical signs of vitiligo but revealed numerous subcutaneous nodular lesions disseminated over the body, particularly on the back, suggesting the possibility of metastatic disease.

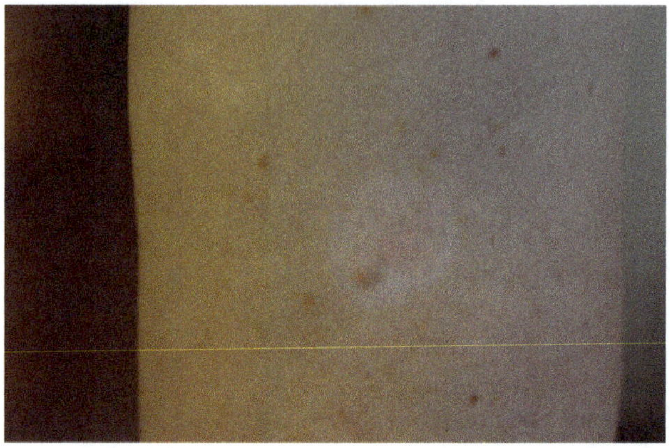

Figure 1: Halo nevus on the left upper arm. The central part shows only a light shadow while the rest of the lesion is depigmented.

Histology of the halo nevus showed intradermal atypical nevus cells but also extensive regression in the superficial dermis (Figures 2 and 3). Histology of the nodular lesion on the back confirmed skin metastases of a melanoma. The suspicion of a regressing melanoma with diffuse metastases (stage IV) with a V600E mutation in the BRAF gene was confirmed. PET-CT demonstrated diffuse metastases near the lungs, adrenal glands, ganglions, peritoneum, retroperitoneum, pericardium, and brain. The patient was referred to oncology for further assessment and therapy but die quickly.

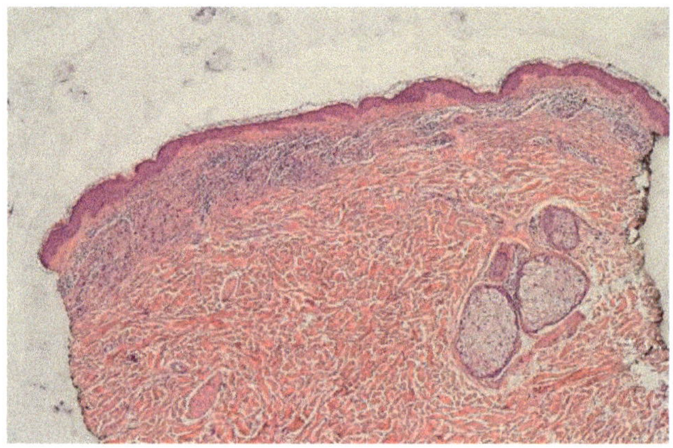

Figure 2: Intradermal atypical nevus cells in the left part of the biopsy, contrasting with regression in the right part (HE 5x).

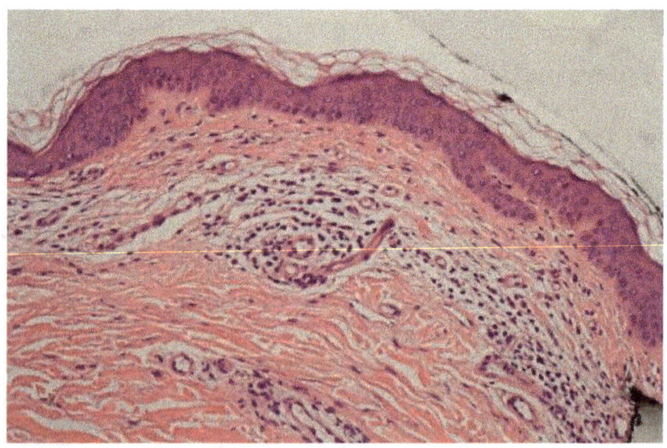

Figure 3: Signs of extensive regression in the superficial dermis, lacking atypical melanocytes (HE 20x).

3. Case Presentation 2

A 21-year-old girl without medical history mentioned having a congenital nevus on the right temple that had started to itch some weeks ago. Clinical evaluation revealed a nevus with a halo of depigmentation measuring six by eight millimetres, with a central zone of homogenic pigmentation (Figure 4). Clinical assessment did not reveal other halo nevi or other diseases, such as vitiligo. Dermatoscopy showed some telangiectasias surrounded by a symmetrical rim of depigmentation. Although there was no clear suspicion of malignancy, excision was performed because the patient was anxious. Histology showed a melanocytic lesion with extensive regression at the margins of the lesion with only a few atypical cells in the dermis (Figure 5). In contrast, the centre of the lesion showed dense melanocytic proliferation with severe atypical features in the dermoepidermal junction as well as in the dermis (Figures 6). This picture confirmed the diagnosis of a superficial spreading melanoma, Breslow 0.70 mm, Clark level three, but no mitoses, ulcerations or invasion into the lymphatics, vasculature, or nerves (pT1a) were observed. Re-excision with large margins was carried out. Follow-up showed no recurrence.

4. Discussion

There is still much discussion about the origin of halo nevi and whether they should be regarded as benign or as a possible reaction to an atypical nevus or melanoma. Weyant et al. sought to determine the frequency of dysplastic nevi and other histologic types of nevi in a series of halo nevi that were diagnosed clinically [7]. They found that out of the 124 halo nevi that were reviewed, 48 (38.7%) were dysplastic nevi, and only 3 (2.4%) were melanomas. Mooney et al. reviewed 142 halo nevi [8]. For 66 cases, the diagnosis of halo nevus was made both clinically and pathologically, and for 76 cases, the diagnosis was based on histological results alone. Among those with a clinicopathological diagnosis of halo nevus, 11% exhibited

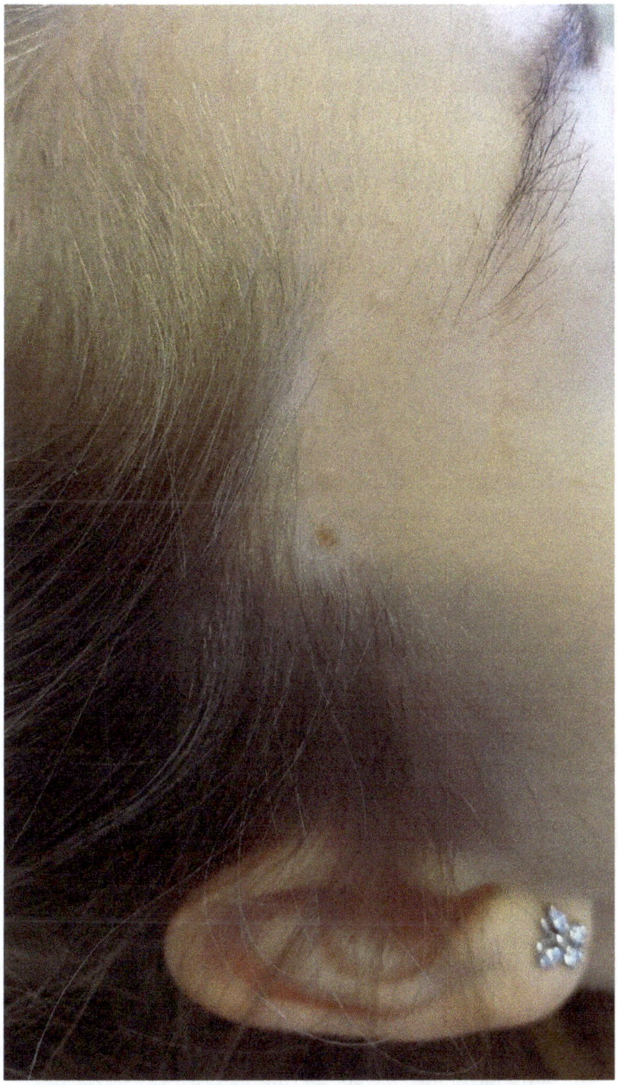

Figure 4: Nevus on the right temporal area surrounded by a symmetrical rim of depigmentation.

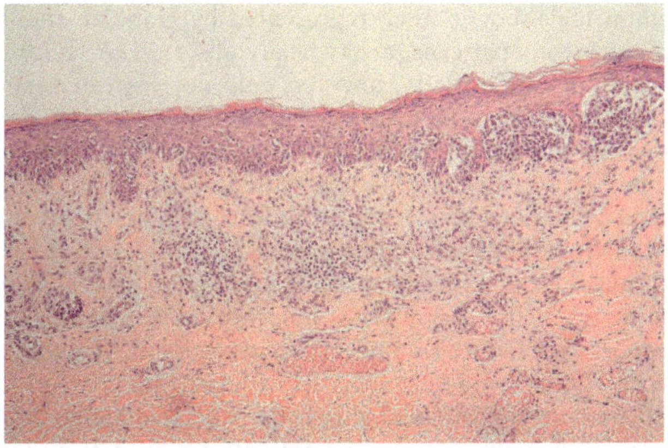

Figure 5: The lesion is characterized by atypical junctional activity and signs of extensive regression in the superficial dermis (HE × 10).

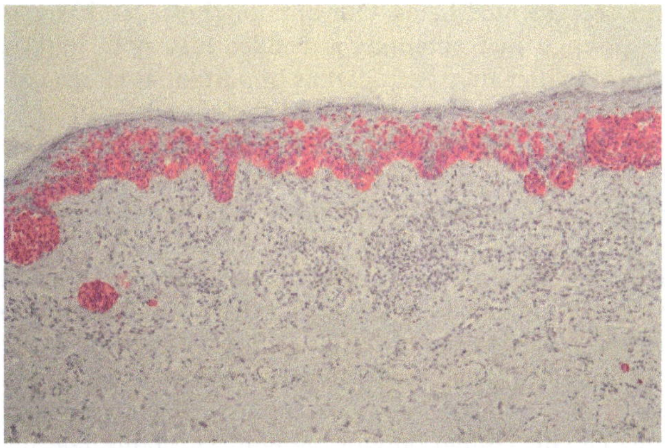

Figure 6: Immunohistochemistry shows bridging and pagetoid spread of atypical melanocytes (Melan A red × 10).

moderate atypia, 16% exhibited minimal atypia to only focally moderate atypia, 24% exhibited minimal atypia, and 49% exhibited no significant atypia. Among patients diagnosed only by pathology, there was also a broad spectrum of atypia, with 8% exhibiting focally severe or severe atypia. This study supports the concept that the halo nevus should not be regarded as a single clinicopathological entity but rather a wide spectrum of histological atypia. For these 142 cases of halo nevi, the authors could not find histology revealing a melanoma. It is important to distinguish halo nevi from regressing melanoma. Therefore, investigators are looking for differences in histopathology between halo nevi seen in benign lesions versus those seen in regressing melanoma. The main differences between the histopathological appearance of a halo nevus and melanoma can be summarized as follows: in the former, nevi cells are arranged in nests, while in melanoma, there are isolated atypical melanocytes in the epidermis and aggregates in the dermis. There is also a well-known difference between the symmetric appearance of nevi and the asymmetric appearance of melanoma. Mature cells with rare or a lack of mitosis are characteristic of a nevus when compared with the numerous mitotic immature cells in melanoma. Even so, in halo nevi, there is a diffuse lymphocytic infiltration throughout the entire lesion, in contrast to melanoma, where the inflammatory infiltrate is concentrated in the periphery. Nevi cell destruction, characteristic of the biological evolution of the halo nevi, has not resulted in the development of fibrosis [9]. On the other hand, the destruction of tumour cells during the regression of melanoma results in papillary dermal fibrosis during the final stage of resorption. Considering all the above, we can state that a depigmented halo must be regarded as a phenomenon that may be associated with different types of melanocytic tumours and with a broad spectrum of histopathological atypia degree. Therefore, investigators should also look for specific characteristics both clinically and dermatoscopically to predict whether the halo nevus is benign or malignant. Blessing et al. considered that halos associated with melanoma have a more asymmetric shape than those associated with melanocytic nevi [9]. Kolm et al. studied the dermatoscopic characteristics of halo nevi and found that the characteristic dermatoscopic features of benign melanocytic nevi, represented by globular and/or homogeneous patterns, are typically observed in children and young adults [10]. However, halo nevi revealed considerable changes in area over time during digital dermoscopic follow-up, albeit their structural patterns remained unchanged. For this reason and because melanoma with halo-like depigmentation, although rare, additionally exhibits melanoma-specific dermoscopic criteria, the authors concluded that the role of digital dermoscopic follow-up in the diagnosis of halo nevi is nonsignificant. Regarding patient age, Rubegni et al. established that patients who have a halo associated with melanoma are older than patients who have a halo nevus associated with benign melanocytic nevi [11]. As our patients are only 21 and 43 years old, we cannot confirm this point of view, and we stress that young age cannot definitively classify the halo nevus as benign. Further studies are expected to add valuable information regarding the features of tumours with depigmented halos. Our opinion, however, based on our cases, is that obtaining a detailed history to look for signs of malignancy is at least as important as clinical and dermatoscopic examinations and therefore cannot be ignored. Halo nevi can also be observed in combination with vitiligo, although the question of whether halo nevi should be considered as a sign of vitiligo or as a risk factor for developing vitiligo is still under debate [12]. Reported incidence of halo nevi in patients with vitiligo ranges between 1% and 48% [4, 13, 14]. Van Geel et al. observed the presence of halo nevi in 31.1% of all patients with vitiligo [12]. They also found that patients with halo nevi only were less likely to experience the Koebner phenomenon than patients with vitiligo only or patients with both halo nevi and vitiligo. Zhou et al. confirmed this conclusion and statistically showed that the presence of the Koebner phenomenon in halo nevi patients is highly suggestive of an increased risk of developing vitiligo. The Koebner phenomenon is often considered a sign of more active or extensive conditions [15]. Therefore, the authors recommend that genetically susceptible individuals avoid any physical or mechanical disturbances, such as scratching or friction on melanocytic nevi, which might lead to the risk of the Koebner phenomenon and subsequent specific immune targeting of melanocytes. Considering all of the above, the concept of a halo around a nevus can be thought of a "pseudo-Koebner" phenomenon. In conclusion, halo nevi are common, especially in children and young adults. Halo nevi develop from a benign acquired melanocytic nevus but can also be seen in dysplastic nevi and even, rarely, in melanoma, which should be emphasized to more to clinicians. Young age does not automatically mean that the halo nevus is of benign origin. Further investigations are necessary to detect clearer-cut clinical and dermatoscopic features to distinguish between benign and malignant origins in halo nevi. However, in our experience, a detailed clinical history and clinical examination (e.g., itchiness and previous dark black pigmentation) are important and can already provide diagnostic clues, especially when there is only one clinical halo nevus. Biopsy is necessary in these cases to avoid missing melanoma, but confocal microscopy can help clinicians to make the decision between excision--biopsy or follow-up [16].

Consent

Patients gave written informed consent to publish the case including clinical image, and they are available on request.

References

[1] A. W. Kopf, S. D. Morrill, and I. Silberberg, "Broad spectrum of leukoderma acquisitum centrifugum," *Archives of Dermatology*, vol. 92, no. 1, pp. 14–35, 1965.

[2] J. K. Rivers, R. MacLennan, J. W. Kelly et al., "The eastern Australian childhood nevus study: prevalence of atypical nevi, congenital nevus-like nevi, and other pigmented lesions," *Journal of the American Academy of Dermatology*, vol. 32, no. 6, pp. 957–963, 1995.

[3] R. A. Zeff, A. Freitag, C. M. Grin, and J. M. Grant-Kels, "The immune response in halo nevi," *Journal of the American Academy of Dermatology*, vol. 37, no. 4, pp. 620–624, 1997.

[4] S. B. Frank and H. J. Cohen, "The halo nevus," *Archives of Dermatology*, vol. 89, no. 3, pp. 367–373, 1964.

[5] M. Aouthmany, M. Weinstein, M. J. Zirwas, and R. T. Brodell, "The natural history of halo nevi: a retrospective case series," *Journal of the American Academy of Dermatology*, vol. 67, no. 4, pp. 582–586, 2012.

[6] C.-H. Lai, S. Lockhart, and S. B. Mallory, "Typical halo nevi in childhood: is a biopsy necessary?" *The Journal of Pediatrics*, vol. 138, no. 2, pp. 283-284, 2001.

[7] G. W. Weyant, C. G. Chung, and K. F. Helm, "Halo nevus: review of the literature and clinicopathologic findings," *International Journal of Dermatology*, vol. 54, no. 10, pp. e433–e435, 2015.

[8] M. A. Mooney, R. J. Barr, and M. G. Buxton, "Halo nevus or halo phenomenon? A study of 142 cases," *Journal of Cutaneous Pathology*, vol. 22, no. 4, pp. 342–348, 1995.

[9] K. Blessing and K. M. McLaren, "Histological regression in primary cutaneous melanoma: recognition, prevalence and significance," *Histopathology*, vol. 20, no. 4, pp. 315–322, 1992.

[10] I. Kolm, A. Di Stefani, R. Hofmann-Wellenhof et al., "Dermoscopy patterns of halo nevi," *Archives of Dermatology*, vol. 142, no. 12, pp. 1627–1632, 2006.

[11] P. Rubegni, N. Nami, M. Risulo, D. Tataranno, and M. Fimiani, "Melanoma with halo," *Clinical and Experimental Dermatology*, vol. 34, no. 6, pp. 749-750, 2009.

[12] N. Van Geel, S. Vandenhaute, R. Speeckaert et al., "Prognostic value and clinical significance of halo naevi regarding vitiligo," *British Journal of Dermatology*, vol. 164, no. 4, pp. 743–749, 2011.

[13] D. M. Wayte and E. B. Helwig, "Halo nevi," *Cancer*, vol. 22, no. 1, pp. 69–90, 1968.

[14] Y. Gauthier, J. E. Surleve-Bazeille, O. Gauthier, and L. Texier, "Ultrastructure of halo nevi," *Journal of Cutaneous Pathology*, vol. 2, no. 2, pp. 71–81, 1975.

[15] H. Zhou, L.-C. Wu, M.-K. Chen, Q.-M. Liao, R.-X. Mao, and J.-D. Han, "Factors associated with development of vitiligo in patients with halo nevus," *Chinese Medical Journal*, vol. 130, no. 22, pp. 2703–2708, 2017.

[16] A. Brugués, S. Ribero, V. Martins da Silva et al., "Sutton naevi as melanoma simulators: can confocal microscopy help in the diagnosis?" *Acta Derm Venereol*, vol. 100, no. 10, p. adv00134, 2020.

52

Isolated Langerhans Cell Histiocytosis of the Vulva in a 28-Year-Old Lady: A Report of a Case and Brief Review of the Literature

Maryam Sadat Sadati,[1,2] **Nafiseh Todarbary**,[3] **Fatemeh Sari Aslani**,[1,4] **and Maryam Hadibarhaghtalab**[1,2]

[1]*Molecular Dermatology Research Center, Shiraz University of Medical Sciences, Shiraz, Iran*
[2]*Dermatology Department, Shiraz University of Medical Sciences, Shiraz, Iran*
[3]*Student Research Committee, Shiraz University of Medical Sciences, Shiraz, Iran*
[4]*Pathology Department, Shiraz University of Medical Sciences, Shiraz, Iran*

Correspondence should be addressed to Maryam Hadibarhaghtalab; maryam_hadibarhaghtalab@yahoo.com

Academic Editor: Alireza Firooz

Langerhans cell histiocytosis (LCH) is a rare, proliferative disorder of Langerhans' cells. The presentation can vary from single organ involvement to multisystem and disseminated in severe cases, affecting children more than adults. Isolated vulvar involvement of LCH in a 28-year-old woman has rarely been described and also there are limited data for diagnosis and treatment. Herein, we report the case of a 28-year-old woman with isolated vulvar LCH, misdiagnosed with herpes simplex infection, successfully treated with thalidomide.

1. Introduction

According to the latest version of the National Comprehensive Cancer Network (NCCN), LCH is categorized to unifocal and multisystem (multifocal single-system or unifocal LCH involving critical organs). Unifocal LCH consists of isolated bone involvement, isolated skin disease, and involvement of other systems, except for critical organs. Multisystem LCH includes asymptomatic with no impending organ dysfunction, symptomatic or impending organ dysfunction, and pulmonary LCH [1].

In medical pieces of literature, only a few cases have been previously reported with vulvar LCH [2]. Primary isolated LCH of the female genital tract is rare, and less than 40 cases have already been reported worldwide [3]. This report presents the clinical and histopathologic features, diagnostic workup, and treatment of a 28-year-old woman as a vulvar LCH case from the Dermatology Department of Faghihi Hospital in Shiraz, Iran.

2. Case Presentation

The patient was a 28-year-old lady admitted to the Dermatology Department of Faghihi Hospital with a chief complaint of small punched-out ulcers located in the genitalia area concomitant with pruritus and posturination dysuria since two years before. Her physical examination was normal except for mild pinkish erosions and two punched-out ulcers in the genital area (Figure 1).

Firstly, the clinical diagnosis was genital herpes simplex and the patient had received several courses of acyclovir and cryotherapy, but she was not cured. Lesion biopsy and immunohistochemistry were done after no improvement in the clinical practice.

Pathology results showed that the collected biopsy was $0.3 \times 0.3 \times 0.3$ cm creamy-gray color skin favoring erosive lichen planus (LP) and lichen simplex atrophicus (LSA). Pathological findings were parakeratosis with some neutrophils and moderate acanthosis with multifocal aggregates

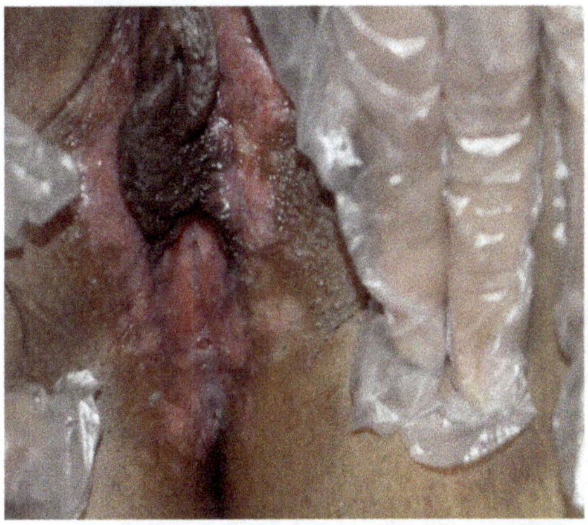

FIGURE 1: Pinkish mild erosions and small punched-out ulcers in genital area.

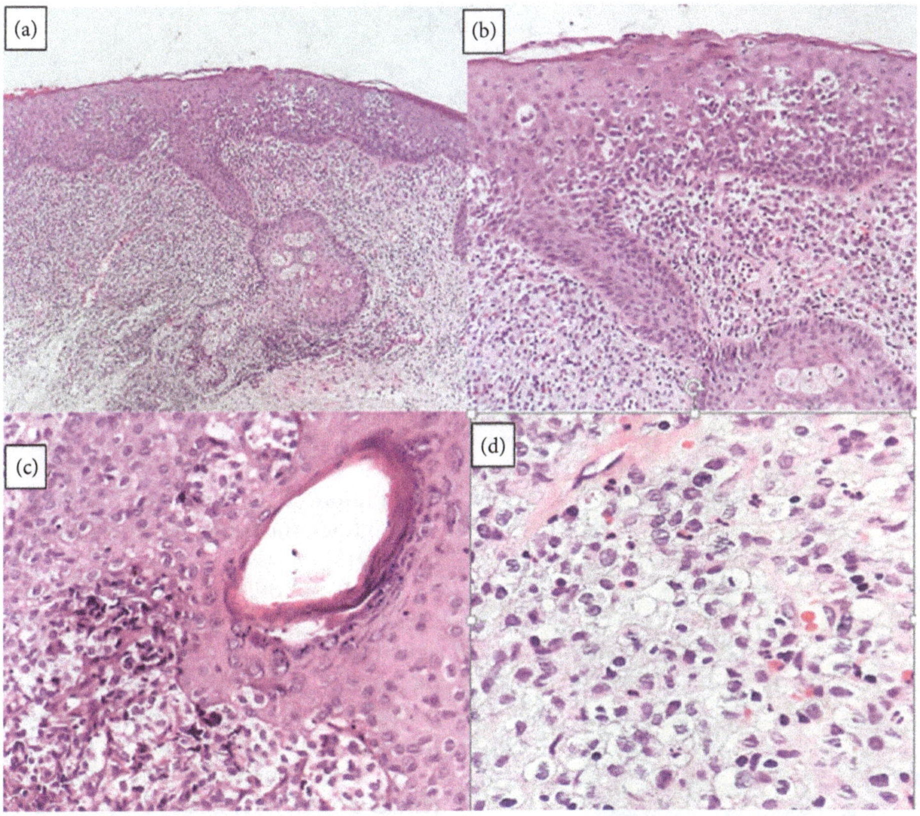

FIGURE 2: (a). There are some aggregates of Langerhans cells in the epidermal layer and diffuse upper and mid-dermal predominantly Langerhans cell infiltration (H&E × 100) (b). There are some aggregates of Langerhans cells in the epidermal layer and diffuse dermal predominantly Langerhans cell infiltration admixed with some eosinophils and few lymphocytes (H&E × 200) (c). Follicular epithelium involved by Langerhans cells (H&E × 400) (d). There is diffuse upper dermal predominantly Langerhans cell infiltration with mitotic figures admixed with some eosinophils and neutrophils and a few lymphocytes (H&E × 400).

of Langerhans cells. The upper and mid-dermis showed sheets of uniform ovoid cells with eosinophilic cytoplasm with a coffee bean or reniform nuclei and eosinophil and lymphocyte infiltration. The follicular epithelium was involved by some aggregates of Langerhans cells (Figure 2).

Based on oncology consultation, brain MRI, PET scan, bone marrow biopsy, skull, and chest X-ray were performed, all of which were normal.

Immunohistochemistry profile on formalin-fixed and paraffin-embedded lesion of genitalia biopsy was CD1a positive, CD68 positive, and S100 positive, and the Langerin marker (CD207) was not available. Finally, the probable diagnosis was LCH (Figure 3).

Treatment was started with the administration of nitrogen mustard and fluocinolone, but she was not cured. Then, thalidomide, 100 milligrams once a day, was prescribed. The patient did not have a pregnancy plan by taking OCP pills and using condoms. Adverse effects and prohibition of pregnancy were explained to her in detail. Finally, the patient's lesions disappeared after one year (Figure 4).

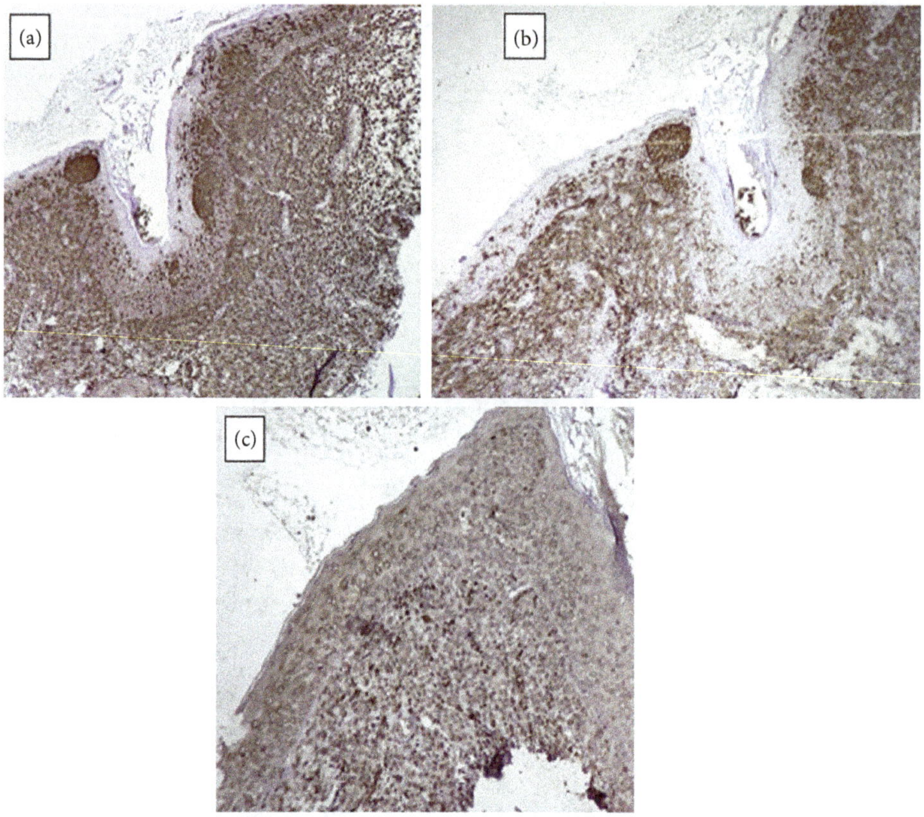

FIGURE 3: (a). S100 immunostaining shows strong diffuse positivity in upper dermis and scattered single as well as aggregates of Langerhans cells in the *epidermis* (×100) (b). CD1a immunostaining of Langerhans cells shows strong diffuse positivity in the upper dermis and scattered single as well as aggregates in the *epidermis* (×100) (c). CD68 immunostaining shows scattered weak positivity upper dermis (×100).

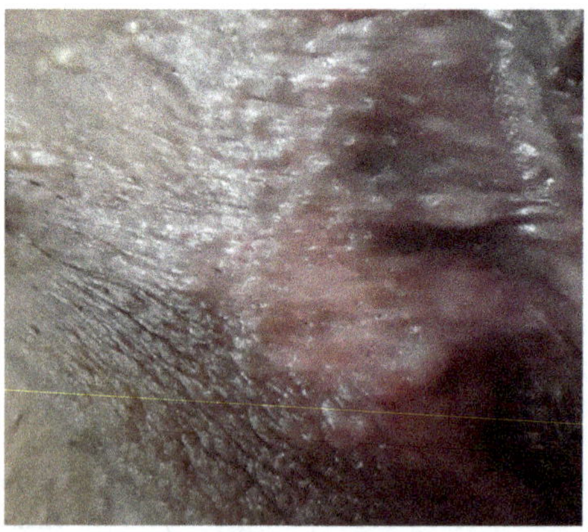

FIGURE 4: Remission after treatment by thalidomide.

The patient was visited every three months for physical examination and checking lab data such as complete blood tests, pregnancy tests, and kidney and liver function tests until the end of treatment; then, she was visited annually.

3. Discussion

LCH is a rare disease, especially among adults, and it can occur at any age [4]. The most common sites of involvement consist of skin, bones, lymph nodes, bone marrow, hypothalamic-pituitary axis, lungs, spleen, liver, bowel, and orbit. In addition, LCH can involve different sites of the female genital tract, including the vulva, vagina, cervix, uterus, and ovaries [5].

In the case of LCH, workups such as full blood count and chemistry, thyroid function tests, urine analysis, and coagulation studies are usually requested. Additionally, radiographic examinations such as skull series and chest radiography should be done depending on the basic diagnostic tests and the 'patient's symptoms [6].

In 1939, Lane and Smith reported the first case of lower female genital tract LCH in a six-year-old child [5]. Herein, we reported a case of adult vulvar LCH with a mimic of herpes simplex lesions which can easily be misdiagnosed; therefore, having this clinical presentation with no response to routine treatment and no risk factor of LCH cannot put LCH off your mind.

Several neoplastic diseases can be mistaken for LCH, such as malignant melanoma, squamous cell carcinoma, sarcoma, and 'Paget's disease of the vulva. Systemic diseases in any patient suspected of vulvar LCH should be evaluated [5].

Although this condition is rare, taking a detailed and accurate medical history, accurate physical examination, and necessary workups like tissue biopsy are strongly recommended to prevent misdiagnosis of the disease and delay in beginning the proper treatment.

Vulvar involvement of LCH can be treated by topical and oral steroids, chemotherapy (vinblastine, vincristine, or 2-

chlorodeoxyadenosine), immune modulators (methotrexate or tacrolimus), radiation, partial or radical vulvectomy with or without lymph node resection, thalidomide, and radiation therapy [7].

Considerably, treatment of isolated vulvar LCH necessitates more investigation, and there is a lack of evidence for standard therapy in patients with pure genital involvement. Santillan et al. reported the first successful administration of thalidomide for genital LCH treatment [5]; it is a successful treatment for localized LCH such as genital, perianal, and disseminated skin lesions [8–10].

The exact mechanism of thalidomide in treating isolated vulvar LCH is not completely recognized. However, recent studies demonstrated anti-inflammatory and antineoplastic features by inhibiting the production of IL-6 and TNF-alpha. These cytokines had expressed extensively within the biopsy of LCH lesions; therefore, they may play a vital role in the tumor cells' relapse, viability, and irregular maturation. In addition, the beneficial effect of thalidomide is possibly due to balancing the expression of pathological cytokines in LCH [11].

Thalidomide is a safe and well-tolerated drug for isolated genital LCH that can cure mucocutaneous LCH and prevent relapse. In our case, our patient's administration of thalidomide, 100 milligrams daily, was effective, easy to administer, and well-tolerated, and lesions were cured.

However, thalidomide is beneficial in vulvar LCH. Due to teratogenic side effects, the patient must have close follow-ups [9]. It could also have a poor response in high-risk multisystem diseases. Generally, thalidomide, 100 mg per day, is used in adults, but monitoring for toxicity with peripheral neuropathy is necessary [12].

References

[1] National Comprehensive Cancer Network (NCCN), "NCCN clinical practice guidelines in oncology," 2021, https://www.nccn.org/professionals/physician_gls/pdf/histiocytic_neoplasms.pdf.

[2] H. Mottl, L. Rob, J. Stary, R. Kodet, and E. Drahokoupilova, "Langerhans cell histiocytosis of vulva in adolescent," *International Journal of Gynecological Cancer*, vol. 17, no. 2, pp. 520–524, 2007.

[3] N. I. Gwacham, D. Ward, and N. D. McKenzie, "Isolated vulvar langerhans cell histiocytosis," *Gynecologic Oncology Reports*, vol. 36, Article ID 100785, 2021.

[4] I. Gurung, Y. Gao, K. Han, and X.-B. Peng, "Adult onset langerhans cell histiocytosis limited to the skin," *Indian Journal of Dermatology*, vol. 64, no. 5, p. 414, 2019.

[5] A. Santillan, A. J. Montero, J. J. Kavanagh, J. Liu, and P. T. Ramirez, "Vulvar langerhans cell histiocytosis: a case report and review of the literature," *Gynecologic Oncology*, vol. 91, no. 1, pp. 241–246, 2003.

[6] R. Subramaniyan, R. Ramachandran, G. Rajangam, and N. Donaparthi, "Purely cutaneous langerhans cell histiocytosis presenting as an ulcer on the chin in an elderly man successfully treated with thalidomide," *Indian Dermatology Online Journal*, vol. 6, no. 6, p. 407, 2015.

[7] R. Wieland, J. Flanagan, E. Everett, and S. Mount, "Langerhans cell histiocytosis limited to the female genital tract: a review of literature with three additional cases," *Gynecologic Oncology Reports*, vol. 22, pp. 4–8, 2017.

[8] M. Shahidi-Dadras, M. Saeedi, S. Shakoei, and A. Ayatollahi, "Langerhans cell histiocytosis: an uncommon presentation, successfully treated by thalidomide," *Indian Journal of Dermatology Venereology and Leprology*, vol. 77, no. 5, p. 587, 2011.

[9] K. L. McClain and C. A. Kozinetz, "A phase II trial using thalidomide for langerhans cell histiocytosis," *Pediatric Blood and Cancer*, vol. 48, no. 1, pp. 44–49, 2007.

[10] S. Saniee, N. Afshari, and S. Kashefi, "Pulmonary langerhans cell histiocytosis with skin involvement; an amazing case report," *Journal of Analytical Research in Clinical Medicine*, vol. 7, no. 1, pp. 32–36, 2019.

[11] C. S. Sander, M. Kaatz, and P. Elsner, "Successful treatment of cutaneous langerhans cell histiocytosis with thalidomide," *Dermatology*, vol. 208, no. 2, pp. 149–152, 2004.

[12] M. Girschikofsky, M. Arico, D. Castillo et al., "Management of adult patients with langerhans cell histiocytosis: recommendations from an expert panel on behalf of Euro-histio-net," *Orphanet Journal of Rare Diseases*, vol. 8, no. 1, p. 72, 2013.

Permissions

All chapters in this book were first published by Hindawi Publishing Corporation; hereby published with permission under the Creative Commons Attribution License or equivalent. Every chapter published in this book has been scrutinized by our experts. Their significance has been extensively debated. The topics covered herein carry significant findings which will fuel the growth of the discipline. They may even be implemented as practical applications or may be referred to as a beginning point for another development.

The contributors of this book come from diverse backgrounds, making this book a truly international effort. This book will bring forth new frontiers with its revolutionizing research information and detailed analysis of the nascent developments around the world.

We would like to thank all the contributing authors for lending their expertise to make the book truly unique. They have played a crucial role in the development of this book. Without their invaluable contributions this book wouldn't have been possible. They have made vital efforts to compile up to date information on the varied aspects of this subject to make this book a valuable addition to the collection of many professionals and students.

This book was conceptualized with the vision of imparting up-to-date information and advanced data in this field. To ensure the same, a matchless editorial board was set up. Every individual on the board went through rigorous rounds of assessment to prove their worth. After which they invested a large part of their time researching and compiling the most relevant data for our readers.

The editorial board has been involved in producing this book since its inception. They have spent rigorous hours researching and exploring the diverse topics which have resulted in the successful publishing of this book. They have passed on their knowledge of decades through this book. To expedite this challenging task, the publisher supported the team at every step. A small team of assistant editors was also appointed to further simplify the editing procedure and attain best results for the readers.

Apart from the editorial board, the designing team has also invested a significant amount of their time in understanding the subject and creating the most relevant covers. They scrutinized every image to scout for the most suitable representation of the subject and create an appropriate cover for the book.

The publishing team has been an ardent support to the editorial, designing and production team. Their endless efforts to recruit the best for this project, has resulted in the accomplishment of this book. They are a veteran in the field of academics and their pool of knowledge is as vast as their experience in printing. Their expertise and guidance has proved useful at every step. Their uncompromising quality standards have made this book an exceptional effort. Their encouragement from time to time has been an inspiration for everyone.

The publisher and the editorial board hope that this book will prove to be a valuable piece of knowledge for researchers, students, practitioners and scholars across the globe.

List of Contributors

Kathleen Herne
Integrated Dermatology of West Palm Beach, West Palm Beach, FL, USA

Robert K. Fabric
Department of Surgery in the Division of Plastic Surgery at the Leonard M. Miller School of Medicine, Miami, FL, USA

Giulia Rinaldi
Guys and St. Thomas' Hospital, NHS Foundation Trust, London, UK

Alisha Chacko and Samira Batul Syed
Great Ormond Street Hospital, NHS Foundation Trust, London, UK

John R. Edminister
University of Toledo College of Medicine and Life Sciences, 3000 Arlington Avenue, Toledo, OH 43614, USA

Nicole Dominiak
Department of Pathology, University of Toledo Medical Center, 3000 Arlington Avenue, Toledo, OH 43614, USA

Lorie D. Gottwald
Department of Dermatology, University of Toledo Medical Center, 3000 Arlington Avenue, Toledo, OH 43614, USA

Chumsaeng Chumsaengsri and Jongjin Suwanthaweemeesuk
Institute of Dermatology, Bangkok, Thailand

Marlyn Wu, Shereen Teymour and Robin Ashinoff
Hackensack Meridian Palisades Medical Center, Palisades, NJ, USA

Hira Ghani
Nassau University Medical Center, Long Island, NY, USA

Guilherme Kuceki
School of Medicine, University of Utah, Salt Lake, UT, USA

Dekker C. Deacon
Department of Dermatology, University of Utah, Salt Lake, UT, USA
Huntsman Cancer Institute, University of Utah, Salt Lake, UT, USA

Aaron M. Secrest
Department of Dermatology, University of Utah, Salt Lake, UT, USA
Department of Population Health Sciences, University of Utah, Salt Lake, UT, USA

Aikaterini Kyriakou, Aikaterini Patsatsi and Elizabeth Lazaridou
Second Department of Dermatology and Venereology, Medical School, Aristotle University of Thessaloniki, Greece

Sofia-Chrysovalantou Zagalioti
Papageorgiou Hospital, Thessaloniki, Greece

Nikiforos Galanis
Department of Orthopedics, Medical School, Aristotle University of Thessaloniki, Greece

A. Walker and J. S. Westerdahl
University of Utah School of Medicine, Salt Lake City, Utah 84132, USA

J. Zussman and J. Mathis
University of Utah, Department of Dermatology, Salt Lake City, Utah 84111, USA

Matthew Lee
Department of Medicine, North Shore University Hospital-Long Island Jewish Medical Center, 300 Community Dr, Manhasset, NY 11030, USA

Nagashree Seetharamu
Department of Oncology, Donald and Barbara Zucker School of Medicine at Hofstra/Northwell, 500 Hofstra Blvd, Hempstead, NY 11549, USA

Abderrahim Sadak
Laboratory of Biodiversity, Ecology and Genome, Faculty of Sciences, Mohammed V University in Rabat, Rabat, Morocco

Hajiba Fellah and Maryam Hakkour
Laboratory of Biodiversity, Ecology and Genome, Faculty of Sciences, Mohammed V University in Rabat, Rabat, Morocco
National Reference Laboratory of Leishmaniasis, National Institute of Hygiene, Rabat, Morocco

Bouchra Delouane and Faiza Sebti
National Reference Laboratory of Leishmaniasis, National Institute of Hygiene, Rabat, Morocco

Asmae Hmamouch
Laboratory of Microbial Biotechnology, Sciences and Techniques Faculty, Sidi Mohammed Ben Abdellah University, Fez, Morocco

Abdelhakim Bouyahya
Laboratory of Human Pathologies Biology, Department of Biology, Faculty of Sciences, and Genomic Center of Human Pathologies, Faculty of Medicine and Pharmacy, Mohammed V University in Rabat, Rabat, Morocco

Mutsuki Hirakawa, Yuki Ishikura, Taketoshi Futatsuya, Reimon Yamaguchi and Akira Shimizu
Department of Dermatology, Kanazawa Medical University, Uchinada, Ishikawa, Japan

Suman Rao, Michelle Bernshteyn, Raman Sohal, Rachael Proumen, Alexandra Goodman and Zachary Shepherd
SUNY Upstate Medical University Hospital, 750 E Adams St., Syracuse, NY 13210, USA

Vikash Paudel
Department of Dermatology and Venereology, National Medical College, Birgunj, Nepal

Deepa Chudal
Nepal Police Hospital, Kathmandu, Nepal

İpek Pınar Aral
Nevsehir Public Hospital, Radiation Oncology Department, Göreme, Turkey

Neşe Göçer Gürok
Elazığ Fethi Sekin City Hospital, Dermatology Department, Elazig, Turkey

Aykut Oğuz Konuk
Elazığ Fethi Sekin City Hospital, Radiation Oncology Department, Elazig, Turkey

Özlem Üçer
Fırat Univercity, Pathology Department, Elazig, Turkey

Leah Cohen
Department of Dermatology, Florida International University HerbertWertheim College of Medicine, Miami, FL, USA

Sonali Nanda
Department of Dermatology and Cutaneous Surgery, University of Miami Miller School of Medicine, Miami, FL, USA

Martin Zaiac
Department of Dermatology, Florida International University HerbertWertheim College of Medicine, Miami, FL, USA
Department of Dermatology and Cutaneous Surgery, University of Miami Miller School of Medicine, Miami, FL, USA
Chairman of the Department of Dermatology, Florida International University HerbertWertheim College of Medicine, Miami, FL, USA

Vikash Paudel, Manish Bhakta Pradhan and Sumit Paudel
Department of Dermatology and Venereology, National Medical College, Birgunj, Nepal

Brijesh Shrestha
Department of Pathology, National Medical College, Birgunj, Nepal

Alireza Firooz
Center for Research & Training in Skin Diseases and Leprosy, Tehran University of Medical Sciences, Tehran, Iran

Fateme Rajabi
Center for Research & Training in Skin Diseases and Leprosy, Tehran University of Medical Sciences, Tehran, Iran
Network of Dermatology Research (NDR), Universal Scientific Education and Research Network (USERN), Tehran, Iran

Kambiz Kamyab
Department of Dermatopathology, Razi Hospital, Tehran University of Medical Sciences, Tehran, Iran

Marta Cassini and Irina Saretzky
University of Buenos Aires, Buenos Aires, Argentina

Julienne Teclessou and Koussake Kombate
Department of, Dermatology and STDs, University Teaching Hospital of Campus, Togo

Bayaki Saka, Séfako Abla Akakpo and Palokinam Pitche
Department of Dermatology and STDs, University Teaching Hospital of Sylvanus Olympio, Togo

Hideyuki Kinoshita, Toshinori Tsukanishi, Takeshi Ishii, Hiroto Kamoda, Yoko Hagiwara and Tsukasa Yonemoto
Department of Orthopedic Surgery, Chiba Cancer Center, 666-2 Nitonacho, Chuo-ku, Chiba 260-8717, Japan

Sumihisa Orita, Kazuhide Inage, Naoya Hirosawa and Seiji Ohtori
Department of Orthopaedic Surgery, Graduate School of Medicine, Chiba University, 1-8-1 Inohana, Chuo-ku, Chiba 260-8670, Japan

Yogesh Poudyal
Sarnath Skin Centre, Shanti Path, Bhairahawa 32900, Nepal

Anita Shah
Department of Pathology, Universal College of Medical Sciences-Teaching Hospital, Ranigaon, Bhairahawa 32900, Nepal

I. Mandekou-Lefaki
Dermatology, Geniki Kliniki–Euromedica Private Hospital, Thessaloniki, Greece

G. Theodosiou
Department of Dermatology, Skåne Univeristy of Skåne, Malmö, Sweden

F.-S. Delli and M. Papageorgiou
State Dermatology Clinic, Hospital for Skin and Venereal Diseases, Thessaloniki, Greece

D. Oikonomou
Plastic Surgery, Private Practice, Thessaloniki, Greece

Brittany Miles and Andrew Armenta
University of Texas Medical Branch, Galveston, Texas, USA

James Mackey
Deja You Medical Aesthetics, League City, Texas, USA

Akiko Yamashita, Misaki Iwashita and Fusanori Nishimura
Department of Periodontology, Division of Oral Rehabilitation, Faculty of Dental Science, Kyushu University, Fukuoka, Japan

Tomomi Sano
Department of Cell Biology and Pharmacology, Faculty of Dental Science, Kyushu University, Fukuoka, Japan

Areti Ganiatsa, Georgios Gaitanis and Ioannis D. Bassukas
Department of Skin and Venereal Diseases, Faculty of Medicine, School of Health Sciences, University of Ioannina, Ioannina, Greece

Constantina Gartzonika and Stamatina Levidiotou-Stefanou
Department of Microbiology, Faculty of Medicine, School of Health Sciences, University of Ioannina, Ioannina, Greece

Paraskevi Voulgari
Rheumatology Clinic, Department of Internal Medicine, Faculty of Medicine, School of Health Sciences, University of Ioannina, Ioannina, Greece

Yousef S. Abuzneid, Hussam I. A. Alzeerelhouseini, Duha Rabi, Ihab Hilail, Hatem Rjoob, Abdelrahman Rabee, Naser Amro and Qutaiba Qafisheh
Al-Quds University Faculty of Medicine, Jerusalem, State of Palestine

Mohammad Kharraz
An-Najah National University Hospital, Nablus, State of Palestine

Jordan N. Halsey
Department of Plastic Surgery, Nationwide Children's Hospital, Columbus, OH, USA

Catherine E. Cottrell
The Ohio State University College of Medicine, Columbus, OH, USA
The Steve and Cindy Rasmussen Institute for Genomic Medicine, Nationwide Children's Hospital, Columbus, OH, USA

Jennifer H. Aldrink
The Ohio State University College of Medicine, Columbus, OH, USA
Department of Surgery, Division of Pediatric Surgery, Nationwide Children's Hospital, Columbus, OH, USA

Gregory D. Pearson
Department of Plastic Surgery, Nationwide Children's Hospital, Columbus, OH, USA
The Ohio State University College of Medicine, Columbus, OH, USA

Esteban Fernandez Faith
Division of Dermatology, Department of Pediatrics, Nationwide Children's Hospital, Columbus, OH, USA
The Ohio State University College of Medicine, Columbus, OH, USA

Suzanna J. Logan and Archana Shenoy
The Ohio State University College of Medicine, Columbus, OH, USA
Department of Pathology and Laboratory Medicine, Nationwide Children's Hospital, Columbus, OH, USA

Kathleen M. Schieffer
The Steve and Cindy Rasmussen Institute for Genomic Medicine, Nationwide Children's Hospital, Columbus, OH, USA

Anna P. Lillis
Department of Radiology, Nationwide Children's Hospital, Columbus, OH, USA

Bhuvana A. Setty
Division of Hematology/Oncology/BMT, Nationwide Children's Hospital, Columbus, OH, USA

Wencilaus M. P. Selvaraj
Dermatology and Venereology Division, University Teaching Hospital, Lusaka, Zambia

Owen Ngalamika
Dermatology and Venereology Division, University Teaching Hospital, Lusaka, Zambia
University of Zambia School of Medicine, Lusaka, Zambia

Fatima K. Yikona
Chelston Level One Hospital, Lusaka, Zambia

Chibamba Mumba
University of Zambia School of Medicine, Lusaka, Zambia
Pathology and Microbiology Department, University Teaching Hospital, Lusaka, Zambia

Kyle Wu, Sara de Menezes and Aaron Robinson
Department of Dermatology, St Vincent's Hospital Melbourne, 41 Victoria Parade, Fitzroy VIC 3065, Melbourne, Australia

Punyawee Ongsri and Supenya Varothai
Department of Dermatology, Faculty of Medicine Siriraj Hospital, Mahidol University, Bangkok, Thailand

Natalie Olson and David Eckhardt
Rocky Vista University, Parker, CO 80134, USA

Angela Delano
St. Anthony North Family Medicine Residency Program, Denver, CO 80208, USA

Vikash Paudel
National Medical College, Birgunj, Parsa, Nepal

Deepa Chudal
Nepal Police Hospital, Kathmandu, Nepal

Mahesh Mathur, Prakash Acharya, Alina Karki, Nisha KC and Jyoti Shah
Department of Dermatology, College of Medical Sciences, Bharatpur 44200, Nepal

Maryam Fattahi
Emergency Medicine Management Research Center, Iran University of Medical Sciences, Tehran, Iran

Alireza Firooz, Mahsa Fattahi and Akram Miramin Mohammadi
Center for Research and Training in Skin Diseases and Leprosy, Tehran University of Medical Sciences, Tehran, Iran

Ensieh Lotfali
Department of Medical Parasitology and Mycology, School of Medicine, Shahid Beheshti University of Medical Sciences, Tehran, Iran

Mahshid Shahrzad Kavkani
Department of Microbial Biotechnology, Islamic Azad University, Damghan, Iran

Ana Thereza Stradioto Casolato
Dermatology Department, University of São Paulo, Medical School, Clinics Hospital, São Paulo, Brazil

Walter Belda Jr.
Dermatology Department, University of São Paulo, Medical School, Clinics Hospital, São Paulo, Brazil
Laboratory of Pathology of Infectious Diseases, Medical School, University of São Paulo, São Paulo, Brazil

Luiz Felipe Domingues Passero
São Paulo State University (UNESP), Institute of Biosciences, São Vicente, Presidente Prudente, Brazil
São Paulo State University (UNESP), Institute for Advanced Studies of Ocean, São Vicente, Presidente Prudente, Brazil

Rajasekar Seetharaman, Anjum Mahmood, Prashant Kshatriya and Divyang Patel
GIOSTAR Research Inc. Pvt. Ltd., Ahmedabad, Gujrat, India

Anand Srivastava
GIOSTAR Research Inc. Pvt. Ltd., Ahmedabad, Gujrat, India
Global Institute of Stem CellTherapy and Research, 4660 La Jolla Village Drive, San Diego, CA 92122, USA

Fatima zahra Elfatoiki , Sophia Capatas, Hayat Dahbi Skali, Fouzia Hali, Hicham Attar and Soumia Chiheb
Department of Dermatology, Ibn Rochd UHC, 1 Quartier des Hopitaux 20000, Casablanca, Morocco

Harsh Patel and William Naber
Ohio University, Heritage College of Osteopathic Medicine, 191 W Union St, Athens, OH 45701, USA

Austin Cusick
Riverside Methodist Hospital, 3535 Olentangy River Rd., Columbus, OH 43214, USA

Craig Oser
Oser Plastic Surgery and Med Spa, 1 Robinson Plaza Suite 230, Pittsburgh, PA 15205, USA

Luiz Alberto Bomjardim Pôrto, Edilamar Silva de Alecrim, Frederico Paiva e Silva, Amalia Sathler Pires, Fabianny Sanglard da Silva and Sandra Lyon
Dermatology Service Eduardo deMenezes Hospital, FHEMIG, Belo Horizonte, Minas Gerais, Brazil

Maria Aparecida de Faria Grossi
Secretary of State for Health, Belo Horizonte, Minas Gerais, Brazil

Marcus Henrique de Souza Brito Xavier
Dermatology Service Alberto Cavalcante Hospi tal, Belo Horizonte, Minas Gerais, Brazil

Jacqueline Deen, Lisa Byrom and Ivan Robertson
Department of Dermatology, Royal Brisbane and Women's Hospital, Brisbane, Queensland, Australia

I. M. Ranaivo
Department of Dermatology, University Hospital Morafeno, Toamasina, Madagascar

L. S. Ramarozatovo, F. A. Sendrasoa, M. Andrianarison and F. Rapelanoro Rabenja
Department of Dermatology, University Hospital Joseph Raseta Befelatanana, Antananarivo, Madagascar

M. Razakanaivo and F. Rafaramino
Department of Oncology, University Hospital Joseph Ravoahangy Andrianavalona, Antananarivo, Madagascar

Farees Saqlain
Harvard Medical School, Boston, MA, USA

Sophia Z. Shalhout
Harvard Medical School, Boston, MA, USA
Department of Medicine, Division of Hematology/ Oncology, Massachusetts General Hospital, Boston, MA, USA

David Michael Miller
Harvard Medical School, Boston, MA, USA
Department of Medicine, Division of Hematology/ Oncology, Massachusetts General Hospital, Boston, MA, USA
Department of Dermatology, Massachusetts General Hospital, Boston, MA, USA

Kevin S. Emerick
Harvard Medical School, Boston, MA, USA
Department of Otolaryngology, Massachusetts Eye and Ear Infirmary, Boston, MA, USA
Department of Otolaryngology, Harvard Medical School, Boston, MA, USA

Tomas G. Neilan
Harvard Medical School, Boston, MA, USA
Department of Medicine, Division of Cardiology, Massachusetts General Hospital, Boston, MA, USA

Tatyana Sharova
Department of Medicine, Division of Hematology/ Oncology, Massachusetts General Hospital, Boston, MA, USA

Franklin R. Blum
UNC Chapel Hill School of Medicine, Chapel Hill, NC, USA

Logan S. D'Souza
UNC School of Medicine Asheville, Asheville, NC, USA

Bayanne Olabi
Department of Dermatology, Lauriston Building, Edinburgh EH3 9EN, UK

Shanti Ayob
Department of Dermatology, NHS Treatment Centre, Nottingham NG7 2FT, UK

Katharine V. Jensen
Department of Psychiatry, Faculty of Medicine and Dentistry, University of Alberta, Edmonton, Alberta, Canada

Adam Abba-Aji
Department of Psychiatry, Faculty of Medicine and Dentistry, University of Alberta, Edmonton, Alberta, Canada
Young Adult Evaluation, Treatment & Reintegration Service, Alberta Hospital Edmonton, Alberta, Canada

Mary Awad, Erik Holzwanger and Sandeep Jubbal
University of Massachusetts Medical School, Worcester, MA, USA

Susan Y. Chon
MD Anderson Cancer Center, Department of Dermatology, 1515 Holcombe Blvd, Houston, TX 77030, USA

Claire J. Wiggins
MD Anderson Cancer Center, Department of Dermatology, 1515 Holcombe Blvd, Houston, TX 77030, USA
Baylor College of Medicine, 1 Baylor Plaza, Houston, TX 77030, USA

Tareq Z. Alzughayyar, Wasim Noureddin Ibrahim Hamad, Eman A. S. Abuqweider, Bilal Nabeel Mohammad Alqam, Sadi A. Abukhalaf and Jihad Samer Zalloum
Al-Quds University, Faculty of Medicine, Jerusalem, State of Palestine

Ali A. Abumunshar, Rami A. Misk and Yousef I. M. Zatari
An-Najah National University, Faculty of Medicine & Health Sciences, Nablus, State of Palestine

Fawzy M. Abunejma
Al-Ahli Hospital, Hebron, State of Palestine

Mohanad Saleh
Intensive Care Unit Al-Ahli Hospital, Hebron University, Hebron, State of Palestine

Bibisha Baaniya and Sudha Agrawal
Department of Dermatology and Venerology, B.P. Koirala Institute of Health Sciences, Dharan, Nepal

Hugues Adegbidi, Bérénice Dégboé, Fabrice Akpadjan, Alida Kouassi and Félix Atadokpede
Dermatology and Venereology Service, National University Hospital CNHU-HKM, University of Abomey-Calavi, Cotonou, Benin

Nadége Agbessi-Mekoun and Christiane Koudoukpo
Dermatology and Venereology Service, Department University Hospital of Parakou (CHUD-Parakou), University of Parakou, Parakou, Benin

S. De Schrijver and O. Vanhooteghem
Dermatology Department, CHU UCL Namur, Site Sainte Elisabeth, Place Louise Godin 15, 5000 Namur, Belgium

I. Theate
Institute of Pathology and Genetics (IPG), Avenue George-Lemaître 25, 6041 Gosselies, Belgium

Maryam Sadat Sadati and Maryam Hadibarhaghtalab
Molecular Dermatology Research Center, Shiraz University of Medical Sciences, Shiraz, Iran
Dermatology Department, Shiraz University of Medical Sciences, Shiraz, Iran

Nafiseh Todarbary
Student Research Committee, Shiraz University of Medical Sciences, Shiraz, Iran

Fatemeh Sari Aslani
Molecular Dermatology Research Center, Shiraz University of Medical Sciences, Shiraz, Iran
Pathology Department, Shiraz University of Medical Sciences, Shiraz, Iran

Index

www.ingramcontent.com/pod-product-compliance
Lightning Source LLC
LaVergne TN
LVHW082207200926
848484LV00008B/2228